Essentials of Public Health Ethics

Ruth Gaare Bernheim, JD, MPH
Chair, Department of Public Health Sciences
School of Medicine
Institute for Practical Ethics and Public Life
University of Virginia
Charlottesville, VA

James F. Childress, PhD
University Professor
John Allen Hollingsworth Professor of Ethics
Institute for Practical Ethics and Public Life
University of Virginia
Charlottesville, VA

Richard J. Bonnie, JD
Harrison Foundation Professor of Law and Medicine
Professor of Public Policy
School of Law
University of Virginia
Charlottesville, VA

Alan L. Melnick, MD, MPH, CPH
Public Health Director/Health Officer
Clark County, WA
Adjunct Associate Professor
Oregon Health & Science University
School of Medicine
Departments of Family Medicine and Public Health & Preventative Medicine
Portland, OR

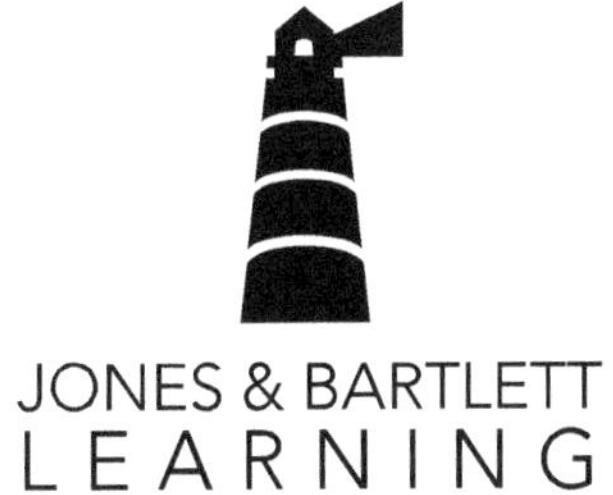

JONES & BARTLETT
LEARNING

World Headquarters
Jones & Bartlett Learning
5 Wall Street
Burlington, MA 01803
978-443-5000
info@jblearning.com
www.jblearning.com

Jones & Bartlett Learning books and products are available through most bookstores and online booksellers. To contact Jones & Bartlett Learning directly, call 800-832-0034, fax 978-443-8000, or visit our website, www.jblearning.com.

Substantial discounts on bulk quantities of Jones & Bartlett Learning publications are available to corporations, professional associations, and other qualified organizations. For details and specific discount information, contact the special sales department at Jones & Bartlett Learning via the above contact information or send an email to specialsales@jblearning.com.

Production Credits
Executive Publisher: William Brottmiller
Publisher: Michael Brown
Associate Editor: Chloe Falivene
Editorial Assistant: Nicholas Alakel
Associate Production Editor: Rebekah Linga
Senior Marketing Manager: Sophie Fleck Teague
Manufacturing and Inventory Control Supervisor: Amy Bacus
Composition: Cenveo® Publisher Services
Cover Design: Kristin E. Parker
Photo Research and Permissions Associate: Ashley Dos Santos
Cover Image: © Portokalis/ShutterStock, Inc.
Printing and Binding: Edwards Brothers Malloy
Cover Printing: Edwards Brothers Malloy

Library of Congress Cataloging-in-Publication Data
Bernheim, Ruth Gaare, author.
Essentials of public health ethics / Ruth Gaare Bernheim, James F. Childress, Richard J. Bonnie, and Alan L. Melnick.
p. ; cm.
Includes bibliographical references and index.
ISBN 978-0-7637-8046-3
I. Childress, James F., author. II. Bonnie, Richard J., author. III. Melnick, Alan L., author. IV. Title.
[DNLM: 1. Public Health Practice—ethics. 2. Public Health—legislation & jurisprudence. 3. Resource Allocation—ethics. WA 21]
R724
174.2—dc23

2013038786

6048

Printed in the United States of America
17 16 15 14 13 10 9 8 7 6 5 4 3 2 1

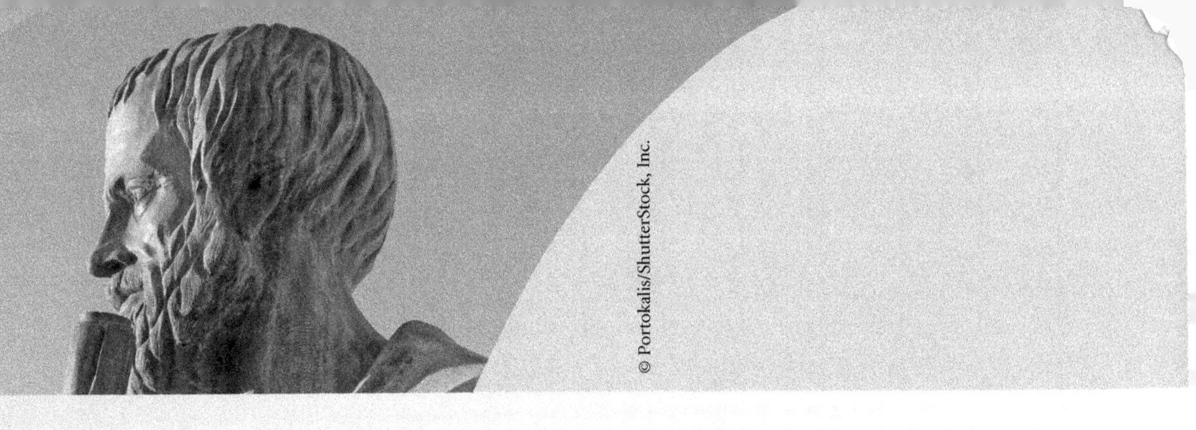

Dedication

To our many students and colleagues, who have taught us so much.

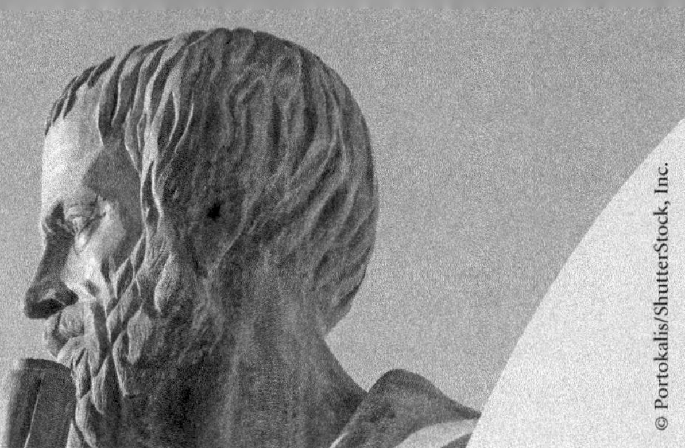

Table of Contents

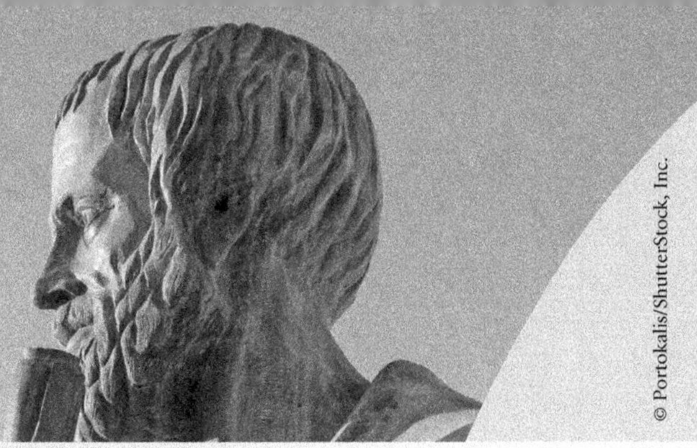

Preface

This book grows out of our interactions in teaching, research and writing, and collaborative projects. Even though this is the first project in which all four of us have collaborated at the same time, we have had many opportunities to work together in various combinations. Those collaborations enabled us to develop the frameworks for this book. This is an integrated book, which grows out of these shared experiences, but we decided it would be useful to list the primary author or authors for each chapter.

We have dedicated this book to our many students and colleagues from whom we have learned so much. Our interactions with students in the classroom as well as those with colleagues in co-teaching, collaborative projects, and conferences have stimulated our reflections and helped us refine our ideas. They have also given us confidence that the frameworks we use in this book can be helpful.

We thank several doctoral students in ethics in the Department of Religious Studies at the University of Virginia for their valuable assistance in the preparation of this book. Laura Alexander, Matthew Puffer, and Mark Storslee provided research assistance on bibliography and arguments for several chapters, and Betsy Mesard, Travis Pickell, and Matthew Puffer prepared the teaching ancillaries. We are also grateful to Aaron Pannone for his help in developing several figures for the book. James Childress wishes to thank his colleagues at the Centre for the Advanced Study of Bioethics at the University of Münster for helpful conversations on John Stuart Mill, public health ethics, and paternalism, in May and June of 2011. Ruth Gaare Bernheim wishes to express her appreciation to Drue Barrett and Leonard Ortmann in the Public Health Ethics Unit at the Centers for Disease Control and Prevention.

Ruth Gaare Bernheim, James F. Childress, Richard J. Bonnie, and Alan L. Melnick

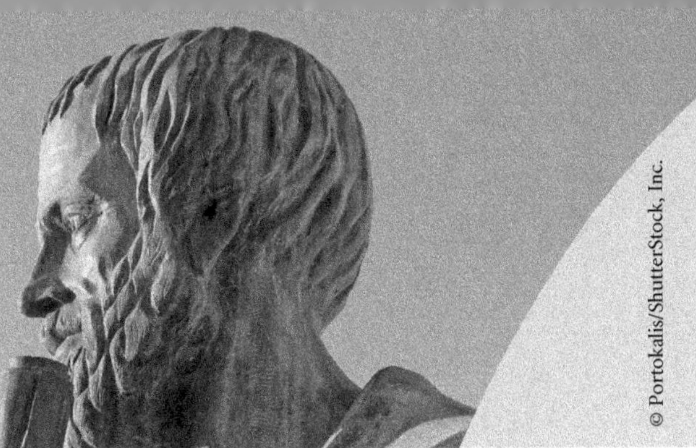

Prologue

As series editor of the *Essential Public Health* series, I am delighted that *Essentials of Public Health Ethics* is now part of our offerings. *Essentials of Public Health Ethics* represents a world-class effort to teach ethics and integrate it into the continuum of public health education. The book reflects the combined efforts of four exceptional authors with decades of experience teaching ethics to a wide range of students in a variety of formats. The authors are all distinguished practitioners, teachers, and scholars in public health ethics and law.

The book begins with a clear, compelling framework for thinking about public health ethics. This framework is integrated throughout the book. Subsequent chapters are devoted to areas of application presented in a logical order, enabling the text to develop an integrated approach. The variety of applications provides flexibility in utilizing the text in course work.

The cases and approach are classroom- and practitioner-tested, having been successfully used to teach students from across the country as well as discussed by practitioners at local and national meetings. Students will find the cases relevant and the analysis insightful. The authors' extraordinary talents and experience allow them to walk students through complex ethical decision making, providing students with progressive ability to tackle new ethical issues on their own.

Take a look at the table of contents and the introductory material, followed by a scan of the chapters. You will find a welcoming yet challenging approach to public health ethics that should appeal to students from a wide range of disciplines headed for diverse careers. Public health ethics has become a key component of public health education. Now there is a text that makes public health ethics come alive.

Richard Riegelman, MD, PhD
Editor, *Essential Public Health* series

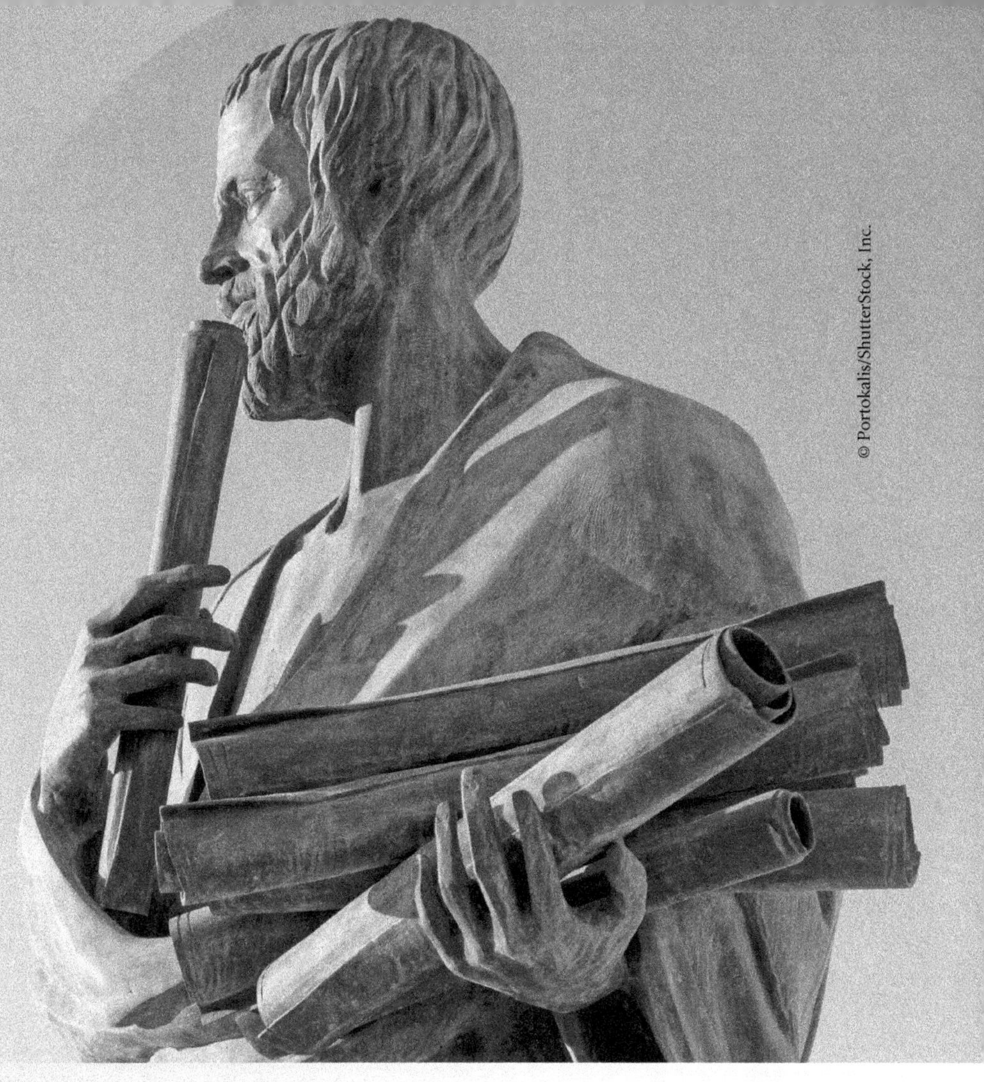

PART I

Foundations

© Portokalis/ShutterStock, Inc.

CHAPTER 1

Introduction: A Framework for Public Health Ethics

by James F. Childress and Ruth Gaare Bernheim

Learning Objectives

By the end of this chapter, the reader will be able to:

- understand public health ethics in the context of public philosophy in the U.S.
- identify several moral norms applicable to public health
- interpret and assess three approaches to ethical conflicts and dilemmas in public health (absolutist, contextualist, and presumptivist)
- utilize justificatory conditions for overriding moral norms in some conflict situations
- appreciate the importance of the process of public justification in public health ethics
- use a set of questions for analyzing ethical dimensions and issues in particular situations
- understand how metaphors shape reflection on ends and means in public health

INTRODUCTION: PUBLIC HEALTH ETHICS: A PRELIMINARY ANALYSIS

This chapter provides an introduction to public health ethics and develops a framework of ethical analysis, deliberation, and justification for public health interventions. Public health officials face myriad decisions as they seek to protect the public's health, prevent illness, disease, injury, and death, and promote the health of the population. Public health is an ethical enterprise, resting on moral foundations, yet some public health interventions appear to threaten or compromise other moral norms, such as liberty, privacy, and confidentiality. Hence public health decisions are sometimes ethically fraught.

Ethical issues may arise on different levels. On the one hand, governmental officials such as legislators, judges, executives, regulators, and health officials frequently recommend or put into place laws and policies regarding public health. For instance, these laws and policies may set the conditions under which it is permissible to impose a quarantine to prevent the spread of a communicable disease, or to notify a person's sexual partners that they are at risk for a sexually transmitted disease. On the other hand, public health officials often must make their own decisions about which goals to pursue and which measures and interventions to undertake, because these laws and policies are usually indeterminate and often authorize actions without prescribing them. Ethical questions and issues arise at both the level of setting laws and policies and the level of deciding what to do where those are indeterminate. For example: Which law or policy regarding justifiable breaches of confidentiality would best protect both the public health and the rights of persons with communicable diseases? And, if the law or policy permits, but does not require, a breach of confidentiality by mandating the disclosure of information to third parties such as sexual partners under certain conditions, what is the ethically justifiable course of action for public health officials? Which ethical and other factors are relevant to these decisions? On what ethical grounds can the public health official justify his or her decisions?

What Is Public Health Ethics?

What, then, is *public health ethics*? About a decade ago, some of the authors of this volume collaborated in an effort to map the terrain of public health ethics.[1] It was not—and is not—an easy task, because of variations in meanings of the terms "public health," "ethics," and the two in combination.

In general, *ethics* refers to the reflective task of interpreting what constitutes moral life and moral actions. We will here concentrate on and engage in normative[a] ethics.[2] In its general sense, normative ethics involves identifying and justifying moral norms regarding right and wrong, good and bad, and determining the meaning, range, and strength of those moral norms for purposes of guiding human action. In its practical or applied mode, normative ethics interprets and guides various domains of life and action, such as business, politics, or public health, in light of moral considerations. Drawing a rough but useful distinction, we can say that *morality* refers more to a social institution or practice—what people believe, value, and do—while *ethics* refers more to the reflective task of interpreting, understanding, and criticizing morality. By contrast, the terms *ethical* and *moral* are often used interchangeably.

The meaning of *public health* may appear to be obvious, but here, too, there are complexities and confusions. According to the now classic definition from the the Institute of Medicine (IOM), public health "is what we, as a society, do collectively to assure the conditions in which people can be healthy."[3] This definition points to a collective activity, but it also refers to the goal of the collective activity—"assur[ing] the conditions in which people can be healthy." We will start with the activity, but our discussion will inevitably incorporate public health goals, such as enabling "healthy people in healthy communities."[3]

Two authors of this book have written elsewhere:[4b]

> ... public health involves not only traditional government action to protect the public from imminent threats, but also, at a more fundamental level, cooperative behavior and relationships of trust in communities, as well as a far-reaching agenda to address complex social, behavioral and/or environmental conditions that affect health.

As a political undertaking, public health includes, at minimum, government's central role, grounded in its police power, to protect the public's health and to provide public goods that would not otherwise be available from individual action alone. Law, with its foundation in a society's political philosophy, provides the framework for the powers and duties of the government to protect public health; sets boundaries on state power to limit individual rights and private interests in order to promote health; and creates incentives and disincentives for individual or organizational activities that affect health.

Government public health actions present at least two types of ethical/political challenges.[5] One set of challenges focuses on the *scope* of public health, e.g., does government have a public health duty to prevent chronic disease by addressing behavioral (sedentary lifestyle) or socioeconomic (poverty) risk factors? Another set of ethical issues involves the appropriate *means* of public health intervention, e.g., should government outlaw risk-taking behavior such as riding a bicycle without a helmet? When is the state justified in isolating a noncompliant patient with tuberculosis? The state's use of its police power, particularly in paternalistic or coercive policies, raises important ethical questions for a liberal, pluralistic democracy and requires moral justification that the public—in whose name the policies are carried out—could reasonably be expected to accept.

As a social endeavor, public health includes many forms of social and community action and increasingly involves overlapping networks of individuals and organizations, including governmental and private agencies, for-profit and nonprofit stakeholders, professionals from many disciplines, and citizens, all working together over time to improve the population's health and the living conditions in the community. Relationship building, whether between public health officials and the public they serve or among community partners, is not merely instrumental, but rather is part of the substance of public health work. Particularly at the local community level, public health interventions, e.g., those that focus on socioeconomic or

[a] Normative ethics is contrasted with both meta-ethics and descriptive ethics. The former analyzes the language, concepts, and methods of ethical reasoning, while the latter studies how people reason and how they act. See Reference 2.

[b] The next four paragraphs are from Childress JF, Bernheim RG. Public health ethics: Public justification and public trust. *Bundesgesundheitsblatt, Gesundheitsforschung, Gesundheitsschutz* 2008;51(2):158–163.

behavioral risk factors, tend to be multidimensional, sustained over months or years, and context-dependent. Community public health campaigns to reduce youth tobacco use are examples of complex, multifaceted programs that depend on community coalition-building and partnerships, as well as numerous social institutions such as the public education system, in order to effect changes in social norms and behaviors related to teen smoking. Ethical analysis in this sphere of public health extends beyond the political to include professional, institutional, and civic duties as well.

Public Philosophy

Public health ethics thus draws on the overlapping domains of formal political, social, and moral philosophy. However, we mainly appeal to an informal or de facto "public philosophy," to use Michael Sandel's language, which refers to "the political theory implicit in our practice, the assumptions about citizenship and freedom that inform our public life."[6] This public philosophy provides an ethical foundation for—and sets limits on—public health laws, policies, and practices and on social institutions and organizations engaged in public health activities. As a normative enterprise, public health ethics can provide a framework to explore the fundamental ethical values that define the relationships of the individual, the state, and social institutions in public health activities aimed at public health goals. It can also provide ways to reason about the conflicts that arise among those ethical values—for instance, in the selection of public health interventions.

MORAL NORMS

Moral Considerations in Public Health

Several moral considerations play important roles in the analysis and assessment of public health activities, including both ends and means. Rather than appearing in a simple code, they emerge from a variety of sources. Some are embedded in our society's public philosophy, as expressed in our laws, policies, practices, and the like. They also appear in the kinds of moral appeals that public health agents make in deliberating about and justifying their actions, as well as in public debates about moral issues in public health. **Table 1.1** captures these "moral considerations in public health."

TABLE 1.1 Moral Considerations in Public Health

1.	Producing benefits
2.	Avoiding, preventing, and removing harms
3.	Producing the maximal balance of benefits over harms and other costs (often called utility)
4.	Distributing benefits and burdens fairly (distributive justice) and ensuring public participation, including the participation of affected parties (procedural justice)
5.	Respecting autonomous choices and actions, including liberty of action
6.	Protecting privacy and confidentiality
7.	Keeping promises and commitments
8.	Disclosing information as well as speaking honestly and truthfully (often grouped under transparency)
9.	Building and maintaining trust

Data from Childress JF, Faden RR, Gaare RD, et al. Public health ethics: mapping the terrain. *Journal of Law, Medicine, & Ethics* 2002;30(2):169–177.

We recognize that these general moral considerations, which we will often call moral norms—but also values, principles, rules, and the like—may have different labels or names and may be interpreted differently in different ethical frameworks. Some frameworks may locate one or more of the above concepts under others. Nevertheless, we contend that the moral content of public health ethics is largely, if not completely, captured by these moral norms. They represent the ethical essentials of public health.

Relations Between Moral Norms and Public Health

Moral norms function in various ways in relation to public health goals and interventions. Several provide warrants for the moral enterprise of public health. Particularly relevant are the norms of benefiting others, preventing and removing harms, utility, and justice. At minimum, "public health" points to a broad and important social benefit that governments and societies generally should and do seek. Public health is both an intrinsic and an instrumental social good; that is, it is good both in itself and for what it enables the society to do. Public health is an intrinsic good because, other things being equal, a healthy society is preferable to an unhealthy one. Public health is an instrumental good because it enables the society to realize other goods it values. For instance, a healthy society is more productive, needs fewer economic resources for health care, and can defend itself better from external threats.

Several norms thus support the enterprise of public health, rendering its achievement an important ideal (but not the only one) and its pursuit an important obligation (within limits). Public health thus falls under the broad norm of beneficence (of producing good), which we have above broken down into (1) producing benefits, (2) avoiding, preventing, and removing harms, and (3) producing the maximal balance of benefits over harms and other costs, the last of which is often referred to as *utility*. This involves governmental and social activities to *protect* the public's health, to *prevent* its ill health, and to *promote* its good health. Justice is also important, because the fair distribution of benefits and burdens in the society requires attention to persons' special vulnerabilities to illness, disease, and injury.

Some general moral norms for societies and governments support at least some public health activities. However, this broad benefit of public health will need to be specified in various ways in different contexts. At this point, we have not indicated exactly how much weight public health goods and goals should have in general and in specific contexts, especially when they conflict with other moral norms. For now, we can affirm that public health is an important value, but not an overarching benefit that always trumps all other goods and norms.

Beyond supporting the governmental and societal pursuit of public health, some norms, as implemented, may actually be a means to or even a precondition for the achievement of public health. There is strong evidence, for instance, that conditions of social injustice contribute significantly to ill health, and that violations of human rights "have adverse effects on physical, mental, and social well-being."[7]

Despite the links between moral norms, including human rights, and public health, conflicts sometimes do emerge in deliberation about whether, to what extent, and how to pursue some specific public health goals. For instance, debates may erupt over how much money should go into public health versus other societal goods when budgets are limited, and about whether the costs or risks of a potentially effective public health intervention are too great to warrant the intervention. In specific contexts, some moral norms, including human rights, may limit and constrain what the state and society may do in pursuit of public health.

If and when moral norms come into conflict, how can we resolve those conflicts? In the remainder of this chapter, we will sketch a framework for resolving ethical conflicts in public health.

ADDRESSING ETHICAL CONFLICTS AND DILEMMAS IN PUBLIC HEALTH

Should the law mandate children's vaccination for certain diseases even against parents' religiously based objections to vaccinations? In seeking to resolve such ethical conflicts and dilemmas—whether in public health or in other domains—we need to attend to two dimensions of ethical norms. One dimension is their range or scope, the other their weight or strength. Reasoning through conflicts and dilemmas requires attention to both dimensions. Sometimes, it may be possible to specify one norm in order to eliminate its conflict with another norm; this occurs by specifying that norm's range or scope of applicability.[2,8] For instance, we might specify the range or scope of privacy, both to make it more concrete for real-life situations and, in the process, to reduce its conflict with some public health pursuits.

However, some conflicts are not amenable to resolution through specification. In such cases, it will be necessary to determine the relative weights or strength of the conflicting norms.[2] In putting forward a framework to address and resolve ethical conflicts and dilemmas in public health, we will first analyze and assess different approaches to determining the weight or strength of conflicting norms and propose justificatory conditions for overriding norms in some situations; then we will focus on a process of public justification.

Absolutist and Contextualist Approaches

There are three basic approaches to formulating the relative weight and strength of conflicting moral norms, and we will seek to determine which approach, or approaches, are the most adequate for deliberating about public health policy and practice in a liberal, pluralistic, democratic society. The first approach is *absolutist*. It asserts that one norm is superior to and always triumphs over all other norms or, in a rank order, over certain other norms. There is general agreement that some norms are absolute—for instance, prohibitions of murder, rape, and cruelty—but few, if any, other norms qualify as absolute. It is implausible to hold that norms such as liberty, privacy, and confidentiality that sometimes conflict with the pursuit of public health are absolute. Absolutist approaches encounter devastating counterexamples and are unable to address ethical complexities in the real world. Consider the following absolutist claims: (1) "liberty (privacy, confidentiality, etc.) should never be sacrificed for public health," or (2) "public health always trumps liberty (privacy, confidentiality, etc.)." Neither absolutist claim is defensible. We can easily think of cases in which individuals' liberties should be overridden to protect the public health—mandatory quarantine in a serious epidemic is a good example. On the other hand, in many cases public health goals may not be clear, specific, or strong enough to override individuals' liberties, or can be realized without compromising those liberties.

At the opposite end of the spectrum from absolutist approaches, we can place contextualist approaches. Contextualist approaches proceed by balancing all relevant factors, including all applicable norms, in a particular context. For instance, officials may balance public health goals against rules of privacy in order to determine which is weightier *in a specific situation*. Advantages of this approach include its flexibility as well as its attention to the particularities of different situations; one disadvantage is its possible arbitrariness and unpredictability. The process of balancing, by itself, seems to make our judgments too intuitive, less reasoned.

A Presumptivist Approach

Falling between absolutist and contextualist approaches is a *presumptivist* approach. It is closer to a contextualist approach in attending to particular circumstances and examining all relevant norms and data, but it also finds bare balancing too unstructured and intuitive to be sufficient. Moreover, in any genuine conflict between the society and the individual, the society tends to win in the process of balancing. Hence, in thinking about *means* to achieve public health goals in a liberal, pluralistic, democratic society, it is important to put more initial weight on the liberty (privacy, confidentiality, etc.) end of the scale, at least to the extent of placing the burden of proof on proponents of policies and actions that infringe upon these personal interests. This also implies a tentative (but nonabsolute) priority for interventions that do not violate liberty and related norms unless necessary and unless other conditions are met. Our "public philosophy" entails this approach. Its presumptions, often expressed in the legal-like language of burden of proof, serve to structure moral deliberation and justificatory arguments in situations of uncertainty and indeterminate norms.[9]

As we have previously argued elsewhere,

> ... a presumptivist framework best structures public health ethics in a liberal, pluralistic, democratic society. A presumptivist framework sets presumptions about means and interventions, but also views these presumptions as rebuttable and identifies the conditions for their rebuttal. Hence, it avoids certain deficiencies of both the absolutist and the contextualist approaches. On the one hand, it is clearly nonabsolutist, since either liberty or public health can take priority in some situations. On the other hand, it moves beyond the contextualist approach's metaphorical balancing by admitting presumptions, burdens of proof, starting points, initial tentative weights, or heuristics in the selection of means to achieve the goal of public health. The presumptions emerge from a society's core values, as expressed and embodied in its constitution, laws, policies, and practices, as well as in its myths and stories, all making up the society's public philosophy. They structure, and should structure, without absolutely determining, the selection of public health interventions.[4]

Interlude: Summary

To summarize and set the stage for a discussion of justificatory conditions, we are focusing on the public philosophy of liberal, pluralistic, democratic societies, a public philosophy that characterizes legal and ethical norms and discourse in the U.S. In addition to the ends of public health that it includes and emphasizes, this public philosophy also attends to means. Following the identification of a public health problem or need that warrants governmental and societal action, the selection of means or modes of intervention becomes crucial. This selection should not treat all potentially effective means, or even all means that would probably produce a net benefit, as equally meritorious, subject only to determining their probable success and balance of good over bad effects. The ends justify the means—what else could?—but not all potentially effective means that would probably produce a net balance of good over bad effects in the particular circumstances. This public philosophy establishes presumptions in favor of means or interventions that respect liberty, privacy, confidentiality, and the like. Hence, our ethical analysis should start with these presumptions. But, as we have argued, these presumptions are nonabsolute and can be rebutted—overridden or outweighed—under certain conditions. Hence, we need to identify rebuttal conditions, what we are here calling "justificatory conditions," that indicate when the presumption in question can be justifiably rebutted.[2,4,10]

JUSTIFICATORY CONDITIONS FOR OVERRIDING NORMS IN CONFLICT SITUATIONS

We now turn our attention to several conditions for justifying infringements of norms such as liberty, privacy, and confidentiality in the selection of public health interventions, as means to achieve public health goals. These conditions can also be viewed as rebuttal conditions because they indicate when the presumption against infringing such norms can be rebutted.

We will explore these several justificatory conditions in part by examining a specific liberty-limiting intervention: mandatory, forcible quarantine. In attempting to slow or

TABLE 1.2 Justificatory Conditions

Justificatory Conditions
Effectiveness: Is the action likely to accomplish the public health goal?
Necessity: Is the action necessary to override the conflicting ethical claims to achieve the public health goal?
Least infringement: Is the action the least restrictive and least intrusive?
Proportionality: Will the probable benefits of the action outweigh the infringed moral norms and any negative effects?
Impartiality: Are all potentially affected stakeholders treated impartially?
Public justification: Can public health officials offer public justification that citizens, and in particular those most affected, could find acceptable in principle?

Data from: Childress JF, Faden RR, Bernheim RG, et al. Public Health Ethics: Mapping the Terrain. Journal of Law, Medicine, & Ethics 2002;30(2):169–177, at 172 and Childress JF and Bernheim RG. Public Health Ethics: Public Justification and Public Trust. Bundesgesundheitsblatt: Gesundheitsforschung, Gesundheitsschutz 2008;51(2):158–163.

stop an outbreak of a serious contagious disease, such as Severe Acute Respiratory Syndrome (SARS), avian influenza, or active tuberculosis (all of which involve airborne transmission), quarantine is recognized as a legitimate public health measure. We will examine forcible quarantine in detail elsewhere; for now, we will use this intervention as a way to illustrate how justificatory conditions work.[10c]

Effectiveness in the Protection or Promotion of Public Health

If there is no reason to believe that a quarantine would be an effective public health measure, then it would be a mistake to impose it. Indeed, not only would forcible quarantine under those circumstances be unwise, it would also be ethically unjustified. Interventions that infringe important social values must have a reasonable prospect of success in order to be justified.

Necessity

Even if forcible quarantine would probably be effective in some cases, it might not be necessary or essential. It might be possible, for instance, to secure voluntary compliance with quarantine requests without resort to the threat or use of force. Liberty and other presumptive values require a search for alternatives before they can be justifiably overridden. In short, a public policy that can accomplish its goals through voluntary cooperation has priority over threat or use of force.

This justificatory condition has implications for different strategies to ensure that persons with, for example, active tuberculosis will complete their treatment until cured, in order to reduce the likelihood of long-term risks to others, particularly from tuberculosis strains that are resistant to multiple drugs. Other things being equal, persuading persons with tuberculosis to complete their treatment until cured, even through the use of financial or other incentives, should have priority over forcible detention. In such a case, proponents of forcible strategies bear the moral burden of proof: They must be able to provide strong reasons for their belief that a coercive approach is necessary and essential.

Least Infringement of Presumptive Value

Suppose that forcible quarantine would satisfy the first two conditions in a particular set of circumstances. Public health officials should still seek the custody alternatives—e.g., confinement at home, admission to a hospital or similar facility, or protective custody in a jail—that are least restrictive and intrusive, yet consistent with obtaining the end that is sought. For some analysts, the condition of least restrictive or intrusive means is a corollary of necessity, in that coercive measures should be necessary in degree as well as in kind. However, it is also helpful to view this condition as a specific requirement to minimize infringements of presumptive values. To take another example, even if it is justifiable to breach privacy or confidentiality in particular circumstances, this third condition places limits on the scope of the infringement, in terms of both the information that is disclosed and the parties to whom it is disclosed.

Proportionality

Some ethicists would fold the previous justificatory conditions into a broader conception of proportionality: If a specific quarantine measure would satisfy the three prior conditions, then it would be a proportionate response to the threat.[11] However, we view proportionality as a separate requirement, because it involves balancing broader considerations. After determining that a proposed coercive intervention such as quarantine would satisfy the first three conditions, we still must ask whether the probable benefits (in risk reduction), minus any probable negative effects, are sufficient to rebut the presumption in favor of freedom from governmental coercion.

[c] The following six paragraphs in the text are from Childress JF, Bernheim RG. Public health ethics: Public justification and public trust. *Bundesgesundheitsblatt, Gesundheitsforschung, Gesundheitsschutz* 2008;51(2):158–163.

Impartiality

Basic standards of fairness apply across public health interventions. More specifically, they require that coercive public health measures, such as quarantine, be imposed impartially. Even though this condition might seem to be unnecessary and even useless, a quick glance at serious outbreaks of infectious disease in the past reveals that victims have been singled out for blame along with others in such broad categories as race, ethnic background, socioeconomic class, or geographical location, and have been subjected to stigmatization and discrimination. Far from being relegated to the past, stigmatization and discrimination occurred in the SARS outbreak in several places, including, for example, in Toronto against the Chinese.[12]

We will examine the sixth condition, public justification, separately because it focuses on the context of justification, indicating to whom the justification must be made as well as the procedures and processes of engagement for creating the social basis for justification.

PUBLIC JUSTIFICATION IN CONTEXT

In making difficult choices in public health that involve important social, cultural, and political norms and values, decision makers at all levels should attempt to act "in ways that preserve the moral foundations of social collaboration" that are at the core of public health.[13] A presumptivist approach for public health ethics, which sets out core moral values and norms as starting points for deliberation, can provide a foundation for social collaboration and for enduring relationships of trust in public health. An explicit acknowledgement of shared core values and common goals and needs in public health can engender trust and support for collective action and even build a community of stakeholders by educating and enabling individuals and entities to see themselves as connected through health.

In a democratic political order, engagement of the public in public health deliberation is an indispensable part of a presumptivist approach because members of society are political and social stakeholders—they themselves have a stake in the ongoing protection of fundamental values such as liberty and privacy that are displayed, embodied, and sometimes overridden for their benefit. Real-time public health decisions are socially situated within particular communities; hence, accountability to and transparency with the public requires that reasons, justifications, and explanations for practices such as quarantine be provided to ensure the public can support such actions. Even forcible quarantine requires considerable voluntary cooperation to be successful. At minimum, justification requires that officials state, "We are choosing to impose quarantine in this context because ..."

Context here includes the particular social, political, and institutional settings in which an action takes place. It also includes such factors as socioeconomic, cultural or demographic features of the population as well as the strength and quality of political and social relationships and discourse in the community. The need for public support directs our attention to relationships—"support from whom to whom for what?"—including, in the case of quarantine, the relationship between public health professionals and community members. Thus, relationships, built on common understandings, developed over time, of roles, obligations, and collaborations, frame the meanings of and justifications for public health decisions and engender the public's trust and willingness to support those decisions.

It is our contention that public health relationships provide a significant context for a framework of core values, presumptions, and justificatory/rebuttal conditions. Because public health is both a political and a social undertaking, we believe public health ethics must include both a framework for deliberation, such as we have proposed, and an explication of the professional and civic roles and relationships that provide the context for public health policies and actions.

The primary public health relationship is between community members (with a background understanding of reciprocal civic obligations of membership in that community) and public health professionals (with their understanding of their authority as government officials established by law, as well as their understanding of their role as health professionals in society). This relationship is complex in that it pulls together many perspectives, languages, and cultures. It includes on the one hand government officials, who are professionals with particular expertise and professional values, and on the other community members with their numerous and simultaneous memberships in diverse groups, families, cultures, and religions.

In addition, the relationship between public health officials and community members is unique: public health officials act as both government agents with police powers, and as health professionals with responsibility for population health, a public good. In a democracy, public health officials might be thought of as physicians to the community, and the process of justification shares some features of a consent process between doctor and patient—one that is framed as a partnership based on voluntary action, with a strong presumption against any "unconsented to" action. Particularly in times of need and vulnerability, health professionals usually are approached as trustworthy because of general societal beliefs about and expectations of health professionals who have ethical commitments to act in the individual's or public's best interests. For instance, a public health code of ethics entitled *Principles of the Ethical Practice of Public Health* that has been adopted by a number of public health professional organizations in the United States explicitly states in Principle 6: "Public health institutions should provide communities with the information they have that is needed for decisions on policies or programs and should obtain the community's consent for their implementation."[14] In a similar vein, the recent IOM report, *The Future of the Public's Health in the 21st Century*, emphasizes the multisectoral dimensions of community health and suggests that a goal of public health is to collaborate with and facilitate the contributions of many community entities: "All partners who can contribute to action as a public health system should be encouraged to assess their roles and responsibilities, consider changes, and devise ways to better collaborate with other partners. They can transform the way they 'do business' to better act to achieve a healthy population on their own and position themselves to be part of an effective partnership in assuring the health of the population. Health policy should create incentives to makes these partnerships easier."[15 (p. 32)]

Public health's emergency preparedness activities illustrate the ways that relationships provide the context for public health ethics. Emergency preparedness, as a community process, requires public health officials to take an active role in building a community of stakeholders prepared to act when an infectious disease or terrorist threat occurs, and in generating community discussions of and deliberations about such policies as rationing scarce resources in an emergency. The fire department metaphor for public health illuminates this role, because fire officials "teach and practice prevention at the same time that they maintain readiness to take on emergencies."[16 (p. 40)] Drills are important not only as instructive devices for practicing activities (such as "know the nearest exit"), but also because, in the context of biopreparedness, we need to "prepare" our civic responses when challenged as a community. The purpose of public debate is not merely to reach a consensus on any one course of action based on fair procedures, but also to build and strengthen our civic commitment to continued cooperation.

Consider, for example, the possible role of the local public health official in preparing a community for hospital triage or quarantine during a public health emergency. At minimum, this role could and should include convening stakeholders such as hospital administrators, community physicians, and community representatives and sponsoring forums for public deliberation to develop and forge professional, institutional, and public support for ethical guidelines. Forms of public engagement and consent could range from providing mere notice to the public through the media, to organizing town hall meetings, to conducting community focus groups and surveys about public values, to establishing an ethics board of community leaders and public representatives. Public health professionals should address which option for community engagement is appropriate, based on contextual factors such as community cohesiveness, expectations, and values. One aim of this activity is to create, over time, a public that cooperates with and trusts each other. The relationships this activity engenders provide the important social context for public deliberation and public justification when public health authorities believe that it is necessary to use liberty-limiting state power, such as forcible quarantine, or must adopt a rationing program because the vaccine supply is limited.

Whatever the governmental public health action—whether the collection of population data during a disease outbreak, or forcible quarantine, or the allocation of scarce vaccines, or an ongoing community program to change social norms—a primary goal should be the development and maintenance of relationships of trust, defined in a report from the IOM as "the belief that those with whom one interacts will take one's interests into account, even in situations in which one is not in a position to recognize, evaluate, or thwart a potentially negative course of action by those trusted."[16,10,d]

ETHICAL CONFLICTS: PERVASIVE OR OCCASIONAL?

Ethical analyses in public health, and elsewhere, often focus on conflicts, dilemmas, and quandaries for obvious reasons: Their difficulties and our perplexities require thoughtful, disciplined, and imaginative responses, as public health officials seek to determine what they should do in such cases. Can they find a way to navigate an apparent conflict, or must they sacrifice some norm or right in order to protect the public's health? For instance, should officials seek a court authorization to confine a recalcitrant tuberculosis patient who refuses to take the medication necessary to achieve a cure in order to protect others?

Ethical Dimensions of Public Health Decisions

While it would be a mistake to ignore such conflicts, it would also be a mistake to reduce public health ethics to these conflicts—public health decisions have ethical

[d] The preceding seven paragraphs in the text are from Childress JF, Bernheim RG. Public health ethics: Public justification and public trust. *Bundesgesundheitsblatt, Gesundheitsforschung, Gesundheitsschutz* 2008;51(2):158–163.

dimensions even if no such difficult conflicts arise. Public health officials often have to determine how best to realize all applicable norms in pursuing public health goals. Their decisions may concern what they should recommend about laws, policies, or regulations on public health or what to do when laws, policies, and regulations permit a range of actions but do not require a specific action. Where indeterminacy and uncertainty exist, decisions have to be made that address the full range of relevant values, including but not limited to public health.

At certain periods, ethical conflicts may seem more salient and unavoidable, depending on the social and political context and the nature and seriousness of public health problems and needs. For instance, since the September 11, 2001 terrorist attack, many in the U.S. have emphasized the strongly felt conflict between public health and liberty as well as between political security and liberty. Liberty is not the only potentially limiting and constraining norm, but we will focus, for illustrative purposes, on the conflict between public health and liberty—or, better, liberties—while keeping in mind and later discussing conflicts between public health, on the one hand, and privacy, confidentiality, private property, and so forth, on the other hand.

Competing Claims about Ethical Trade-offs in Public Health

For some interpreters of public health law and ethics, conflicts between public health and norms protecting individual liberties are not only common, but also inevitable. It is harmony that is atypical and exceptional.[17,18] For other interpreters, such conflicts are unusual and generally avoidable; trade-offs are not usually necessary.[7] For instance, lawyer/bioethicist George Annas denies that "in a public health emergency, there must be a trade-off between effective public health measures and civil rights."[19,20] Public health, in this view, does not typically conflict with norms protecting individual liberties but generally presupposes those norms in the effective pursuit of its ends and goals. Indeed, respecting the relevant norms and presumptions regarding public health interventions will generally provide a basis for public trust and cooperation, which are essential for the success of most public health activities.

Scope of Societal Values: Inclusion of Personal Values

In addressing this debate, it is important not to view "ethical problems" in public health policy and practice only in terms of conflicts between the individual on the one hand, and the state or society on the other—or put another way, between collective interests and individual interests. Such formulations are unsatisfactory, flawed, and indefensible. A society or state may have a strong commitment to the values associated with individuals and their lives and activities. These include individuals' liberties, privacy, confidentiality, and other rights. In the U.S., the society and the state have such high regard for these individual values that they are, in fact, social values; they are embedded in our de facto public philosophy, represented in the constitution, laws, judicial decisions, professional codes, public discourse, and the like—all important points of reference. It is thus a mistake simply to set unspecified collective interests over against individual interests.

Those individual values are shared social values that are embodied in American myths and narratives that feature individuals and their actions. They are constitutive values that shape and express our national identity. If civil liberties and rights are values and norms within our communal identity, and even partially constitutive of that identity, then they represent collective interests too, just as public health does. This leads to an important shift in perspective: Trade-offs occur not simply *between* individual interests and collective interests, as though only the latter really constitute societal identity, but rather *within* and *among* our social values. Our collective interests, properly understood, include civil liberties and rights as well as public health, among other values.

Historical Perspective on Conflicts in Public Health

Historical perspective may be useful. It is plausible to view the conflict between liberty and public health as common in public health law and policy until the last 60 years or so. Two co-authors of this volume have sometimes taught a course entitled *Confronting Plagues: Historical and Contemporary Responses to Epidemics*. In doing so, they have observed recurrent conflicts during major outbreaks of diseases such as plague, cholera, tuberculosis, and sexually transmitted diseases. In part because of limited scientific knowledge (at least in some of these outbreaks) and human tendencies to seek scapegoats in crises, individual liberties commonly have been sacrificed. The last half of the 20th century saw a clearer and firmer legal recognition in the U.S. of rights to liberty, privacy, and due process, in general and in relation to health and health care. These rights were increasingly recognized in legislation and judicial opinions regarding contraception, abortion, life-sustaining treatment, and the detention and treatment of persons with mental illness.

Another development helped to alter the overall perspective on conflicts between public health and liberty: By the last third of the 20th century, to many observers the major threats from contagious diseases appeared to be largely under control. Major achievements included vaccines for several contagious diseases, such as polio, and effective treatments for such contagious diseases as tuberculosis. In some ways, public health itself languished for a time because it was deemed to be less necessary and less important in view of these achievements.

Then came acquired immunodeficiency syndrome (AIDS), caused by human immunodeficiency virus (HIV) infection, in the early 1980s, followed over subsequent years by threats from other infectious and communicable agents, such as avian influenza, and from possible terrorist attacks that might use biological agents (e.g., anthrax) as well as other weapons of mass destruction. When HIV/AIDS emerged, the structure of civil rights and liberties, the modes of transmission of HIV/AIDS, the social groups in which these infections first appeared led to what some call "AIDS exceptionalism."[21] This phrase suggests that HIV/AIDS was largely exempted from some traditional public health measures such as named reporting and quarantine. HIV's mode of transmission was certainly a factor in such exemptions: HIV was soon understood to be transmitted only through the exchange of bodily fluids, either directly or indirectly, through sexual contact, sharing needles and syringes, or contaminated transfused blood or blood products. In the context of and as a result of this experience, claims of harmony between public health and liberty, and other norms and rights, became even more dominant. According to Ronald Bayer and James Colgrove, both major figures in public health ethics,

> Given the unique biological, epidemiological, and political factors that shaped the public policy discussion, it became possible to assert that there was no tension between public health and civil liberties, that policies that protected the latter [civil liberties] would foster the former [public health], and that policies that intruded on rights would subvert the public health.[22]

To take one example: Since HIV-infected patients' voluntary cooperation was needed to identify and notify at-risk sexual partners, assurance of the protection of their privacy and confidentiality was deemed important to public health.

From this perspective, then, conflicts between public health and individual liberties and rights generally do not erupt, though exceptional and difficult cases flare up on occasion. For the most part, effective public health measures and civil liberties and rights can and do coexist. On the one hand, as previously suggested, civil liberties and rights—as well as human rights more broadly—contribute to public health and, in some cases, are indispensable to the effective pursuit of public health, as the above example indicates. On the other hand, it is usually possible to find—and certainly important to seek—methods, measures, and interventions that are effective and, at the same time, that do not infringe these rights and liberties. Hence, it is important to reject two extremes—either (1) that trade-offs between public health and various liberties and rights are omnipresent and inevitable, or (2) that protecting liberties and rights will never impede effective public health measures. Instead, it is essential to examine particular situations and cases to determine whether there is a conflict, whether it can be avoided or mitigated, and so forth. Take the following example: if public health officials can persuade individuals who have active tuberculosis to undergo directly observed treatment until cured, no individual liberties are violated, whether the effective persuasion comes through rational appeals about individuals' health and the health of others or through incentives for compliance. In either case, liberty is not compromised.

ANALYZING ETHICAL ISSUES IN PARTICULAR SITUATIONS

Policy makers and public health officials have to analyze ethical issues in particular situations, whether in making decisions

TABLE 1.3 Analyzing Ethical Issues in Public Health

What public health problems, needs, concerns are at issue?
What are appropriate public health goals in this context?
What is the source and scope of legal authority, if any, and which laws and regulations are relevant?
What are the relevant norms and claims of stakeholders in the situation and how strong or weighty are they?
Are there relevant precedent legal and ethical cases?
Which features of the social-cultural-historical context are relevant?
Do professional codes of ethics provide guidance?

Data from Bernheim RG, Nieburg P, Bonnie RJ. Ethics and the practice of public health. In Goodman RA (ed): *Law in Public Health Practice*, 2nd edn. New York: Oxford University Press, 2007.

or recommendations about laws and policies, or about courses of action when laws and policies are indeterminate. In either of these situations, the previous table provides helpful questions for rigorously and imaginatively analyzing ethical issues in public health.

We will use this analytic framework to examine a range of problems and cases in subsequent chapters. We will start with an examination of legal authority for public health in its protective, preventive, and promotive modes. Then we will examine several clusters of moral norms related to utility, justice, and respect for personal liberties and other interests; in the process we will consider more closely how both to specify and to weight these norms in order to guide public health decisions. Subsequently, we will turn to a series of public health interventions, using case studies to open up the range of ethical issues. This analytic framework will be used to illuminate these issues and to reach ethically defensible decisions, in light of the justificatory conditions previously explicated.

THE ROLE OF THE PUBLIC HEALTH CODE OF ETHICS

We now turn to the *Public Health Code of Ethics* and its dozen principles of the ethical practice of public health.[23] This code was developed in 2002, under the auspices of the Public Health Leadership Society, with input from representatives of several organizations involved in public health. The aim, indicated by the Preamble, was to "highlight the ethical principles that follow from the distinctive characteristics of public health." Hence, it was not intended to be novel or to exhaust the content of public health ethics. Underlying several of the code's ethical principles is a fundamental belief in human interdependence as "the essence of community." This belief is expressed in the public health effort "to assure the health of whole communities," but also in recognition of the inextricable tie between individual health and communal life.

The authors of the code intended it primarily "for public and other institutions in the United States that have an explicit public health mission" but also stressed that it could be pertinent and helpful to institutions and individuals whose work has effects on the health of the community even though they do not have an "explicit public health mission." As we will see, physicians and other health professionals outside the conventional public health structure often have a role, sometimes even legally mandated, in public health—for instance, to report certain conditions to public health authorities.

The following table presents the 12 principles of the code.

TABLE 1.4 Principles of the Ethical Practice of Public Health (Public Health Leadership Society)

1	Public health should address principally the fundamental causes of disease and requirements for health, aiming to prevent adverse health outcomes.
2	Public health should achieve community health in a way that respects the rights of individuals in the community.
3	Public health policies, programs, and priorities should be developed/evaluated with community members' input.
4	Public health should advocate and work for the empowerment of disenfranchised community members, aiming to ensure that the basic resources and conditions necessary for health are accessible to all.
5	Public health should seek the information needed to implement effective policies and programs that protect and promote health.
6	Public health institutions should provide communities with the information they have that is needed for decisions on policies or programs and should obtain the community's consent for their implementation.
7	Public health institutions should act in a timely manner on the information they have within the resources and the mandate given to them by the public.
8	Public health programs and policies should incorporate a variety of approaches that anticipate and respect diverse values, beliefs and cultures in the community.
9	Public health programs/policies should be implemented in a manner that most enhances the physical and social environment.
10	Public health institutions should protect the confidentiality of information that can bring harm to an individual or community if made public. Exceptions must be justified based on the high likelihood of significant harm to the individual or others.
11	Public health institutions should ensure their employees' professional competence.
12	Public health institutions and their employees should engage in collaborations and affiliations in ways that build the public's trust and the institution's effectiveness.

Reproduced from: Public Health Leadership Society (2002). *Principles of the ethical practice of public health* version 2.2. New Orleans, LA. PHLS.

These principles operate on several levels. Some of them specify the broad ethical values and norms we have already. Hence, there is substantial overlap between our framework and the ethical principles articulated in the code. Some of them are much more specific as befits a professional code—for example, #11: "Public health institutions should ensure their employees' professional competence." This is obviously a precondition of the ethical practice of public health but is not something we will discuss here.

As we proceed, we will note the overlap, convergence, and interaction between the principles stated in this code and the clusters of ethical values and norms that we present, and we will at times show how the code's principles apply to particular cases. However, an appeal to the code by itself—"This is what the code says"—will not provide a sufficient public justification for public health policies and practices. Such justifications will come from appeal to broad, shared ethical values and norms, embedded in the society's institutions including the law, as well as in the code's ethical principles. However, the ethical principles in the code provide helpful guidance in practical decision making in public health.

METAPHORS IN PUBLIC HEALTH ETHICS

In this final section we consider the role of metaphors in public health ethics.[24,25,e] Metaphors involve seeing something as something else—for example, seeing human beings as wolves or life as a journey. "The essence of metaphor," according to George Lakoff and Mark Johnson in *Metaphors We Live By* (p. 5), "is understanding and experiencing one thing through another."[26]

Metaphors are unavoidable, and they frame and shape what we see and experience even when we are not consciously aware of them. They are sometimes dismissed as merely decorative when they are noticed at all. However, they do have cognitive significance, and attending to them may enable us to make better ethical judgments about policies, practices, and actions in public health. Some metaphors may even be "generative metaphors" that produce significant ethical insights into situations we confront and relevant norms.[27] For instance, the metaphor of the ladder in the Intervention Ladder proves to be an illuminating way to think through various public health interventions in relation to respect for autonomous choices and liberties. Earlier we suggested that the metaphor of fire officials illuminates public health's dual roles in prevention and in preparation for emergencies

We can evaluate metaphors not only by their decorative and rhetorical significance—for instance, how they stir people's emotions—but also by how well they illuminate what is going on and what should go on. These are the descriptive and prescriptive uses of metaphor. The metaphor of the parent-child relationship in the model of paternalism accurately describes some public health practices, but elsewhere we test its adequacy for ethical guidance in public health. In addition, we will consider the metaphor or analogy of the lifeboat when we examine the ethics of rationing or triage, and several other metaphors when we consider public health surveillance.

Evaluating metaphors' descriptive function (helping us see what is going on) requires attention to accuracy and adequacy. Evaluating their prescriptive function, their adequacy to guide and motivate policies and actions in public health, requires attention to the ethical principles and values they highlight and hide. Which do they illuminate and which do they obscure? Do they adequately account for the full range of general moral considerations for the analysis and assessment of public health policies and actions? This, for instance, is what we will do in our examination of paternalism. For now, we will focus on two current metaphors for public health: public health as warfare and public health as stewardship.

Public Health as Warfare

We often think of policies and actions, even nonmilitary ones, through metaphors of warfare. This has been particularly true in medicine and public health, at least since the emergence in the late 19th century of the germ theory of disease, which identified biological agents that invade the human body and threaten its defenses. Our conversations and debates in both medicine and public health frequently resort to military metaphors, which both illuminate and distort descriptions of and ethical guidance in medicine and public health. Our language tips us off to the prevalence of military metaphors, even when we are not fully aware that we are using them because they seem so natural to us. Childress points to several war-related metaphors in written and oral descriptions of modern biomedicine:

> The physician as the captain leads the battle against disease; orders a battery of tests; develops a plan of attack; calls on the armamentarium or arsenal of medicine; directs allied health personnel; treats aggressively; and expects compliance. Good patients are those who fight vigorously and refuse to give up. Victory is sought; defeat is feared. Sometimes there is even hope for a "magic bullet" or a "silver bullet."[24]

[e] Metaphors and analogies have substantial overlap. Analogies focus on similarities between two entities, such as a lifeboat situation and the intensive care unit. There is a rough consensus that, while metaphors presuppose some similarities, they also enable us to see similarities in entities that appear to be dissimilar.

We fight against illness, disease, and trauma as immediate enemies and against death as our ultimate enemy. Practicing medicine requires being "on the firing lines" or "in the trenches," and practitioners often have "war stories" to share. Moreover, the lens of military training and hierarchy can illuminate demanding medical training and structures of authority in medicine.[28] Furthermore, "[a]s medicine wages war against germs that invade the body and threaten its defenses, so the society itself may also declare war on cancer or on AIDS under the leadership of its chief medical officer, who in the United States is the Surgeon General."[24] Susan Sontag's point applies directly to public health: "Where once it was the physician who waged *bellum contra morbum*, the war against disease, now it's the whole society."[29]

The complex of military metaphors has positive, negative, and ambiguous implications in medicine, health care, and public health. On a personal level it can empower resistance and support courageous, vigorous efforts to combat disease and death.[28] However, it can also lead to futile and counterproductive actions. Some persons coping with chronic, debilitating diseases have found military metaphors unhelpful and even harmful, and as a result, have resorted to other metaphors—for instance, one young patient found a better life in viewing diabetes as a *teacher* rather than, as previously, an *enemy* to be conquered.[30]

Following are some common practical implications of the military metaphor. These are tendencies in ethical interpretation and application rather than necessary implications. First, the metaphor of medicine as warfare tends to underwrite overtreatment, even in the face of imminent death, since death is the ultimate enemy. Second, military metaphors tend to frame the society's healthcare budget as a defense budget in the war against morbidity and mortality. These metaphors may support a larger allocation of funds for the societal defense represented by medicine, health care, and public health than might otherwise be warranted. And, within health care, they suggest a set of priorities: critical care over preventive and chronic care; lethal diseases, such as some forms of cancer, over chronic diseases; acute technological interventions, such as intensive-care units, over less technological modes of care.[24]

Some of the negative or ambiguous implications of military metaphors could be corrected, at least partially, if we understood and conducted warfare in health care and public health not as a total war, but rather in line with the "just-war" or "limited-war" traditions, which stress limited objectives and limited means. In the just-war tradition, for example, waging a war is not ethically justifiable unless there is a reasonable prospect of success, the probable positive effects of the intervention outweigh the risks, the distinction between enemy combatants and noncombatants is maintained, and so forth.

The military metaphor has been sharply challenged in medicine and health care, but it has continued to flourish in public health, in part because of its function in describing and guiding society's responses to contagious diseases that threaten the public's health. This is not surprising because, after all, the spread of severe infectious diseases across borders can pose threats to a state's stability and security as much as military aggression across those borders.[31] Hence, as Mark Hall notes, "[t]he metaphors of public health strategy are war-like."[32]

In our sociocultural context, the metaphor of war is almost expected when a serious threat to a large number of residents requires the mobilization of societal resources, particularly when that threat comes from biological organisms that attack the body. It provides a way to galvanize the society and to marshal its resources for an effective counterattack. The ambiguous and negative implications previously noted need resistance and correction in this context too. Furthermore, the war metaphor is perhaps even more dangerous, both rhetorically and practically, when the war on terror becomes the model for the war on infectious diseases.[33] Limits are even more difficult to maintain in such a war.

Another serious ethical ambiguity in society's war against contagious diseases emerges in the identification of the enemy, such as a threatening virus. This process of identification is an important and necessary part of the battle. Once this occurs, it is possible to identify human vectors who may "harbor" the virus, "infect" others, and even become public "enemies." When AIDS appeared in the early 1980s, the society undertook what was described as a "war against AIDS." As part of this war, researchers vigorously sought to pinpoint the responsible biological agent, soon identified as HIV. Once tests were developed to detect the virus—the immediate "enemy"—in human beings, it was possible to identify individuals who were "carriers" of the virus, who "harbored" the virus, and who supposedly endangered others. Not surprisingly—but nonetheless problematically—many proposed draconian policies to identify HIV-infected individuals, perhaps even through mandatory screening and testing. Such "carriers" tended to become "enemies" in social discourse and practice as much as the virus itself.[34] Despite warnings by the Surgeon General and others that the war against HIV was not a war against people with HIV, this distinction was too subtle for many.

As already noted, military metaphors would be less problematic if the society followed the constraints of the just-war tradition in waging war, by pursuing limited objectives and using limited means, rather than being tempted by a total war or crusade stoked by rampant and often uninformed or ill-informed fears. Since we are not likely to eliminate the war metaphor in public health—nor should we try to do so—it is important that we use it selectively, when the situation warrants, and with due regard to ethical limits.

Public Health as Stewardship

A creative proposal to interpret and even reorient public health appeared in the Nuffield Council on Bioethics' 2007 report *Public Health: Ethical Issues*, which proposed the metaphor of *stewardship*. The report argues that a state, guided by the metaphor or model of stewardship, should act as a steward—an agent or overseer—of the health of its population. It stresses the state's duty to "look after" the population's important needs, including their individual and collective health needs. Even if the state views the public's health as an intrinsic value, a value in and of itself, it can also protect and promote the public's health as a "primary asset" because "higher levels of health are associated with greater overall well-being and productivity."[35] Its obligations include providing the conditions that permit people to be healthy and taking steps to reduce health inequalities, with special attention to disadvantaged and vulnerable groups. In emphasizing the state's stewardship of public and population health, the report does not assign sole responsibility to the state or preclude various public-private collaborations. Far from it—there are also corporate responsibilities for public health. According to the report, several goals and constraints flow from the stewardship model, as indicated in the following two tables.

TABLE 1.5 The Stewardship Model: Goals of Public Health Programs

Aim to reduce the risks of ill health that people might impose on each other.
Aim to reduce causes of ill health by regulations that ensure environmental conditions that sustain good health, such as the provision of clean air and water, safe food, and appropriate housing.
Pay special attention to the health of children and other vulnerable people.
Promote health not only by providing information and advice, but also by programs to help people overcome addictions and other unhealthy behaviors.
Aim to ensure that it is easy for people to lead a healthy life, for example, by providing convenient and safe opportunities for exercise.
Ensure that people have appropriate access to medical services.
Aim to reduce health inequalities.

Modified from the Nuffield Council on Bioethics. Public health: ethical issues (November 2007), published by the Nuffield Council on Bioethics, London, England. Available at: http://www.nuffieldbioethics.org/sites/default/files/Public%20health%20-%20ethical%20issues.pdf (accessed May 3, 2013).

TABLE 1.6 The Stewardship Model: Constraints on Public Health Programs

Not attempt to coerce adults to lead healthy lives.
Minimize interventions that are introduced without the individual consent of those affected, or without procedural justice arrangements (such as democratic decision-making procedures) which provide adequate mandate.
Seek to minimize interventions that are perceived as unduly intrusive and in conflict with important personal values.

Modified from Nuffield Council on Bioethics, *Public Health: Ethical Issues* (November 2007), published by the Nuffield Council on Bioethics, London, England. Available at: http://www.nuffieldbioethics.org/sites/default/files/Public%20health%20-%20ethical%20issues.pdf (accessed May 3, 2013).

Critics of the stewardship metaphor make several points. A main criticism—one we share—is that it is difficult to see how these several goals and constraints, as important as they are in public health, are systematically related to the metaphor itself. At most this very broad metaphor provides a general orientation for public health rather than operational guidance. According to critics, it is a "rather muddled metaphor," one that is inadequately explored in the report.[36] As a result, its substantive content is limited. Some developers of the stewardship model insist in response that it provides "an explicitly value-rich framework against which policy makers and others can assess existing policy, and develop new policy, by determining to what degree they achieve its goals, while minimizing unnecessary burdens and constraints."[37]

What is more crucial than finding the best possible metaphor for public health is recognizing that our views about public health goals and means, as well as the situations in which we have to make decisions, are often shaped by metaphors that we may not explicitly recognize and that may have positive, negative, or ambiguous implications we fail to see. We need to attend to those metaphors (whether they are functioning descriptively or prescriptively), assess their adequacy, and correct, constrain, and supplement them as needed. Public health officials may not be able to decisively shape or reshape the systems of metaphors that guide the society's response to public health needs and threats. Those metaphorical systems may be too deeply embedded in the society and culture to allow significant alterations. Despite such barriers, it is important, in public communication and public engagement, to attend to those embedded metaphors and address their positive, negative, and ambiguous implications, sometimes by invoking alternative metaphors. (See our discussion of health communication in Chapter 9.)

CONCLUSIONS

In this chapter, we developed a framework for examining ethical and legal values and norms and for evaluating the use of several tools and interventions in public health. We examined the public philosophy that marks legal and ethical norms and discourse in the U.S. These include attention to the end(s) of public health and also the means, in the form of various tools and interventions, which are used to realize the end(s). Effective means are crucially important but not all potentially effective means can be ethically justified. This public philosophy sets (rebuttable) presumptions in favor of interventions that respect liberty, privacy, confidentiality, and so forth. Hence, our ethical analysis of means should start with these presumptions that can be overridden or outweighed, if certain "justificatory conditions" are met in the process of public justification for public health policies, practices, and actions. We should not exaggerate ethical conflicts and dilemmas in public health because there are often ways to avoid or reduce tensions. One helpful step is to analyze situations and decisions in public health in a systematic way, through a variety of questions, including the ones we identified. Another valuable step is to consider situations and prospective decisions in light of the *Principles of Ethical Practice of Public Health*. Finally, it is also important to attend to the metaphors that often subconsciously guide our reflections about ends and means in public health and to consider their strengths and weaknesses as well as possible alternative metaphors.

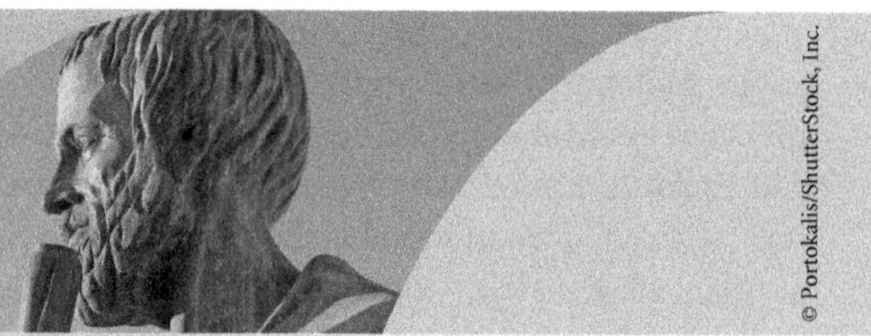

Discussion Questions

1. What is distinctive about a presumptivist approach to public health ethics (in contrast to contextualist and absolutist approaches)? And what are its advantages and disadvantages?
2. Do you believe that public justification is important in public health policies, practices, and actions? Why or why not?
3. Suppose a public health policy, such as quarantine, violates individuals' liberty. Do you believe that it must satisfy all of the justificatory conditions identified in this chapter to be ethically acceptable? Why or why not?
4. From your perspective, do you believe that conflicts between moral norms and the realization of public health goals are (a) common and unavoidable for the most part, or (b) uncommon and avoidable for the most part? Explain your answer.
5. Can you think of other metaphors than the ones discussed in this chapter for guiding reflections about public health goals and means?

REFERENCES

1. Childress JF, Faden RR, Gaare RD, et al. Public health ethics: mapping the terrain. *Journal of Law, Medicine & Ethics* 2002;30(2):169–177.

2. Beauchamp TL, Childress JF. *Principles of Biomedical Ethics*, 7th edition. New York: Oxford University Press, 2013.

3. Institute of Medicine. *The Future of Public Health*. Washington, DC: National Academy Press, 1988.

4. Childress JF, Bernheim RG. Public health ethics: public justification and public trust. *Bundesgesundheitsblatt, Gesundheitsforschung, Gesundheitsschutz* 2008;51(2):158–163.

5. Bernheim RG, Nieburg P, Bonnie RJ. Ethics and the practice of public health. In: Goodman RA (ed). *Law in Public Health Practice*, 2nd edition. New York: Oxford University Press, 2007.

6. Sandel MJ. *Democracy's Discontent: America in Search of a Public Philosophy*. Cambridge, MA: Harvard University Press, 1996.

7. Mann JM. Medicine and public health, ethics and human rights. *The Hastings Center Report* 1997;27(May-June):6–13.

8. Richardson HS. Specifying, balancing, and interpreting bioethical principles. *Journal of Medicine and Philosophy* 2000;25:285–307.

9. Gaskins RH. *Burdens of Proof in Modern Discourse*. New Haven, CT: Yale University Press, 1992.

10. Childress JF, Bernheim RG. Beyond the liberal and communitarian impasse: a framework and vision for public health. *Florida Law Review* 2003;55(6):1191–1219.

11. Working Group of the University of Toronto Joint Centre for Bioethics. *Ethics and SARS: Learning Lessons from the Toronto Experience*. Toronto, Canada: The University of Toronto Joint Centre for Bioethics, 2003. This report is available at http://www.yorku.ca/igreene/sars.html (accessed July 31, 2007).

12. Schram J. Personal views: how popular perceptions of risk from SARS are fermenting discrimination. *BMJ* 2003;326(7395):939.

13. Calabresi G, Bobbitt P. *Tragic Choices*. New York: W.W. Norton & Co., 1978.

14. Public Health Leadership Society. *Principles of the Ethical Practice of Public Health*, 2002. http://www.phls.org/home/section/3-26/ (accessed July 31, 2007).

15. Institute of Medicine. *The Future of the Public's Health in the 21st Century*. Washington, DC: The National Academies Press, 2003.

16. Soto MA, Abel C, Dievler A. *Healthy Communities: New Partnerships for the Future of Public Health: A Report of the First Year of the Committee on Public Health,* Institute of Medicine. Washington, DC: National Academy Press, 1996.

17. Gostin LO. When terrorism threatens health: how far are limitations on personal and economic liberties justified? *Florida Law Review* 2003;55:1105–1170.

18. Gostin LO. Public health law in an age of terrorism: rethinking individual rights and common goods. *Health Affairs* 2002;21(6):79–93

19. Annas GJ. Bioterrorism, public health, and civil liberties. *New England Journal of Medicine* 2002;346:1337–1342.

20. Annas GJ. Bioterrorism, public health, and human rights. *Health Affairs* 2002;21:94–97.

21. Bayer R. Public health policy and the AIDS epidemic: an end to HIV exceptionalism? *New England Journal of Medicine* 1991;324:1500–1504.

22. Bayer R, Colgrove J. Bioterrorism, public health, and the law. *Health Affairs (Project Hope)* 2002;21(6):98–101.

23. Public Health Leadership Society. *Principles of the Ethical Practice of Public Health* 2002. Available at: http://phls.org/CMSuploads/Principles-of-the-Ethical-Practice-of-PH-Version-2.2-68496.pdf (accessed April 15, 2013).

24. Childress JF. Metaphor and analogy. In: Post SG (ed), *Encyclopedia of Bioethics*. New York: Macmillan Reference USA, 2003.

25. Childress JF. Metaphor and Analogy. *Practical Reasoning in Bioethics*. Bloomington, IN: Indiana University Press, 1997.

26. Lakoff G, Johnson M. *Metaphors We Live By,* 2nd edition. Chicago: University of Chicago Press, 2003.

27. Schön DA 1979. Generative metaphor: A perspective on problem-setting in public policy. In: Ortony A (ed), *Metaphor and Thought*. Cambridge, UK: Cambridge University Press, 1979:254–268.

28. Reisfield GM, Wilson GR. Use of metaphor in the discourse on cancer. *Journal of Clinical Oncology* 2004;22(19):4024–4027.

29. Sontag S. *Illness as Metaphor* and *AIDS and Its Metaphors*. New York: Doubleday Anchor Books, 1990.

30. Pray L, Evans, R III. *Journey of a Diabetic*. New York: Simon and Schuster, 1983.

31. De Grandis G. On the analogy between infectious diseases and war: how to use it and not to use it. *Public Health Ethics* 2011;4(1):70–83.

32. Hall MA. The scope and limits of public health law. *Perspectives in Biology and Medicine* 2003;46(Suppl):S199–S209

33. Mongoven A. The war on disease and the war on terror: a dangerous metaphorical nexus? *Cambridge Quarterly of Healthcare Ethics* 2006;15:403–416.

34. Childress JF. Mandatory HIV screening and testing. In: Reamer FG (ed), *AIDS & Ethics*. New York: Columbia University Press, 1991:50–76.

35. Nuffield Council on Bioethics. *Public Health: Ethical Issues*. London: Nuffield Council on Bioethics, 2007. Available at: www.nuffieldbioethics.org (accessed January 17, 2013).

36. Dawson A, Verweij M. The steward of the Millian state. *Public Health Ethics* 2008;1(2):193–195.

37. Baldwin T, Brownsword R, Schmidt H. Stewardship, paternalism and public health: further thoughts. *Public Health Ethics* 2009;2(1):113–116.

© Portokalis/ShutterStock, Inc.

CHAPTER 2

Moral Considerations: Bases and Limits for Public Health Interventions

by James F. Childress

Learning Objectives

By the end of this chapter, the reader will be able to

- Understand how general moral considerations function in deliberation about and justification of ends and means in public health
- Understand the principle of utility and its applications in public health, including the distinction between social utility and medical or health utility
- Explain the formal and material criteria of justice and how different theories of justice present different material criteria
- Understand how utility and egalitarian justice sometimes conflict in triage in public health crises and possible ways to resolve these conflicts
- Describe and use the Intervention Ladder
- Understand the place and function of respect for autonomous choices and liberties in assessing interventions in public health
- Distinguish and assess strong paternalism and weak paternalism
- Distinguish and relate privacy and confidentiality

TABLE 2.1 Moral Considerations in Public Health

1. Producing benefits
2. Avoiding, preventing, and removing harms
3. Producing the maximal balance of benefits over harms and other costs (often called utility)
4. Distributing benefits and burdens fairly (distributive justice) and ensuring public participation, including the participation of affected parties (procedural justice)
5. Respecting autonomous choices and actions, including liberty of action
6. Protecting privacy and confidentiality
7. Keeping promises and commitments
8. Disclosing information as well as speaking honestly and truthfully (often grouped under transparency)
9. Building and maintaining trust

Data from Childress JF, Faden RR, Gaare RD, et al., et al. Public Health Ethics: Mapping the Terrain. Journal of Law, Medicine, & Ethics 2002;30(2):169–177.

INTRODUCTION

Public health ethics rests upon a set of general moral considerations (GMCs) that have been widely discussed in the literature. These general considerations include the following:

Our task in this chapter is to further develop these GMCs in several clusters. First, we will consider (#1) producing benefits in conjunction with other connected moral considerations: (#2) avoiding, preventing, and removing harms, and (#3) producing the maximal balance of benefits over harms and other costs. We will examine all of these under the heading of utility, with particular attention to applying the principle of utility in public health through cost-effectiveness analysis, cost-benefit analysis, and risk-benefit analysis. We conclude that these formal, analytic techniques are useful with qualifications and within limits, including limits set by principles of justice.

The next section investigates (#4) distributing benefits and burdens fairly (*distributive justice*) and ensuring public participation, including the participation of affected parties (*procedural justice*). It outlines competing criteria of justice for determining what is due to individuals and groups. It further considers how to allocate resources in a public health crisis, such as a bioterrorist attack or pandemic influenza, as well as how to incorporate both utility and egalitarian justice in substantive criteria, public participation, and procedural fairness in determining ethically justifiable triage in such contexts.

We then turn to (#5) respecting autonomous choices and actions, including liberty of action. The chapter to this point will have considered how in public health to formulate goals and benefits, balanced against costs and harms, and how to distribute benefits and burdens fairly. In this section, it turns to potentially limiting moral considerations that may put some presumptive—i.e., nonabsolute—obstacles in the way of producing maximum benefit. Which means may public health officials ethically use in getting individuals to act in ways that will prevent personal and societal ill health or promote good health? Here we will start from and modify the Intervention Ladder proposed by the Nuffield Council on Bioethics to explore different interventions and the circumstances under which they can be ethically justified. We will also consider the conditions under which specifically paternalistic interventions, i.e., interventions aimed at the welfare of the individual himself or herself, can be ethically justified.

Privacy and confidentiality (#6) are two moral considerations that may create important but nonabsolute obstacles to the pursuit of public health through gathering and sharing personal information. We will closely examine their meaning, scope, and weights. Surveillance and notification of others at risk, such as an HIV-infected individual's sexual partners, are two areas of public health practice that, in some cases, require determining whether and when it is justifiable to override privacy and confidentiality.

We will not devote specific sections of this chapter to the last three GMCs in **Table 2.1**: (#7) keeping promises and commitments, (#8) disclosing information as well as speaking honestly and truthfully (often grouped under transparency), and (#9) building and maintaining trust. Instead, we will note their implications at different points in this chapter.

Three other preliminary notes: First, we refer to these general moral considerations in various ways: as *GMCs*, sometimes as *norms*, *principles*, or *values*, and, occasionally, as *rules*. Second, we refer to the moral requirements they entail both as *obligations* or *duties*, from the standpoint of the agents, and as *rights*, from the standpoint of those affected. For most moral obligations or duties in this volume, there are generally correlative rights. So, for the most part (but not always), we can say either (1) "A" has an *obligation* or *duty* to "B," or (2) "B" has a *right*, by which we mean a *justified claim*, against "A." Third, we do not develop these clusters of GMCs in a systematic moral, social, or political theory. Rather, we will view these as embedded in our liberal, democratic society (where "liberal" refers to the commitment to liberty). We focus mainly on obligations to pursue public health within a country without developing our important responsibilities for global public health. Within a liberal, democratic society, such as the U.S., particular public health programs and interventions must satisfy principles of utility, justice, and the others we examine in this chapter.

UTILITY: BALANCING PROBABLE BENEFITS, COSTS, AND RISKS

Utility

The principle of utility has had various interpretations over the last few centuries, as philosophers and others have filled out the normative phrase: "do the greatest good" or "do the greatest good for the greatest number." It provides a way to determine right and wrong, or justified and unjustified, policies, practices, and actions by determining whether they "do the greatest good." However, there are sundry interpretations of the values that enable us to appraise a state of affairs as good or bad. Historically, many utilitarians have appealed to subjective values, such as pleasure, happiness, or satisfaction of desires, but some have appealed to objective values viewed as intrinsically good, such as health, knowledge, and beauty.[1] Categories like welfare may have subjective or objective formulations. We do not need to attempt to resolve these debates but only to stress the importance of attending to the values operative in different assessments of states of affairs, effects, and consequences.[a]

In this chapter, the principle of utility is understood as the principle of producing the maximal balance of good over bad effects or maximum net benefits. We will examine a few

[a] These debates about values have led many in recent years to prefer the label consequentialism to utilitarianism, enabling them better to separate the disputes about value from the judgments about producing the net balance of good over bad consequences. But the question of value has still to be resolved. See Driver J, "The History of Utilitarianism," *The Stanford Encyclopedia of Philosophy* (Summer 2009 Edition), Zalta EN (ed). http://plato.stanford.edu/archives/sum2009/entries/utilitarianism-history/ and Sinnott-Armstrong W, "Consequentialism," *The Stanford Encyclopedia of Philosophy* (Winter 2012 Edition), Zalta EN (ed). http://plato.stanford.edu/archives/win2012/entries/consequentialism/

of the controversies about defining and measuring benefits when we consider how public health benefits are specified through such measures as lives or life–years or quality-adjusted life–years.

Recognizing the GMC—norm or principle—of utility does not commit us to utilitarianism as an overall framework. Utilitarians tend to make utility the foundational principle from which all other moral norms are derived or the dominant principle that overrides all other moral considerations. It is not necessary to affirm either of these views in order to use the principle of utility as we do—that is, as one among several principles that must be considered in making ethical judgments in public health.

Utility-based judgments about policies, practices, and actions in public health from the standpoint of the principle of utility may proceed informally or formally. We make informal judgments about balancing benefits, costs, and risks all the time, but sometimes we use formal analytic techniques in balancing them. We will start with the latter.

Cost-Effectiveness and Cost-Benefit Analyses

In public health, health policy, and health care, considerations of utility are often specified and applied through tools of formal analysis, especially cost-effectiveness analysis (CEA) and cost-benefit analysis (CBA).[2,3,4] We are viewing all of these as efforts to maximize societal welfare, often expressed as the principle of utility.

In public health policy and practice, formal, analytic, economic methods have been employed as a way to improve decision making particularly when trade-offs are involved, for instance, between costs and benefits. Their proponents contend that these tools can aid decisions by providing more systematic, quantitative, comparative input about programs and interventions. These tools enable us to state more formally and systematically what we ordinarily consider in less formal and systematic ways.

CEA, CBA, and similar assessments can play important roles in setting and determining how best to pursue specific public health goals. A good example comes from the debate over several years about whether the human papillomavirus (HPV) vaccine should be recommended for males as well as for females in order to reduce the HPV-associated conditions for both. (The societal debate about the HPV vaccine is discussed elsewhere.) At one point, after reviewing further data about the effects of HPV infections on males, the Advisory Committee on Immunization Practices considered the cost-effectiveness of a strategy of adding HPV vaccinations for males to the programs then targeted at females. Following is its assessment:

> Mathematical modeling suggests that adding male HPV vaccination to a female-only HPV vaccination program is not the most cost-effective vaccination strategy for reducing the overall burden of HPV-associated conditions in males and females when vaccination coverage of females is high (>80%). When coverage of females is less than 80%, male vaccination might be cost-effective, although results vary substantially across models. Because the health burden is greater in females than males, and numerous models have shown vaccination of adolescent girls to be a cost-effective use of public health resources, improving coverage in females aged 11 and 12 years could potentially be a more effective and cost-effective strategy than adding male vaccination.[5]

Reproduced from Licensure of Quadrivalent Human Papillomavirus Vaccine (HPV4, Gardasil) for Use in Males and Guidance from the Advisory Committee on Immunization Practices (ACIP). Morbidity and Mortality Weekly Report. 2010;59:630–632.

CEA is obviously not the only consideration in setting a vaccination policy but it is, in our judgment, a relevant one. However, considerations of justice are also important in setting vaccine policy regarding males and females.

One major difference between CEA and CBA is how each presents the benefits that are incorporated into its analysis. CEA states the benefits it measures in various ways. For instance, public health officials might use measures such as years of life (life-years or LYs), quality-adjusted life–years (QALYs), number of cases prevented, or number of persons screened for the outcomes of its programs and interventions. CEA eschews the use of money in stating the benefit that is being balanced against costs. Its conclusions appear in formulations such as "cost per QALY." Public health officials can use CEA to compare different public health programs or interventions only if they have the same endpoint, such as life-years saved. It is not possible to compare different public health programs or interventions if their endpoints are different—for instance, life-years saved versus reduction in the days of work lost to influenza.

By contrast, CBA may begin with nonmonetary quantitative units, such as cases prevented, statistical deaths, or QALYs, but it typically moves beyond these units. It attempts to restate the benefits in ways that will facilitate a direct comparison between the benefits and the costs as well as between different programs and interventions that may have different outcomes such as saving life–years or reducing days lost from work. CBA accomplishes this by using monetary figures for both the benefits and the costs. Hence, it can present benefit-cost ratios that can then be compared.

Both of these methods have their defenders and their detractors. A major line of defense focuses on their value in providing quantitative input for decision makers in public health and elsewhere. This defense holds that these methods can reduce the need to rely on assigning intuitive weights to different options and can help avoid the vagaries of a political process marred by conflicting ideologies, competing interest groups, and an uniformed public. Critics, however, charge that these techniques sometimes are used as a way to bypass rather than inform democratic public engagement. In such cases, they may be employed by persons with technical expertise but with only a narrow vision and limited understanding of the legitimate ethical, legal, social, and political constraints on the use of such methods. Furthermore, critics charge, these methods are not broad enough to capture the entire range of relevant values and options and, in particular, may not adequately consider and may even conflict with principles of justice.

Many of the harshest criticisms are directed at CBA's effort to translate the range of possible goals and benefits being sought into dollar figures. It appears to reduce what is valuable and valued to dollar amounts—even to state the value of life in monetary terms—and thus to screen out much that is important in public health as well as in the society at large. It might appear useful to develop consistent valuations of human life across different programs, such as public health, environmental protections, and transportation, but it is not easy to do. In particular, all of the methods used to assign a dollar value to life seem unsatisfactory and perhaps even seriously flawed.[6] This is one reason CBA is generally less important than CEA in public health. In addition CEA also requires less time and fewer resources, is generally clearer and easier to grasp, and, as a result, is better suited to informing decision making.[7]

It is beyond our task in this chapter to offer a full-scale evaluation of CEA and CBA from an ethical standpoint. Since CEA is more widely used in public health, we will attend to some of its limitations. One concern is that it tends to focus on the costs and benefits that can be measured fairly easily.[8] Ethically, it is important to attend to the range of relevant benefits and costs in conducting analyses of programs and interventions. For instance, the Varicella (chickenpox) vaccine was not deemed to be cost saving for the healthcare system when only the cost per life-year gained was considered; however, on a broader analysis that considered the loss of parental work time in caring for children, it turned out to be cost effective.[8]

At first glance it might appear implausible to challenge one premise of QALY-based CEA—that a healthy life-year has equal value for everyone. The CEA slogan is that a QALY is a QALY whoever possesses it. Nevertheless, there are legitimate challenges, particularly from the standpoint of justice. First, CEAs based on QALYs may in fact discriminate against older persons because, in general, an intervention that prevents the death of younger people will probably produce more QALYs than an intervention that prevents the death of older people. Other things being equal, older people will have fewer life-years ahead of them to be saved. Sometimes it is justifiable to give priority to younger people over older people in allocation decisions, but by focusing on life-years, QALY-based CEAs tend to hide this trade-off rather than enabling us directly to wrestle with it. Second, public health programs and interventions built on CEAs based on QALYs or life-years may not give enough attention to the number of different individual lives that could be saved. After all, if the goal is production of QALYs, then there is no ethical difference between an intervention that saves one person with 60 expected QALYs and another intervention that saves three different people each with 20 expected QALYs. This runs counter to our ordinary ethical intuitions about and expectations regarding public health policies—it lets a mathematical approach trump human solidarity, beneficence, and justice. In short, the preference of QALY-based CEA for life-years over individual lives and for the number of life-years over the number of individual lives is ethically problematic.[6] Finally, and also problematically, QALYs operate with an assumption that there is "a lower utility to society of prolonging life for individuals with preexisting disability than for people without disability." This raises another justice question about discrimination against persons with disabilities.[8]

Graham and colleagues stress an "obvious but sometimes forgotten" point—CEA is not the only consideration in decision making in public health and other areas: "Other important factors include notions of justice, equity, personal freedom, political feasibility, and the constraints of current law."[9] As we will see in the next section, how much value is attached to the reduction of particular risks, for example, may depend on the nature of those risks, such as whether they are voluntarily assumed or out of our control. For all their problems, these formal analytic methods can be ethically used not to make ethical decisions but, within limits, to inform such decisions. While recognizing that "CEA methods pose ethical challenges," Grosse and colleagues are right to stress that "excluding cost-effectiveness as a consideration is also ethically problematic."[8] We should use these methods within limits and without assuming that they will produce complete answers for public health policy and practice.

Risk Assessment

In addition to examining public health programs and interventions through a systematic analysis of their costs, effectiveness, and benefits, another important application of utility focuses on risks and benefits. Sometimes benefits themselves are construed in terms of risk reduction—for instance, a public health program may be designed to achieve the goal (benefit) of reducing the risk of an outbreak of an infectious disease.

Risk assessment features the analysis and evaluation of probabilities of certain negative outcomes, particularly harms. (Following Feinberg, we understand harms as "setbacks to interests."[10]) The process of risk assessment involves several stages.[11] The first is *identifying* risks through locating dangers or threats, for instance, of an outbreak of a deadly avian influenza. Second is the task of *estimating* the risk, which entails determining, to the greatest extent possible, the probability and the magnitude of the harms associated with those dangers or threats. To continue the example of avian influenza: Based on early reports about recent cases, public health officials will seek to estimate the probability of pandemic influenza, in light of what is known about the ease of bird-to-human transmission and human-to-human transmission, as well as the severity (morbidity and mortality) of the infections that have occurred. A third step is *evaluating* the risk. This evaluation seeks to determine whether the identified and estimated risks are acceptable. Acceptability may hinge on balancing the risks and probable benefits of different courses of action in this context.[6] Risk is an inherently probabilistic term, whereas benefits need to have qualifiers to indicate they are not certain or definite. Examining risks, that is, the probability and severity of harms, in relation to various objectives may involve *risk-benefit analysis* (RBA).

These three stages of risk assessment may be followed by a fourth stage involving actions to control and manage risks depending on the cost-effectiveness ratios of different possible actions to reduce risks. Risk-reduction itself may be viewed as a benefit and various interventions may be evaluated in light of their effectiveness and cost-effectiveness in reducing risks of morbidity and mortality from, say, an avian influenza outbreak (**Figure 2.1**).

FIGURE 2.1 Risk Analysis and Assessment

		Severity of Harm	
		Trivial	**Serious**
Probability of Harm	**Low**	1	2
	High	3	4

Variations in Risk Perception

Public health policies and practices are often contested because of significant variations in people's perceptions of risk. It is tempting to assume that expert risk analysts and the general public will have substantially different perceptions of risks, in part because the general public may not adequately appreciate statistical probabilities. This may in part be true, but differences can also be expected across both groups because a number of factors influence perceptions of risk, both the probability of harm's occurrence (low to high) and the severity of that harm (trivial to serious). Perceptions of risk reflect several factors beyond the relevant numbers, such as the harm's severity in terms of morbidity and mortality or its statistical probability. For instance, risk perceptions may be influenced by whether the agent voluntarily assumes the risks rather than having them imposed by others, and whether he or she has some control over them (for example, by driving an automobile rather than flying commercially). They may also be influenced by whether the risks are new rather than familiar, and whether they are dreaded because of some associated conditions such as stigmatization.[12,13] The stigma associated with HIV infection in its early years led people to fear the risks associated with accidental HIV infection more than other comparable risks, such as accidental infection with hepatitis B prior to the development of an effective vaccine.

The public's perception of risk, even if its estimate of probabilities or severities is distorted, forms an important part of the context of public health policies and practices. The complexities indicate both the necessity and the difficulties of public communication and engagement around perceived risks and risk reduction strategies.

DISTRIBUTIVE JUSTICE

In the context of public health, justice is one of the core GMCs, which we stated as distributing benefits and burdens fairly (distributive justice) and ensuring public participation, including the participation of affected parties (procedural justice).

Justice is one of the most widely invoked and protean principles in public health ethics. A cluster of terms appears in formulations of justice, terms such as equality, equity, fairness, and impartiality.[14,15] However defined, justice frequently indicates one important basis of public health, as reflected in the goal of just health. For most frameworks of justice, public health is not only a maximization model, such as might develop from the standpoint of the principle of utility, which, on some interpretations, seeks the maximization of public or population health without regard to its distribution. Distributive justice approaches attend to whose health is involved, i.e., how health is distributed in a society, its patterns of distribution. In a public health context, it frequently attends to the vulnerable and disadvantaged as well as to the social determinants of health. Principle #4 of the *Principles of the Ethical Practice of Public Health* stresses both the egalitarian thrust and the concern for the vulnerable: "Public health should advocate and work for the empowerment of disenfranchised community members, aiming to ensure that the basic resources and conditions necessary for health are accessible to all."

Historically, the term justice has had both broad and narrow meanings. For instance, in the Biblical context, justice is usually viewed as roughly equivalent to righteousness. Instead of viewing justice as covering all of morality, we define it as giving each person his or her due and each group its due. Then it becomes necessary to determine the criteria for specifying what is due to persons and groups.

Formal Justice and Material Justice

One place to start is the distinction between formal justice and material justice or between a formal criterion of justice and material criteria of justice. At least since Aristotle, the formal criterion of justice has been to treat equals equally, or similar cases similarly. At first glance, this might not appear to be very helpful, since as a formal criterion, it is empty—it does not specify the relevant respects in which people must be equal or cases similar. Nor does it indicate how those who are equal in relevant respects should be treated, only that they should be treated equally. Nevertheless, the formal criterion of justice plays an important role in challenging various forms of discrimination and unequal treatment based on arbitrary differences.

Because of the emptiness of formal justice, it is necessary to specify material criteria that identify relevant characteristics for determining equals and unequals. These material criteria may be specified in different ways in different contexts of justice. They may look different depending on whether we are considering, for instance, distributive justice, retributive or criminal justice, commutative justice (contracts), or compensatory justice (rectifying past injustices). Our primary focus is distributive justice, that is, justice in the distribution of benefits and burdens, costs, and risks, coupled with justice in procedures and processes, such as public participation, often crucial in specifying what is due individuals and groups under conditions of scarcity, such as a public health crisis (which we will focus on in the excursus that follows this section).

Examples of material criteria include "to each according to his/her need," "to each according to achievement," "to each according to effort," "to each according to ability to pay," and so forth. These and other material criteria are defensible in certain contexts but not others. The just distribution of grades in an academic course should track students' achievements, rather than their need or their ability to pay. However, the distribution of expensive automobiles justly follows the material criterion of ability to pay. In the context of health care, distribution according to need is recognized as an important requirement of justice, but it may be combined with other criteria as well, such as the probability of a successful outcome; or, in a two-tiered system, such as operates in the U.S., ability to pay (or to have insurance pay) may play a role as well.

Consistent with our overall approach, we are not going to develop a full-blown theory of justice to compete in the marketplace of theories of justice, but we will identify several contending theories that take specific material criteria (sometimes in combination) as largely determinative of what is due individuals and groups. These theories are useful as "ideal types" that indicate the presuppositions and implications of taking one or more material criteria as far as they can be taken in a systematic framework. Hence, they provide helpful points of reference in societal conversations about what is due individuals and groups, what constitutes just public health. Readers will recognize versions of these theories in those conversations.[b]

Theories of Distributive Justice

Libertarian Justice Theory

As its name suggests, a libertarian theory of justice, influenced by philosophers such as John Locke and Robert Nozick, focuses on individuals' liberties, and so emphasizes our duties to respect others' liberties and the state's duty to protect our liberties, conceived as rights, when they are threatened. This often leads to a conception of the "minimal state," sometimes

[b] We are largely limiting our attention to the public health within the United States rather than globally. Global responsibilities are important, but beyond the scope of our discussion here, other than in passing.

TABLE 2.2 Types of Theories of Distributive Justice

Libertarian
Utilitarian
Egalitarian
Communitarian

called the "night watchman state," designed to prevent or punish transgressions of individual boundaries, including individuals' property rights. Taxation, as emphasized by the Tea Party in the U.S., is generally opposed as an unjust violation of liberty rights, especially if it goes beyond what is necessary for the minimal state to protect liberty rights. On this view, health care is not a right, but people may voluntarily choose to act charitably and contribute to health care for others and may within a community even voluntarily consent to some form of healthcare distribution. Public health may be legitimate particularly if it focuses on protecting individuals against contagious diseases—a form of boundary violation—rather than on broader conceptions of health promotion that mark much contemporary public health.

Utilitarian Justice Theory

Utilitarian theories of justice, historically shaped by such figures as Jeremy Bentham and John Stuart Mill, ground conceptions of justice in the principle of utility, which requires, as we saw in the previous section, actions, policies, or rules that produce maximal net benefits. According to Mill, "justice is a name for certain moral requirements, which, regarded collectively, stand higher in the scale of social utility, and are therefore of more paramount obligation, than any others; though particular cases may occur in which some other social duty is so important, as to overrule any one of the general maxims of justice."[16 (p. 259)] Justice, which involves correlative duties and rights, is not independently warranted but is rather derivative from utility. In this framework, duties and rights in just health care or just public health presuppose a foundation in net social utility. Health care and public health can be valued at least to the extent that they contribute to net social utility.

Communitarian Justice Theory

Like utilitarian theories, communitarian theories of justice, drawing on a number of philosophical perspectives, do not assign independent significance to individual rights, such as liberty, in contrast to libertarians (and to proponents of egalitarian justice). Rather, their conception of just health care and public health depends on the community's conception of the good of health, in relation to other goods, and the contributions of health care and public health to all those goods, not simply to health. Daniel Callahan, a representative of this perspective, approaches the allocation of health care from a putative shared substantive consensus about the good society. Hence, his questions for judging just allocations in health care and public health focus on their contributions to a good society: "Just what is it that good health brings to a society and how much and what kind of it are necessary for a good society? What is the common good it will bring us, and what is the public interest that it serves?"[17 (p. 105–106)] However elusive a substantive consensus may be—and it appears to be more elusive in a pluralistic society than Callahan and many communitarians suppose—this approach resonates with public health ethics, in viewing the community as both a *source* of insight into values and as a *target* (beyond the aggregation of individuals) for just health care and public health.

Egalitarian Justice Theory

Egalitarian theories of justice draw on philosophical and religious perspectives that recognize the equality of persons in at least some respects and the importance of treating them as equals in certain respects. Although there are a number of different versions of egalitarian theories, many of those in the last several decades have been influenced by the magisterial theory of justice propounded by John Rawls.[14] These generally recognize equalities in certain basic social goods but allow for other inequalities as well, and most of them recognize the possible legitimacy of a two-tiered system, with the lowest tier being a decent minimum or adequate level of health care (to be set in a deliberative democratic way). Among those influenced by Rawls' work, Norman Daniels, building on Rawls' conception of "fair equality of opportunity," argues that justice requires a society to remove or reduce obstacles that prevent fair equality of opportunity. This includes providing programs that compensate for persons' disadvantages such as their health disadvantages.[18,19] Egalitarian theories differ depending on whether they emphasize more equal opportunities, more equal capabilities, more equal welfare, or some combination of these.[20,21]

Certainly if we focus on opportunities and seek to ensure fair equality of opportunity, in combination with the formal criterion of justice, this will provide a reason for criticizing the use of several characteristics as bases for distributing benefits and burdens. We can start with obvious characteristics that are not relevant to the distribution of health care or health and that are not under the control of individuals—these include gender, race, and ethnicity. Their use as criteria in public health is generally discriminatory (unless, perhaps, as correctives to counter previous discrimination). Studies indicate that there are numerous racial and ethnic disparities in health care for a range of medical conditions and that these disparities lead to worse health outcomes for individuals and groups—a situation that an Institute of Medicine report rightly labels "unacceptable."[22]

At a broad level, egalitarian principles of justice feature equal regard for all persons and the treatment of each person as an equal, according to fair procedures, in the distribution of goods. This does not preclude rationing health care and other contributors to good health but sets constraints on how that rationing can proceed. It will regularly require fair participation in decisions that affect the distribution of such goods, and it will generally require fair procedures, such as ways to appeal adverse decisions. In the excursus that follows, we will consider whether and how egalitarian justice (in distribution, procedures, and participation) can be combined with utility in triage in a public health crisis.

EXCURSUS: JUST CARE IN A PUBLIC HEALTH CRISIS: UTILITY AND EGALITARIAN JUSTICE

What is just care in a public health crisis? We continue to explore the principles of utility and egalitarian justice by considering their place in the allocation of resources in a public health crisis. Several societal macro-allocation decisions determine, by default if not by design, how many doses of vaccine and antiviral medications and how many ventilators and intensive care beds will be available in a crisis. They thus determine the extent of scarcity of needed resources in a public health crisis and the intensity of the dilemmas that arise. In this section we will not focus on such macro-allocation decisions but instead will examine just care in a public health emergency or crisis, such as a deadly pandemic influenza or bioterrorist attack.

Triage in a Public Health Crisis

Let's imagine a public health crisis of the magnitude of the 1918–1919 pandemic influenza, which is estimated to have killed over half a million people in the U.S. and as many as 40 million worldwide. In such a crisis, which criteria and procedures should we use to allocate vaccines (if a vaccine is ready for use), antiviral medications, ventilators, and access to intensive care? We will consider several proposals based on utility and see whether and how far they can satisfy the requirements of egalitarian justice, and where they may need to be modified or rejected from that standpoint. The perspective of egalitarian justice, as we interpret it, requires that each person be treated as an equal but not necessarily identically; that unequal distributions of goods, including medical care, can sometimes be justified, particularly in public health crises; but that the criteria and processes of distribution in such contexts must themselves be fair, provide fair equality of opportunity, sometimes represented in lotteries, recognize the transcendence of persons over their social roles and functions, and involve the participation of affected stakeholders. Not all utility-based systems of allocation are equally problematic or satisfactory from an egalitarian perspective.

Several different terms have been used to describe and direct the process of distributing scarce preventive, prophylactic, and therapeutic resources in a public health crisis. These include distribution, (micro)allocation, selection, triage, rationing, and the like. However much they point to the same process, some of their connotations are different enough to affect public communication and public justification. "Selection" evokes conflicting images. On the one hand, it seems neutral and descriptive; on the other hand, many recall its use in Nazi Germany's extermination programs. The terms "distribution" and "allocation" offer more neutral descriptions and do not immediately evoke the harsh circumstances and hard choices suggested by "rationing" and "triage." "Triage" usually implies systematic "rationing" using classifications and categories that are efforts to "do the greatest good for the greatest number" (utility). It is often used to describe rationing medical and other goods in military contexts, civilian emergency responses—for example, to earthquakes or a mass casualty shooting—and emergency units in hospitals. A system of triage grades people according to needs and probable outcomes, and it seeks to maximize utility.[23,24] We will use the terms "triage" and "rationing" most of the time.

Types of Utility-based Triage

When we presented the principle of utility earlier in this chapter, we did not stress that it is often applied within certain boundaries rather than universally. For instance, when we talk about utility in public health, we often are thinking within our national boundaries, even though the principle's logic is universal. In approaching triage or rationing in a public health crisis, several possible boundaries of utility need attention.

Health or *medical utility* focuses on what would produce the greatest benefit among those already suffering from the serious effects of a natural or human-made public health crisis or at high risk of suffering such effects. The first step in triage is to determine medical utility, but it often extends beyond medical utility to include *social utility*, sometimes characterized as the social value or worth of the individuals who might be salvaged. It is very important to draw distinctions within

TABLE 2.3 Utility-Based Triage in a Public Health Crisis

Health or medical utility
Social utility
• Narrow social utility
• Broad social utility

social utility, between what we might characterize as *broad social utility* and *narrow social utility*. Broad social utility considers the overall value or worth of the individual to the society. By contrast, narrow social utility focuses on specific valuable (and perhaps essential) social roles that an individual fills or social functions that he or she discharges.[24]

Rationing based on medical utility does not necessarily violate the requirements of egalitarian justice. Take, for instance, medical utility focused on saving lives. As Derek Parfit notes, we try to save more lives "[b]ecause we do give equal weight to saving each. Each counts for one. That's why more count for more."[25] Here judgments of utility and egalitarian justice overlap, but we will raise some questions later about efforts to further specify and operationalize medical utility.

Social utility is more complicated. Both broad and narrow versions of social utility are in tension with egalitarian justice, but it may be possible to justify one but not the other in a public health crisis. In our view, it is not justifiable to ration resources in such a crisis by appeal to broad social utility, worth, or value, based on a judgment of people's lives viewed as a whole. However, a limited appeal to narrow social utility in triage—to save lives, to protect the fabric of the social order—in a public health crisis may be ethically acceptable. In recognizing limited, narrow social utilitarian exceptions to his egalitarian framework, ethicist Paul Ramsey focused on specific functions highly valued by the community in an emergency or crisis, such as an earthquake, and considered such functions similar to those performed by sailors on a lifeboat after a shipwreck—it is ethically justifiable to save some sailors in order to increase the chances of the lifeboat's endurance until help can arrive.[26] In such contexts, rationing by narrow "comparative social worthiness" can be ethically justified.

Applications of Medical and Social Utility

We can further explore the distinction between medical and social utility (both broad and narrow) by considering a proposal by Pesik, Keim, and Iserson for the ethical allocation of emergency care following a terrorist attack with weapons of mass destruction. Their arguments are not limited to such terrorist attacks but extend to other public health crises too.[27] Following are their lists of acceptable and unacceptable criteria for allocating scarce medical care in that context.

TABLE 2.4 Acceptable and Unacceptable Criteria for Allocating Scarce Medical Care in an Emergency Following a Terrorist Attack

Should Consider	Should Not Consider
Likelihood of benefit	Age, ethnicity, or sex
Effect on improving quality of life	Talents, abilities, disabilities, or deformities
Duration of benefit	Drug or alcohol abuse
Urgency of the patient's condition	Antisocial or aggressive behaviors
Direct multiplier effect among emergency caregivers	Socioeconomic status, social worth, or political position
Amount of resources required for successful treatment	Coexistent conditions that do not affect short-term prognosis

Modified from Pesik N, Keim ME, Iserson KV. Terrorism and the ethics of emergency medical care. *Annals of Emergency Medicine* 2001;37:642–646 with permission from Elsevier.

As indicated in this table, Pesik and colleagues identify a range of factors that should and should not be considered in rationing scarce resources in such an emergency. All the criteria they propose for use rest on judgments of medical utility and one criterion also incorporates narrow social utility—"direct multiplier effect among emergency caregivers" because of their ability to help others.[27] By contrast, the criteria they oppose generally reflect broad social utility—stated in either positive or negative terms—or, independently of broad social utility, violate standards of egalitarian justice: discrimination based on age, ethnicity, or sex, or on talents, abilities, disabilities, or deformities, or on coexistent conditions that do not affect short-term prognosis. In general, their list is reasonable. However, as we will see below, it overlooks some potentially important social functions that probably should receive priority in some public health crises.

Triage systems based on medical utility generally attend to persons' degrees of need and probabilities of successful treatments. Not surprisingly, Pesik and colleagues' material criteria focus, specifically, on likelihood of benefit, effect on quality of life, duration of benefit, and urgency of need. They also incorporate a criterion of amount of resources required. This criterion, which is sometimes called a "principle of conservation," recognizes that it is important not to exhaust large amounts of limited resources on a few persons. Pesik and colleagues state the point this way: "the likelihood of benefit using minimal resources takes precedence [in order] to maximize the efficient use of scarce medical supplies."[27] Moreover, "practitioners must prioritize intervention to those who will benefit most from the fewest resources."[27] These criteria are ethically justifiable from the standpoint of medical utility.

The criterion of "direct multiplier effect among emergency caregivers" clearly seeks to maximize medical utility, but insofar as it attends to the value of a specific social function, it also represents narrow social utility or instrumental value. Triage in military and civilian disaster contexts has often included narrow social utility, along with medical utility. For instance, it has been common to include in conceptions of salvageability in military triage not only saving individual lives but also "returning the wounded to duty and the earlier the better."[23 (p. 11)]

In a severe public health crisis, stemming from pandemic influenza or a bioterrorist attack, social functions other than the one Pesik and colleagues identified probably will also be important, whether to save more lives or maintain the social order. These crucial social functions almost certainly will not favor only those of higher socioeconomic status or broad social value. Many of the crucial social functions will include tasks such as transportation, supplying food, providing security, maintaining electrical power, and burying the dead.

We may be able to identify some crucial social roles and functions with confidence in advance of a particular public health emergency, but it may be difficult to predict with great precision which social roles and functions will be essential and will lack sufficient personnel. Hence, some ethicists suggest that we publicly debate the ethical rationale for the narrow social utility or instrumental value exception and then "hold it in reserve" depending on the circumstances that emerge.[28] Nevertheless, it is reasonable to assign priority for distribution of vaccinations to workers in vaccine production and to physicians and healthcare professionals with direct patient contact because of the multiplier effect we noted previously. However, the criterion of narrow social utility or instrumental value will probably not be appropriate in the distribution of ventilators in an influenza pandemic because of the difficulty of restoring persons who require ventilator use to functional capacity during the pandemic.[28,29]

Public Participation, Public Trust, and Social Stability

Social utilitarian systems of allocation, according to some ethicists, are so unstable by their very nature that they cannot endure if they are transparent but, instead, will require either deception or coercion.[30] They believe that at-risk individuals simply will not consent to a social utilitarian system, but only to one based on egalitarian justice. They may be right about this for a strictly social utilitarian system. However, a richer and fuller interpretation of utility is available. We are proposing a system that combines medical utility with narrow social utility, tempered throughout by egalitarian concerns for equal respect, fair procedures, and fair opportunity. We believe that such a system for a public health crisis can be ethically justified to the public and can garner public support.

There have been several efforts to formulate ethically justifiable and operational systems of triage in advance of a public health crisis. These usually involve multiple criteria, including specifications of what we have called medical and narrow social utility along with egalitarian considerations. Specifications of medical utility have taken several directions, some of them evident in our discussion of utility earlier in this chapter. The specification of medical utility in terms of saving lives, in the context of decisions about ventilator use, has too often been limited to survival to discharge from the hospital.[28] Countering this tendency is one reason Pesik and colleagues emphasized duration of benefit. If duration is emphasized, then it may be useful to focus on life-years, rather than on lives; but as we saw earlier in this chapter, this also raises serious questions of distributive justice—even more so if these life-years are adjusted for quality or disability. Still another approach stresses the life-cycle criterion, which calls for providing each individual with an equal or fair opportunity to live through the various stages of life.[31] According to White and colleagues, even though this criterion gives priority to the young, it does not unjustly discriminate against older people; rather, it "is inherently egalitarian because it seeks to give all individuals equal opportunity to live a normal life span."[28]

Recent proposals for allocation systems in a public health emergency have rightly recommended several substantive or material criteria. These multi-criteria systems do not yield algorithms for decision making, and the criteria frequently require further specification and balancing. White et al propose an allocation system that "incorporates and balances multiple morally relevant considerations."[28] These considerations are (1) saving the most lives, (2) maximizing the life-years saved, and (3) prioritizing young patients who have not had an opportunity to live a full life.[28] In another multi-criteria proposal, Persad et al recommend what they call a "complete lives system" for "very scarce medical interventions." This system gives priority to younger people who have not yet had the opportunity to live a complete life, but it also incorporates other criteria: prognosis (potential life-years), saving the most lives, lottery, and instrumental value (narrow social utility).[32] The first several are morally relevant in all allocation decisions, while the last (instrumental value) could be justifiable in situations such as pandemic influenza.

Such multi-criteria proposals, involving ethicists and professionals, help us see more clearly the ethical issues involved in different systems of triage. As helpful as these proposals are, we need public engagement and participation in developing, specifying, balancing, and implementing multi-criteria systems for triage for several reasons. First, throughout we have emphasized not only the public's right to justification—that is, to publicly articulated reasons for triage decisions—but also the importance of public participation in the process of setting allocation standards and procedures. Second, among the basic GMCs identified as foundational to public health ethics is the concept of building and maintaining public trust. This is important throughout public health ethics, but it is particularly important here. According to Bailey and colleagues, "In working towards a just distribution, we must engage the public. What will and will not be accepted by our communities will largely depend upon whether individuals understand the basis for the schemes, and whether they agree with the ethical underpinnings."[33] The public's trust cannot be blind; it *must* be informed and engaged trust. And without public trust, a society will not be able to handle a public health crisis very well.

In a time of crisis, public health and other public officials, as well as healthcare professionals, understandably may consider members of the public to be (at best) passive nonparticipants or (at worst) major obstacles to an effective public health response. Hence, they may be reluctant to be transparent, to communicate effectively, and to engage the public. A more defensible approach views the public as a capable partner and ally. Glass and Schoch-Spana contend that "generally effective and adaptive collective action" is possible, and that "failure to involve the public as a key partner in the medical and public-health response could hamper effective management of an epidemic and increase the likelihood of social disruption."[34] They propose several guidelines for integrating the public into planning responses to an epidemic resulting from a bioterrorist attack; these guidelines, with appropriate modifications, apply to other public health crises too.

TABLE 2.5 Guidelines for Integrating the Public into Planning for Public Health Crises

Treat the public as a capable ally in the response to an epidemic
Enlist civic organizations in practical public health activities
Anticipate the need for home-based patient care and infection control
Invest in public outreach and communication strategies
Ensure planning that reflects the values and priorities of affected populations

Data from Glass TA, Schoch-Spana M. Bioterrorism and the people: how to vaccinate a city against panic. *Clinical Infectious Diseases* 2002;34:217–223.

This last guideline is very important for public engagement and public trust, not only in specifying and balancing criteria of medical utility but also, and perhaps especially, in specifying and balancing criteria of narrow social utility—these cannot stray too far from the affected populations' "values and priorities," or trust and cooperation will evaporate. And, at minimum, the public's trust and cooperation are essential. In particular, the public needs to have confidence in the procedures and standards of triage because some, perhaps many, will not receive the vaccination, prophylaxis, or treatment they need and want. Hence, it is crucial that the criteria be developed in public with public participation and justified publicly, in advance of the crisis and as it continues to evolve.

We are emphasizing public participation as a corrective, intended to counter the tendency to exclude the public or to involve the public too little and too late.[28] In no way do we minimize the indispensable participation of public health professionals, physicians, other healthcare professionals, and the like, in planning for a public health crisis. Decisions in a public health crisis must be made in light of the best available scientific evidence at the time and revised in light of the developing information.[33]

FAIR PROCEDURES AND PROCESSES

In a number of works, Norman Daniels, sometimes in collaboration with James Sabin, has argued for the importance of fair procedures and processes in priority setting in health care and public health. Fair process is a form of procedural justice. One of Daniels' articles is entitled "Establishing a fair process for priority setting is easier than agreeing on principles."[35] He emphasizes that "the moral legitimacy of limits and priorities ... involves not just who has moral authority to set them, but how they are set." Moral legitimacy or authority is not equivalent to legal authority, though it often presupposes legal authority. "In the absence of consensus on principles, a fair process allows us to agree on what is legitimate and fair."[35]

TABLE 2.6 Conditions of Fair Process: Accountability for Reasonableness

Publicity Condition
Relevance Condition
Revisability and Appeals Condition
Regulative Condition

Data from Daniels N. *Just Health: Meeting Health Needs Fairly*. Cambridge, UK: Cambridge University Press, 2008, pp. 118–119.

Following is a table of Daniels' four conditions of fair process, which are designed to ensure accountability for reasonable decisions in priority setting.

The *publicity condition* requires a transparent process with publicly available rationales that articulate the grounds for priorities. The *relevance condition* requires that stakeholders affected by priority decisions concur that the grounds—normative, scientific, empirical—for priorities be recognized as relevant to fair decisions. The third condition, the *revisability and appeals condition*, provides for a way to revisit and revise decisions as new evidence and arguments emerge, and for an appeals process for those who believe they merit an exception to the priority policies. Finally, the *regulative condition*, which Daniels also calls the enforcement or regulation condition, requires some mechanism to ensure that the first three conditions are being met.[36]

Another important question is how much consistency there must be across geographical areas even within the same country. Obviously, fair processes in particular communities may produce considerably different approaches to rationing—this was certainly evident in the criteria and methods for rationing influenza vaccine in the U.S. in 2004–2005. While operating within some broad federal guidelines, different communities supplemented their priority schemes based on risks to the individual and risks the individual might create for others with lotteries and first-come, first-served. Moreover, some formal and informal prioritization occurred on the basis of social function. That particular crisis was overblown, but the question remains how much variation can be tolerated in rationing schemes in a national public health crisis. To be more specific: during a public health crisis, how much variation can a community of, say, 100,000 people tolerate in the criteria employed for access to intensive care and ventilators by a community hospital versus the criteria used by a university-based tertiary care hospital?

Ultimately, the public health crisis, whatever it is, will pass. Whether and how the pieces can be picked up and public life can resume will depend in part on how tragic choices were handled. As Calabresi and Bobbit remind us, when societies confront tragic choices that involve fundamental social-cultural values, they must "attempt to make allocations in ways that preserve the moral foundations of social collaboration."[37 (p. 18)]

RESPECT FOR AUTONOMOUS CHOICES AND LIBERTIES

One of the basic GMCs in public health ethics is *respecting autonomous choices and actions, including liberty of action.* This is a presumptive principle or value, but one that can sometimes be rebutted in the name of public health. It is important that public health be specified in particular circumstances, rather than presented as a vague, univocal goal that trumps all principles and values that might set limits on means to realize it. Yes, some public health goals will override autonomous choices and liberties, but not all will, especially the goals that are largely if not exclusively paternalistic. Hence, specification is required to determine exactly which goals in which circumstances will triumph over these presumptive constraints. In any event, as we show in this section, many interventions in the name of public health do not seriously compromise autonomous choices and liberty of action, and, because of the importance of respect for autonomy and liberty, they should have priority in the selection of interventions. Nevertheless, in some circumstances, coercive and other measures that restrict or eliminate individuals' choices in the name of public health can satisfy the justificatory conditions we have sketched: effectiveness, necessity, least infringement, proportionality, and impartiality in the context of public justification.

The Intervention Ladder

In its important report on public health ethics, the Nuffield Council on Bioethics proposed what it called an "intervention ladder" to help us think through the various ways public health policies and practices can affect people's choices.[38] The report contends that interventions "higher up the ladder are more intrusive and therefore require a stronger justification."[38] Following are the steps or rungs of the "intervention ladder."

This proposed Intervention Ladder is a helpful starting point, but it is problematic in some ways and incomplete in others. The steps or rungs are not always separate and even the lower interventions may be unjustifiable in some circumstances. Much again will depend on the public health goal that is sought as well as on the other GMCs. In using the

TABLE 2.7 Intervention Ladder

Intervention Ladder
8. Eliminate choice
7. Restrict choice
6. Guide choice by disincentives
5. Guide choice by incentives
4. Guide choice by changing the default policy
3. Enable choice
2. Provide information
1. Do nothing

Data from: the Nuffield Council on Bioethics report, *Public Health: Ethical Issues* (London: Nuffield Council, November 2007) Available at: http://www.nuffieldbioethics.org/sites/default/files/Public%20health%20-%20ethical%20issues.pdf Accessed January 17, 2013.

Intervention Ladder for heuristic or exploratory purposes, we will also indicate possible expansions of or developments off different rungs.

The language of the first step, "do nothing," is potentially misleading because taking no specific action against the threat does not preclude the possibility of monitoring the situation. Monitoring, surveillance, and the like can provide data that may be useful in taking other steps. Even though the justificatory burden increases as we climb the Intervention Ladder, doing nothing or only monitoring can also require ethical justification, for instance, in view of the deaths that occur as a result of not intervening to get motorcyclists to use helmets. Moreover, we should note, doing nothing or simply monitoring the situation also affects individuals' choices; it is part of what is called "choice architecture," which we will discuss below, and it influences individual choices.[39]

The second step involves providing information—for instance, about the value of exercise or certain diets. It is hard to see ethical problems with providing accurate, truthful information to make informed choices possible and even to shape personal choices in the direction of a public health goal, such as a healthier diet. This rationale, for example, is behind labels providing information about calories in different foods. In its simplest formulation (provide information), this step may not adequately stress the place and value of rational persuasion—i.e., the provision of reasons to try to persuade the individual to act in the desired ways. Whether the information is provided in a neutral way to create the possibility of informed choices, or in a persuasive way with reasons offered for the benefits of certain actions, this step in no way compromises autonomy.

In addition to rational persuasion, there is also the possibility of presenting both information and reasons in graphic ways to appeal to the public's imagination and emotions. So, for instance, in addition to providing information about the health impact of smoking cigarettes, and offering reasons individuals should not start smoking or should stop if they have started, the government and private groups could present images that graphically depict the terrible health consequences for many smokers. Such a presentation of information attempts to stoke viewers' imaginations and emotions in order to lead them to the desired behaviors.[40] **Figure 2.2** is one example from the Centers for Disease Control and Prevention's campaign to warn people about the terrible health effects of smoking.

Such advertisements go well beyond the provision of information to ensure informed choices and beyond efforts at rational persuasion. They seek to change behavior by appealing to the imagination and the emotions through graphic and powerful images. In combination with other efforts, they also seek to alter social norms, in part by stigmatizing and shaming conduct. In a 2013 opinion piece in *The New York Times*, Richard Reeves writes: "New York is deploying a powerful weapon to reduce teen pregnancy: shame. New advertisements around the city dramatize the truncated life chances of children born to teenagers; in one, a tear-stained toddler stares out, declaring: 'I'm twice as likely not to graduate high school because you had me as a teen.'"[41] Critics of this campaign against teen pregnancy decry the effort to shame communities and individuals as ineffective, counterproductive, and hurtful to communities and individuals. By contrast, Reeves defends it on the grounds that even in a liberal society, shame can function as "a form of moral regulation, or social 'nudge,' encouraging good behavior while guarding individual freedom."[41]

Even though stigmatizing conduct can be effective in some contexts, it raises important ethical issues. Its use requires thoughtful justification, and it must be used in ways that are likely to be effective without being harmful. This will require attention to other factors; for instance, in a campaign against teen pregnancy, both education and the availability of contraception will also be important. Furthermore, Reeves emphasizes, "it is equally important that shame not be used as an excuse for lack of support. Once prevention, including moral pressure, has failed, and a child is born to a teenager, the overriding priority must be to provide as much help as possible."[41]

It is also important to distinguish stigmatizing *conduct* from stigmatizing *persons* who engage in that conduct. This is at best very difficult. Campaigns against smoking, as

FIGURE 2.2 A Tip from a Former Smoker (CDC advertisement)

In March 2012, the Centers for Disease Control and Prevention (CDC) "launched the first-ever paid national tobacco education campaign–*Tips From Former Smokers (Tips)*." This campaign seeks to get people to quit smoking "by highlighting the toll that smoking-related illnesses take on smokers and their loved ones." These "hard-hitting ads showed people living with the real and painful consequences of smoking. Many of the people featured in the ads started smoking in their early teens, and some were diagnosed with life-changing diseases before they were age 40. The ads featured suggestions or 'tips' from former smokers on how to get dressed when you have stoma or artificial limbs, what scars from heart surgery look like, and reasons why people have quit smoking." The accompanying print advertisement—there are also videos—presents Terrie, age 52, from North Carolina, whose throat cancer is blamed on smoking that led to a laryngectomy. According to the CDC, the effect of the *Tips* campaign was "immediate and intense."
See http://www. cdc.gov/tobacco/campaign/tips/about/campaign-overview. html

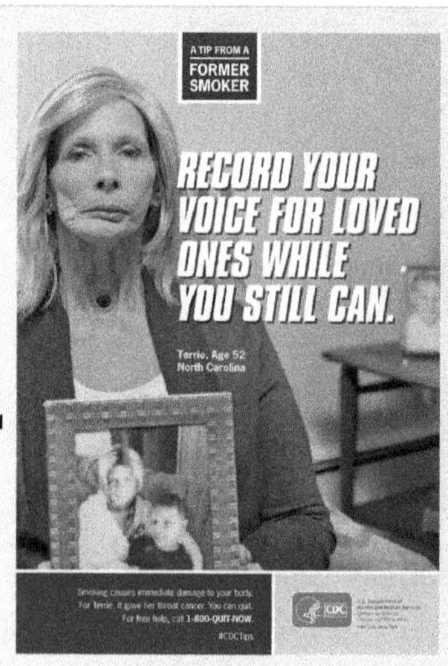

Reproduced from: CDC. Tips From Former Smokers: Terrie's Story. http://www.cdc.gov/tobacco/campaign/tips/resources/ads/tips-2-ad-terrie-full.pdf. Accessed June 27th, 2013.

represented in the advertisements noted above and in policies such as increased taxation of cigarettes, often have the effect, if not the intention, of stigmatizing smokers as well as smoking, and this can lead to smokers becoming targets of resentment and hostility.[42] In the U.S., smoking is more prevalent among lower socioeconomic groups, and ethical questions, including questions of justice, arise about stigmatization of socially vulnerable persons. Similar points apply to teen pregnancies, where there is the additional problem of effectively stigmatizing the conduct of males—the focus has been primarily on teen girls who become pregnant.

For all efforts to persuade or motivate through the presentation of information, in whatever form, a fundamental ethical requirement is truthfulness, a component of one of our GMCs (#8). Indeed, one possibility not included in the Intervention Ladder would not be ethically justifiable in the pursuit of public health—the manipulation of information through deception or lying. Some manipulations that might be effective would simply not be ethical. For instance, exaggerating risks could motivate behavior. Or, to take an even more dramatic example, manipulating persons' memories, by creating false beliefs, may be effective in behavior modification in some contexts. One team of researchers found that it could get individuals to avoid certain foods by manipulating them to believe a lie—that those foods had actually made them sick when they were young. It could also lead individuals to eat asparagus by convincing them to believe falsely that they had once really liked asparagus.[43] These experiments thus involved creating false bad memories of unhealthy foods to avoid and false good memories of healthy foods. In one experiment, Loftus and colleagues had 131 students complete forms that indicated their food experiences and preferences; these forms included some questions about strawberry ice cream. These students then received a fake computer analysis of their forms that allegedly indicated what they really and truly liked and disliked. However, the computer reports for 47 of the students indicated, again falsely, that they had been sickened by eating strawberry ice cream when they were young. Later, close to 20% of these students indicated on a questionnaire that strawberry ice cream had made them sick, and that they were not going to eat it in the future.[43] However, for whatever reason, researchers were not able to engender false beliefs about the consumption of chocolate chip cookies and potato chips![43] Moreover, it is not known how long such false memories endure. However useful the creation of false memories might be in engendering healthy behavior, it transgresses important ethical barriers and violates respect for persons, their dignity, and their autonomy. It would be morally perilous for a democratic society even to contemplate such manipulations as options.

The third rung on the Intervention Ladder is to enable choices. Individuals may not pursue healthy options for themselves or for others because of the difficulties of doing so, perhaps because of a lack of capacity or resources to carry them out or because of the costs of doing so. Consider a person who has tuberculosis and for whom the recommended approach is Directly Observed Therapy (DOT) for treatment until noncontagious or cured. One way to secure the person's compliance with DOT may be to enable his or her choice by providing vouchers for transportation to a center for DOT. Reducing parents' out-of-pocket costs for their children's recommended vaccinations has also been effective in the U.S. Other examples include providing free fruits in school cafeterias, funding participation in "stop smoking" programs, and building lanes for bicycles.[38] This rung on the Intervention Ladder poses no ethical concerns from the standpoint of respect for autonomous choices and liberties; however, it may raise important issues of utility and distributive justice.

Guiding choices by altering the defaults (step #4 on the Intervention Ladder) is an often effective way to shape conduct without undermining individuals' liberty to choose.[44] It is a "nudge" that leaves the final choice with the individual. In *Nudge: Improving Decisions about Health, Wealth, and Happiness*, Thaler and Sunstein define a "nudge" as "any aspect of the choice architecture that alters people's behavior in a predictable way without forbidding any options or significantly changing their economic incentives."[39 (p. 6)]

More broadly, "choice architecture" organizes "the context in which people make decisions," and it is ubiquitous and never purely neutral.[39] In reviewing and evaluating a proposed policy that would affect persons' decisions in one direction or the other, we may worry about whether a nudge is warranted. However, even if unnoticed, the existing policy itself constitutes a "choice architecture" that affects individuals' decisions. For instance, if the U.S. were to attempt to increase the supply of organs available for transplantation by adopting an "opt-out" policy, it would not be establishing a "choice architecture" where none existed. Rather, it would be replacing one kind of "choice architecture" with another.

The current U.S. policy for obtaining organs for transplantation is an "opt-in" policy: If individuals while alive do not take steps, such as signing a donor card or checking "donor" on their driver's license or entering a donor registry, they will not be considered donors (although U.S. law allows the next of kin to donate the decedent's organs if he or she did not indicate an objection to donation). By contrast, in an "opt-out" system, which is common in Europe, an individual's nonobjection to organ donation while alive will be counted as consent to organ donation after his or her death. In both systems, a little effort will be required to take an action that differs from the default. In an "opt-in" system, the default is nondonation unless the individual takes an action to signify donation; in an "opt-out" system, the default is donation unless the individual takes an action to indicate objection to donation. In either system, the final decision about organ donation rests with that individual—he or she has the liberty to say "yes" or "no" to organ donation. An Institute of Medicine Committee on Increasing Rates of Organ Donation held that in order for an "opt-out" policy of organ donation to be ethically acceptable, there must be public understanding and clear, easy, nonburdensome, reliable, and widely available ways for individuals to indicate their refusal.[45]

In this regard, Thaler and Sunstein argue that if an intervention is to count as a "mere nudge," it "must be easy and cheap to avoid."[39 (p. 6)] While placing fruit at eye level in a school cafeteria nudges students to select the fruit, rather than something else that is also available, a school's ban on junk food would not count as a nudge.[39] Furthermore, "nudges"—e.g., guiding behavior by changing the default policy—need to be distinguished from interventions that significantly change individuals' "economic incentives."[39 (p. 6)] Hence, there is often an important distinction between changing the default option and taking the next two steps on the Intervention Ladder: guiding choice by incentives or by disincentives, at least if these incentives or disincentives are significant. To be sure, setting the defaults in certain directions works in part because of the "costs" involved in taking the nondefault option, such as signing a donor card or registering as a nondonor. Often there are also cognitive and psychological costs, but they too must be low for the altered default to count as a nudge.[39]

The next rung (#5) on the Intervention Ladder is guiding choices by incentives. For instance, in securing the compliance with DOT by a person with tuberculosis, it might be possible not only to enable his choice by providing vouchers for transportation but also to motivate compliance by providing incentives, such as money he can spend however he chooses. In addition, there is evidence (discussed elsewhere) that incentive awards to clients or families can effectively increase rates of vaccination.

While some view the use of incentives as potentially coercive ("Cash might coerce some people into changing behavior...."[46]), others insist that providing incentives cannot be considered coercive because it expands rather than restricts options.[47] We take the latter perspective, but we concede that providing incentives can still be morally problematic in some circumstances. On the one hand, if the amount of the incentive falls below an acceptable threshold it may be exploitative in that it takes unfair advantage of a person's situation. On the other hand, if the amount is too large, it may constitute an undue inducement.

Still another concern is the stigmatization associated with conditional cash transfers—i.e., conditional on behavioral changes—directed at disadvantaged persons. Some also argue that cash payments can change behavior without making behavioral change a condition for the transfer; they contend that payments to poor mothers generally end up being used for their children's health and well-being.[46] Even defenders lay down some stringent requirements for justification of incentives for people to care for their health: "They should be used only when the program is likely to do more good than harm to disadvantaged individuals, taking account of compliance costs, stigma, and stress to recipient; the behavior change is sufficiently verifiable to deter fraud and gaming; and the program is likely to be cost effective, taking account of all benefits and costs, including administration and monitoring."[48]

Critics also register their concern about the deleterious impact of incentives on a person's character. Incentives are directed at conduct not character, but some worry that they may also damage character. "Incentive programs," Ruth Grant argues, "ought to come with a 'caution' label" because they "have been shown repeatedly to undermine motivation and performance, as well as to corrode character."[49 (p. 122)] Furthermore, their effects tend to be limited to the short term.[49] However, if the short-term public health goal is to get parents to have their children vaccinated, then the use of effective financial incentives may be more important (for the children and for others) than strengthening the parents' character or other long-term goals.

The next rung on the Intervention Ladder is guiding choices through disincentives, especially but not only financial disincentives. Obvious examples include increasing taxes on cigarettes to discourage smoking, or fining people for failing to get recommended vaccinations—the last was the penalty in the famous early 20th century case *Jacobson v. Massachusetts.* Depending on the kind and level of the disincentive involved, disincentives can be effective in some circumstances. In the U.S. we do use (and generally find acceptable) the nonmonetary disincentive or sanction of not allowing children to attend school if they have not had certain vaccinations. In addition to being a disincentive or sanction, this also functions to protect other children in the school context. Elsewhere, we will consider the use of monetary sanctions, such as the distribution of fewer food vouchers, following parental or guardian failures to adhere to the schedule for their children's vaccinations. While there is some evidence that these disincentives were effective in the short run, major concerns arose about justice and fairness in the distribution of burdens and benefits and about the harm to the children who may have been deprived of needed food (see Chapter 7).

The Intervention Ladder's penultimate rung is restricting choice. The Nuffield Council gives examples of regulating so as to restrict the options available to consumers by requiring the removal of unhealthy ingredients from foods.[38] Another example is New York City Mayor Michael Bloomberg's proposed ban on the sale of sugared drinks over 16 ounces in certain contexts. This ban would restrict and constrain individuals' choices about drinks but, in the final analysis, would not totally rule out those choices, because individuals could simply buy more than one smaller-size beverage. However, they would end up paying more—another disincentive. The final rung on the Intervention Ladder is eliminating choice. One example is forcible quarantine of people who have been exposed to certain infectious diseases or forcible isolation of people who have begun to show the symptoms of those diseases.

The Nuffield Council's Intervention Ladder does not use the label of coercion for any of its steps, and most of the interventions listed are not properly considered coercive. Some of them may be ethically problematic or even wrong in some circumstances for other reasons. Nevertheless, some forms of the final three interventions are or may be coercive. The paradigm situation of coercion is evident when the robber confronts the victim: "Your money or your life." Years ago, a notoriously stingy comedian could garner some laughs by saying, "Let me think about it." This is a coercive situation, but many of the actions that influence choices one direction or another are not coercive, even though careless discussants may label them as such.

The term "coercion" has been overused and overextended in critiques of different interventions in public health as well as in critiques of policies, practices, and actions in therapy and research. Hawkins and Emanuel offer a helpful examination of this often misused concept. For them, "coercion involves a threat that makes a certain choice irresistible."[47] Their further explication softens the notion of irresistibility: "A person is coerced when her choices are unfavorably narrowed by someone who is trying to get her to do something she would not otherwise do."[47] An intervention can be unsuccessfully coercive or incompletely coercive—in that the coerced choice turns out not to be an irresistible one after all.

Coercive acts, Hawkins and Emanuel argue, have two features. The first is the type of choice a coerced individual faces: narrowed, constricted options. This feature is not sufficient for coercion because not all situations of narrowed, constricted choice are coercive. For instance, an individual may face a set of choices that are *all* bleak or dire, such as deciding among (choice 1) extreme radiation or (choice 2) massive chemotherapy for a cancer that is likely to be deadly without treatment (choice 3)—certainly a narrow set of options, but the individual may still make his or her own choice about which treatment to undertake, if any. A second feature is thus also indispensable for a situation to be coercive: others' purposeful actions created the situation of narrowed, constricted choice.[47] An example might be confinement (or the threat of confinement) of a person who is not complying with the therapeutic requirements for tuberculosis; such tactics represent a coercive effort to get him or her to comply.

The top three rungs of the Intervention Ladder need to meet a higher bar of justification in light of the justificatory conditions we identified (effectiveness, necessity, least infringement, proportionality, impartiality, all to be met in the context of public justification). And they can be met under certain conditions, as the examples suggest. We have also attempted to show in this section that many of the other interventions are often ethically justified but that they also frequently raise ethical issues that need to be addressed.

Moreover, we should not overemphasize the limits placed on public health interventions by respect for autonomous choices and various liberties. These are important presumptive limits that may direct public health officials to find ethically preferable interventions rather than limiting potentially effective interventions. Furthermore, it is often important in public health to *express community* rather than merely to *impose community*. Certainly the imposition of community, in the sense of imposing communal obligations in the name of protecting or promoting public health, is ethically justifiable in some circumstances. Forcible isolation of an uncooperative patient with tuberculosis who is putting others at risk is a good example, as we have seen. However, in many contexts, expressing community and solidarity by providing resources and support may also be as effective—or even more effective—than imposing community through manipulation or coercion.[50]

Paternalistic Interventions

Our examination of the Intervention Ladder used a variety of examples and arguments for and against different interventions in those examples. We did not distinguish the several types of reasons for those interventions: public health, population health, financial and other costs to the society, and the individual's own welfare. The heading for this section is "paternalistic interventions," but an equally good heading would be "paternalistic reasons for interventions."

Paternalistic actions have two characteristic features: (1) they aim to protect or promote the welfare of individuals themselves (rather than others or the society), and (2) they seek to accomplish this goal by overriding some of the individuals' choices and actions.[51,52] The metaphor back of paternalistic actions is that of father-child relationships, particularly as those relationships were portrayed in the late 19th century, when the term paternalism appeared. This metaphor was alive in the language of "paternal government" that John Stuart Mill and others used to criticize governmental policies even before the term "paternalism" came on the scene.[53 (p. 94)] It still accurately describes the rationale for some interventions by public health officials, physicians, and others, but it is normatively problematic because it highlights the value of benefiting the individual while obscuring or downplaying the principle of respecting their autonomous choices and liberties.

We need to distinguish *weak* and *strong* paternalism, a distinction apparently first drawn by Feinberg and subsequently developed by others.[54] (The terms *soft* and *hard* are also sometimes used in their place.) In strong paternalistic actions, the intended beneficiary is a person who is considered to be autonomous or substantially autonomous but whose choices and actions put him or her at risk. Such actions infringe the intended beneficiary's autonomy, and, hence, are at least presumptively wrong. As Ronald Dworkin suggests, paternalistic interventions are disrespectful, demeaning, and insulting to the beneficiary whose autonomy they violate.[55 (pp. 262–63)] There are also consequentialist reasons to challenge such paternalistic interventions. According to John Stuart Mill, "[t]he strongest of all the arguments against the interference of the public with purely personal conduct, is that when it does interfere, the odds are that it interferes wrongly, and in the wrong place."[53 (p. 78)] For all these reasons, it is hard to justify taking the final three steps on the Intervention Ladder—the three steps that most compromise autonomy—to secure health and other benefits for the autonomous individual who resists those interventions. By contrast, it is justifiable to take those steps under some conditions to protect or promote public health, as distinguished from the health of the autonomous individual. However, the "libertarian paternalism" advocated by Thaler and Sunstein accepts interventions below the top three rungs, which leave the individual free to resist and which can be more easily justified even for paternalistic reasons.[39]

In *weak* paternalism, by contrast, the intended beneficiary is considered to be nonautonomous or substantially nonautonomous. Consequently, his or her choices and actions do not warrant the respect and noninterference the autonomous person can claim. The principle of respect for autonomous choices and actions does not stand in the way of interventions to protect or promote the interests of the nonautonomous or substantially nonautonomous person, who may have significant mental deficiencies, serious psychiatric problems, drug addiction, and so forth. Justice and fairness as well as public beneficence warrant such interventions. However, it is not easy in public health policy and practice to determine when people are substantially nonautonomous and thus may be coerced for their own benefit—for instance, is a person's obesity the result of substantially autonomous or substantially nonautonomous choices?

Proponents of governmental interventions into personal choices and actions rarely defend those interventions as paternalistic, or at least as purely paternalistic. Usually, they argue that the interventions are also necessary to protect other individuals, the public health, public resources, particularly financial resources, and so forth. It is sometimes plausible, in view of public expenditures on health care and other goods and services, to point to the societal impact of individuals' actions that may initially appear only to harm themselves.

The debates about laws that require motorcyclists to wear helmets are instructive. Some arguments for mandatory helmet laws are clearly paternalistic—the goal is to protect the motorcyclists themselves. Other arguments seek, sometimes with difficulty, to demonstrate that motorcyclists who do not wear helmets increase risks and costs to others. For instance, they may create hazards for passing vehicles and may impose excessive burdens on rescue teams, physicians, nurses, and other health professionals as well as on medical institutions. The public may also complain about bearing some or all of the costs of the motorcyclist's care.

One report indicates that in 2010, "helmet use saved the lives of 1,544 motorcyclists, and an additional 709 lives might have been saved if all motorcyclists had worn helmets... Helmets are proven to save lives and money, and universal helmet laws are the most effective way to increase helmet use."[56] Another study similarly concludes: "Examination of individual state experiences with motorcycle helmet legislation demonstrates that universal motorcycle helmet laws effectively promote helmet use compliance, reduce morbidity and mortality in motorcycle crashes, and lower the healthcare costs and associated societal burdens of these crash victims."[57] It is important to consider, in view of the best available evidence, the strengths and weaknesses of different arguments about protecting individuals' best interests, public and population health, and the public treasury. Most often paternalistic arguments will be mixed with other kinds of arguments as this example indicates—the reasons for intervention, in this case a coercive intervention, are directed at the individuals affected and at the impact their actions have on other individuals or on the society.

PRIVACY AND CONFIDENTIALITY

In the context of public health as well as health care, the protection and nondisclosure of individuals' personal information is an important—though nonabsolute—ethical obligation. Disclosures of a patient's personal information by healthcare professionals without the patient's authorization may be decried as a breach of privacy, or as a breach of confidentiality, or both. There is a close relationship between privacy and confidentiality, but it is also essential to distinguish them. Despite their partial overlap in protecting personal information, their differences also need attention. Privacy emerged centuries after confidentiality became prominent, but we will start with privacy because it is the broader category.

Privacy

We define privacy as a state or condition of limited access, including nonaccess, to a person.[6] Access to a person may occur in any one of a number of ways—for instance, through looking at, listening to, or touching the person, or through receiving information about the person from others' reports or from laboratory data. We follow Anita Allen's characterization of four dimensions of privacy, each of which involves limited access to a person, and we add a fifth dimension: relational or associational privacy (**Table 2.8**).[58]

Informational privacy, which is most commonly emphasized in public health ethics, particularly in the context of surveillance, involves limited access or nonaccess to personal

TABLE 2.8 Dimensions of Privacy

Informational privacy
Physical privacy
Decisional privacy
Propriety privacy
Relational/associational privacy

Data from Allen A. Genetic privacy: emerging concepts and values. In: Rothstein MA (ed). *Genetic Secrets: Protecting Privacy and Confidentiality in the Genetic Era*. New Haven, CT: Yale University Press, 1997:31–59.

information and protection and nondisclosure of any personal information acquired by public health officials. *Physical* privacy concerns access to persons and their personal spaces, *decisional* privacy encompasses personal choices and zones or spheres of such choices, and *propriety* privacy includes property interests, such as interest in a person's DNA or image.[58] The fifth dimension of privacy, which we have added to Allen's list, is *relational* or *associational* privacy. This last dimension includes various personal relations or associations with others as well as individuals' decisions with others in those relations or associations. Examples include family life and friendship as well as less intimate associations. While identifying these various dimensions is useful, the lines between them are far from clear cut and impermeable. And there is substantial overlap between some of these dimensions of privacy and other moral notions, for instance, between decisional privacy and autonomy.

Another valuable distinction is between *having privacy* and *having a right to privacy*. A person may have privacy—in the sense that others do not access that person in any of the several ways noted—without having a right to privacy, that is, a justified claim against others that they not infringe that person's privacy. Conversely, a person may have a right to privacy but still lack privacy if others violate her right. Many factors may determine whether a person has privacy—perhaps others are indifferent to her or have no effective way to access her, or perhaps they respect her enforceable right to privacy. Whatever the reason for a person's state or condition of limited access, that person has privacy whether or not she has a right to privacy.

Several dominant metaphors for public health surveillance, an indispensable tool in public health, suggest its risk to privacy, especially informational privacy. Whether surveillance is viewed as "the eyes of public health" or the "radar" for public health or a way to keep "a finger on the pulse of the health of a community," it involves access to individuals or at least to information about them. Surveillance thus entails the reduction or loss of privacy at least to some extent.

The distinction between anonymous (or anonymized) information and personally identified (or identifiable) information is crucially important in analyzing and evaluating uses of surveillance as a tool in public health. Anonymous information does not sacrifice individual privacy, and thus does not create psychosocial or other risks for individuals from whom it is derived. Similarly, informational privacy is not threatened if personal identifiers have been removed and there is adequate security for the anonymized information. Data for epidemiological purposes, such as determining pockets of influenza in different communities, may not need personal identifiers, but public health surveillance sometimes requires individuals' names or other personal identifiers for effective action. Tracking persons exposed to an infectious disease is one example.

How strong or weighty are privacy and the right to privacy? As important as privacy and the right to privacy are in our society, they represent only one value or moral consideration among many. In considering public health tools and interventions, privacy and the right to privacy set only presumptive, though nonetheless important, limits, and can be overridden when the justificatory conditions we have identified are met.

Confidentiality

Confidentiality overlaps with informational privacy—both involve limited access to information about a person. While informational privacy has a more recent pedigree, emerging a little over a century ago, confidentiality is arguably one of the oldest and most prevalent rules in medical ethics. Confidentiality can be viewed as a way to protect informational privacy within a specific set of relationships.

Suppose a person seeks health care and voluntarily enters into a relationship with one or more healthcare professionals. That person willingly surrenders much of his or her privacy in order to gain the benefits of that relationship through accurate diagnosis, informed prognosis, and efficacious treatment. In a confidential relationship in health care, the information generated about a patient is protected, within limits, by rules of confidentiality. A patient has reasonable and legitimate expectations that the information generated in this relationship (generally) will not be disclosed to others without his or her consent or authorization. Of course, these expectations are set in different ways by different institutions, societies, and legal systems. For instance, a patient seeking care in a hospital can expect—and may even have explicitly or implicitly consented to—further disclosures of personal information to a variety of health professionals and ancillary staff contributing to her care. In addition, the law sets certain limits on these expectations, requiring healthcare professionals to disclose, depending on the state, epilepsy, gun-shot wounds, suspected child abuse, certain contagious diseases, and the like. Moreover, the Privacy Rule implementing the Health Insurance Portability and Accountability Act of 1996 (HIPAA) allows the disclosure of personally identifiable health information for public health purposes even if the individual has not specifically authorized it.[59]

One big ethical question is where the legal and policy boundaries should be set for protected information in health care. Physicians and other health professionals have considerably more latitude to disclose information without personal identifiers than information with personal identifiers, such as name, social security number, etc. As we noted above, much public health surveillance, particularly for epidemiological purposes, can be conducted without personal identifiers. However, sometimes it is crucial to have access to personal identifiers—for instance, to determine the source of an outbreak of food poisoning.

A further clarification of the distinction between privacy and confidentiality may be useful. Only someone who is in a confidential relationship with another person can infringe, breach, or violate that person's right to confidentiality. Years ago, when newspaper columnist Jack Anderson reported that the well-known and controversial lawyer Roy Cohn was enrolled in a National Institutes of Health experimental trial of the drug AZT for the treatment of AIDS, critics charged that some healthcare professionals had violated Cohn's rights of confidentiality and privacy by passing on this information to Anderson, who in turn had violated Cohn's right to privacy by publishing it. Only those in a confidential relationship with Cohn could have violated his right to confidentiality or failed to protect his confidentiality; others not involved in a confidential relationship may have violated his privacy, but they could not have violated the confidentiality of the relationship.[60]

In short, "[c]onfidentiality is present when one person discloses information to another, whether through words or other means, and the person to whom the information is disclosed pledges, implicitly or explicitly, not to divulge that information to a third party without the confider's permission."[6 (p. 318)] If the patient from whom the information was derived consents to the release of that information to third parties, there is no breach of confidentiality. Consent to disclosure cancels the obligation to respect confidential information at least to the extent of the consent.

The presumptive duty to protect confidential information thus hinges in part on the implicit or explicit pledge by the health professional or the larger context in which the care is provided, such as institutional or legal requirements. So it in part rests on promise-keeping. There are also other possible grounds for this duty. One of these is already evident: patients' autonomy and their privacy rights. Another is based on the probable consequences of having rules of confidentiality that patients can rely on when they seek help. Without a reasonable and legitimate expectation of confidentiality, within certain limits, people would be reluctant to yield their privacy to health professionals because of fears of harm, such as embarrassment and stigmatization, from unauthorized disclosures of their personal information. This reluctance would compromise effective health care.

This consequentialist argument does not establish how narrow or broad, how strong or weak, or how exception-less rules of confidentiality need to be in order to ensure effective health care. A version of the debate about such questions was evident in the legal decisions in the famous *Tarasoff* case and in the commentary surrounding that case.[61] In this case, a male patient in therapy confided in his therapist that he wanted to kill a young woman who had rebuffed his romantic interest in her. The therapist was concerned enough that he alerted the university police, who, after talking with the young man, determined that he was not a sufficient threat to require further detention. The therapist's patient killed the young woman when she returned to the area. Her family filed a lawsuit contending that the therapist did not do enough to prevent their daughter's death and that he should also have warned the intended victim of his patient's threatened violence.

This lawsuit eventually led to a California Supreme Court decision on the bases and limits of rules of confidentiality.[61] In an important, precedent-setting opinion, the majority held that therapists have an affirmative obligation to warn the intended victims of a patient's or client's threatened violence, while the minority opinion rejected such an affirmative obligation. Both opinions appealed to consequentialist/utilitarian arguments in assessing a rule that would require therapists to warn third parties based on information gained in the therapeutic relationship, thus breaching the confidential relationship. The consequentialist/utilitarian questions about rules of confidentiality include: Would requiring therapists to warn prospective victims in such cases save more lives? Or would a stronger protection of confidentiality save more lives by encouraging and enabling troubled individuals to disclose their deepest, darkest desires and fantasies so they could be effectively addressed in the therapeutic relationship? It is by no means clear which side has stronger evidence for these speculative consequences.

A similar debate has surrounded rules of confidentiality in the care of HIV-infected patients who have sometimes been reluctant or even refused to disclose their positive HIV status to their sexual partners. On the one hand, there are concerns that specific, identifiable individuals might become infected because they do not know their partner's positive HIV status and thus are unaware of some of the risks involved in the relationship. On the other hand, there are concerns that requiring healthcare professionals to warn sexual partners in such cases could lead people to avoid testing and thus prevent them from obtaining information, counseling, etc., that could help them protect their partners as well as themselves. In short, the debate concerns which rule of confidentiality would save the most lives. This debate has shifted more in the direction of disclosure as

HIV/AIDS has come to be viewed as a "chronic" disease rather than a "lethal" disease as a result of advances in antiretroviral treatment—because of the need to start treatment as early as possible, because the disease is less stigmatized, and so forth.

Physicians and other healthcare professionals may, in effect, find themselves in a public health role, with a public health task to discharge, when their patients are exposing others to significant risks, that is, a high probability of serious harm. They may, and sometimes should, breach confidentiality in order to protect identifiable third parties at risk—for instance, in the case of a recalcitrant patient who refuses to inform his sexual partner of his positive HIV status and refuses to engage in safer sexual practices. The strategy proposed by American Medical Association's Council on Ethical and Judicial Affairs for such a case is a reasonable one: "Physicians must honor their obligation to promote the public's health by working to prevent HIV-positive individuals from infecting third parties within the constraints of the law." It then indicates three interrelated steps the physician *should* take "if an HIV-positive individual poses a significant threat of infecting an identifiable third party."[62]

TABLE 2.9 Steps Physicians Should Take when an HIV-Infected Patient Endangers a Third Party: Recommended by the AMA

(a)	notify the public health authorities, if required by law;
(b)	attempt to persuade the infected patient to cease endangering the third party; and
(c)	if permitted by state law, notify the endangered third party without revealing the identity of the source person.

Data from *Recommendations in Code of Medical Ethics of the American Medical Association*, 2010–2011 Edition. Chicago, IL: American Medical Association, 2010;2:23 (issued June 2008), p. 127.

Two of these steps—(a) and (c)—depend on what the law requires or permits and so raise again the question about which laws and policies are ethically justifiable. The other step (b)—"attempt to persuade the infected patient to cease endangering the third party"—does not indicate how far the physician must go to confirm the patient's cessation of endangerment.

CONCLUSIONS

This chapter has explored four major clusters of GMCs: utility; distributive justice; respect for autonomous choices and actions, including liberty; and privacy and confidentiality, along with ample illustrations of their implications for goals and means, programs and interventions, in public health. Some of these GMCs (e.g., utility and justice) serve as grounds for public health, while some serve as potentially limiting principles (e.g., respecting autonomous choices and actions and privacy and confidentiality). The latter should not be viewed as mere obstacles, because in many contexts public health can best be protected and promoted by respecting autonomous choices, including liberty of action, or by guarding privacy and confidentiality. As the Intervention Ladder suggests, these presumptive obstacles may even lead us to find alternative interventions that are effective but that do not seriously compromise autonomy or liberty (or privacy or confidentiality, for that matter). Nevertheless, in some cases these GMCs remain obstacles, presumptive rather than absolute ones, which can sometimes be justifiably overridden in the name of public health, not as a vague category but as a specific set of concrete and important goals.

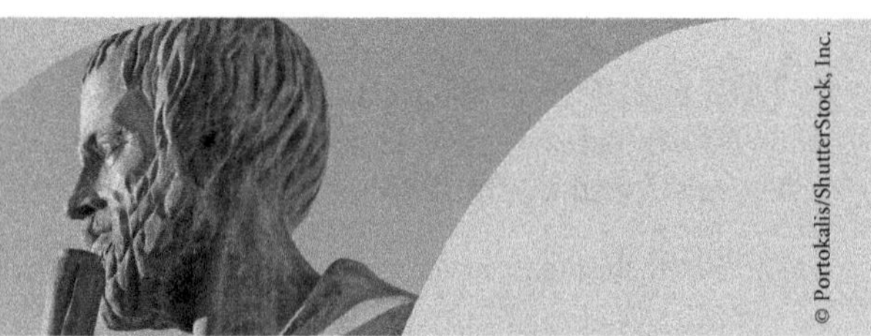
© Portokalis/ShutterStock, Inc.

Discussion Questions

1. Do you believe that utility and egalitarian justice can be successfully combined in a system of substantive criteria and processes for triage in a public health emergency? If so, how? If not, what alternative do you propose?
2. Do you find any moral issues in the lower rungs of the Intervention Ladder? Do you agree that the higher rungs of the Intervention Ladder must meet a higher burden of justification?
3. What is your view about the use of stigmatization and shaming in the context of campaigns to reduce teen pregnancies and cigarette smoking?
4. Define a paternalistic intervention and distinguish strong and weak versions. Can you think of cases in which strong paternalistic interventions would be ethically justified?
5. What is the distinction between privacy and confidentiality? How much weight should they have when information about individuals could protect other individuals or public health?

REFERENCES

1. Driver J. The history of utilitarianism. In: Zalta EN (ed). *The Stanford Encyclopedia of Philosophy* (Summer 2009 Edition). http://plato.stanford.edu/archives/sum2009/entries/utilitarianism-history/

2. Gold MR, Siegel JR, Russell LB, Weinstein MC (eds). *Cost-Effectiveness in Health and Medicine*. New York: Oxford University Press, 1996.

3. Miller W, Robinson LA, Lawrence RS (eds). *Valuing Health for Regulatory Effectiveness Analysis*. Washington, DC: National Academies Press, 2006.

4. Neumann PJ. *Using Cost-Effectiveness Analysis to Improve Health Care: Opportunities and Barriers*. New York: Oxford University Press, 2005.

5. Licensure of Quadrivalent Human Papillomavirus Vaccine (HPV4, Gardasil) for Use in Males and Guidance from the Advisory Committee on Immunization Practices (ACIP). *Morbidity and Mortality Weekly Report*. 2010;59:630–632.

6. Beauchamp TL, Childress JF. *Principles of Biomedical Ethics*, 7th edition. New York: Oxford University Press, 2013.

7. Centers for Disease Control and Prevention. Economic Evaluation of Public Health Preparedness and Response Efforts: Tutorial. Cost Effectiveness Analysis: Introduction. Available at http://www. cdc. gov/owcd/eet/CostEffect2/Fixed/1. html. (accessed May 1, 2013).

8. Grosse SD, et al. Lessons from cost-effectiveness research for United States public health policy. *Annual Review of Public Health* 2007;28:365–391.

9. Graham JD, Corso PS, Morris JM, et al. Evaluating the cost-effectiveness of clinical and public health measures. *Annual Review of Public Health* 1998;19:125–152.

10. Feinberg J. *Harm to Others: The Moral Limits of Criminal Law,* Vol I. New York: Oxford University Press, 1984.

11. Yoe C. *Primer on Risk Analysis: Decision Making under Uncertainty*. Boca Raton, FL: CRC Press, 2012.

12. Slovic P. *The Perception of Risk* (Earthscan Risk in Society). New York: Routledge, 2000.

13. Slovic P. *The Feeling of Risk: New Perspectives on Risk Perception* (Earthscan Risk in Society). New York: Routledge, 2010.

14. Rawls J. *A Theory of Justice*. Cambridge, MA: Harvard University Press, 1971; revised edition, 1999.

15. Barry B. *Justice as Impartiality*. New York: Oxford University Press, 1995.

16. Mill JS. *Utilitarianism*. In: Robson JM (ed). *Collected Works of John Stuart Mill*. Indianapolis, IN: Liberty Fund, 2006 [reprint of the original published by the University of Toronto Press in 1969]

17. Callahan D. *What Kind of Life: The Limits of Medical Progress*. New York: Simon and Schuster, 1990.

18. Daniels N. *Just Health Care* (Studies in Philosophy and Health Policy). Cambridge, UK: Cambridge University Press, 1985.

19. Daniels N. *Just Health: Meeting Health Needs Fairly*. Cambridge, UK: Cambridge University Press, 2008.

20. Nussbaum MG. *Creating Capabilities: The Human Development Approach*. Cambridge, MA: The Belknap Press of Harvard University Press, 2011.

21. Powers M, Faden R. *Social Justice: The Moral Foundations of Public Health and Health Policy*. New York: Oxford University Press, 2006.

22. Smedley BD, Stith AY, Nelson AR (eds), for the Committee on Understanding and Eliminating Racial and Ethnic Disparities in Health Care, Institute of Medicine. *Unequal Treatment: Confronting Racial and Ethnic Disparities in Health Care*. Washington, DC: National Academies Press, 2003.

23. Winslow GR. *Triage and Justice: The Ethics of Rationing Life-Saving Medical Resources*. Berkeley, CA: University of California Press, 1982.

24. Childress JF. Triage in response to a bioterrorist attack. In: Moreno JD (ed), *In the Wake of Terror: Medicine and Morality in a Time of Crisis*. Cambridge, MA: The MIT Press, 2003;77–93.

25. Parfit D. Innumerate ethics. *Philosophy and Public Affairs* 1978;7:285–301.

26. Ramsey P. *The Patient as Person: Exploration in Medical Ethics*. New Haven, CT: Yale University Press, 1970; second edition, 2002.

27. Pesik N, Keim ME, Iserson KV. Terrorism and the ethics of emergency medical care. *Annals of Emergency Medicine* 2001;37:642–646.

28. White DB, Katz MH, Luce JM, Lo B. Who should receive life support during a public health emergency? Using ethical principles to improve allocation decisions. *Annals of Internal Medicine* 2009;150:132–138.

29. Ventilator Document Working Group, Ethics Subcommittee of the Advisory Committee to the Director, Centers for Disease Control and Prevention. *Ethical Considerations for Decision Making Regarding Allocation of Mechanical Ventilators during a Severe Influenza Pandemic or Other Public Health Emergency*. July 1, 2011. Available at http://www.cdc.gov/od/science/integrity/phethics/docs/Vent_Document_Final_Version.pdf (accessed May 15, 2013).

30. Baker R, Strossberg M. Triage and equality: An historical reassessment of utilitarian analyses of triage. *Kennedy Institute of Ethics Journal* 1992;2:103–123.

31. Emanuel EJ, Wertheimer A. Public health. Who should get influenza vaccine when not all can? *Science* 2006;312:854–855.

32. Persad G, Wertheimer A, Emanuel EJ. Principles for allocation of scarce medical interventions. *Lancet* 2009;373:423–431.

33. Bailey TM, Haines C, Rosychuk RJ, et al. Public engagement on ethical principles in allocating scarce resources during an influenza pandemic. *Vaccine* 2011;29:3111–3117.

34. Glass T, Schoch-Spana M. Bioterrorism and the people: how to vaccinate a city against panic. *Clinical Infectious Diseases* 2002;34:217–223.

35. Daniels N. Accountability for reasonableness [editorial]. *BMJ*. 2000;321:1300–1301.

36. Daniels N. How to achieve fair distribution of ARTs in 3 by 5: Fair process and legitimacy in patient selection. Background paper for the consultation on equitable access to treatment and care for HIV/AIDS, Geneva, Switzerland, 26–27 January 2004. Available at http://www.who.int/ethics/en/background-daniels.pdf (accessed May 15, 2013).

37. Calabresi P, Bobbitt P. *Tragic Choices*. New York: W. W. Norton & Company, 1978.

38. Nuffield Council on Bioethics. *Public Health: Ethical Issues* (London: Nuffield Council on Bioethics, November 2007). Available at: www. nuffieldbioethics.org (accessed January 17, 2013).

39. Thaler RH, Sunstein CR. *Nudge: Improving Decisions about Health, Wealth, and Happiness*. New Haven, CT: Yale University Press, 2008.

40. Blumenthal-Barby JS. Between reason and coercion: Ethically permissible influence in health care and health policy contexts. *Kennedy Institute of Ethics Journal* 2012;22(4):345–366.

41. Reeves RV. Shame Is Not a Four-Letter Word. *The New York Times*, March 15, 2013.

42. Bayer R, Stuber J. Tobacco control, stigma, and public health: Rethinking the relations. *American Journal of Public Health* 2006;96:47–50.

43. Mestel R. Swallowing a Lie May Aid in Weight Loss, Research Suggests. *Los Angeles Times*, August 2, 2005.

44. Johnson EJ, Goldstein D. Do defaults save lives? *Science* 2003;302(5649):1338–1339.

45. Childress JF, Liverman CT (eds) for the Committee on Increasing Rates of Organ Donation, Board on Health Sciences Policy. *Organ Donation: Opportunities for Action* (Washington, DC: The National Academies Press, 2006).

46. Popay J. Should disadvantaged people be paid to take care of their health? No. *BMJ* 2008;337:141.

47. Hawkins JS, Emanuel EJ. Clarifying confusions about coercion. *Hastings Center Report* 2005;35(5):16–19.

48. Cookson R. Should disadvantaged people be paid to take care of their health? Yes. *BMJ* 2008;337:140.

49. Grant RW. *Strings Attached: Untangling the Ethics of Incentives.* New York: Russell Sage Foundation; Princeton, NJ: Princeton University Press, 2012.

50. Childress JF. *Practical Reasoning in Bioethics.* Bloomington, IN: Indiana University Press, 1997.

51. Childress JF. *Who Should Decide? Paternalism in Health Care.* New York: Oxford University Press, 1982.

52. Childress JF. Paternalism in health care and public policy. In: Ashcroft RE, Dawson A, Draper H, McMillan J (eds). *Principles of Health Care Ethics*, 2nd edition. Chichester, UK: John Wiley & Sons, Ltd., 2007: 223–231.

53. Mill JS. *On Liberty.* David Spitz (ed). New York: W. W. Norton & Company, Inc., 1975.

54. Feinberg J. Legal paternalism. *Canadian Journal of Philosophy* 1971;1:105–124.

55. Dworkin R. *Taking Rights Seriously.* Cambridge, MA: Harvard University Press, 1977.

56. Helmet Use Among Motorcyclists Who Died in Crashes and Economic Cost Savings Associated With State Motorcycle Helmet Laws — United States, 2008–2010. *MMWR* 2012;61(23):425–430.

57. Derricka AJ, Faucherb LD. Motorcycle helmets and rider safety: A legislative crisis. *Journal of Public Health Policy* 2009;30:226–242.

58. Allen AL. Genetic privacy: Emerging concepts and values. In *Genetic Secrets: Protecting Privacy and Confidentiality in the Genetic Era*, ed. Mark A. Rothstein. New Haven, CT: Yale University Press, 1997;pp. 31–59.

59. U.S. Department of Health and Human Services. Health Information Privacy, 45 *C. F. R.* 160 and 164. Available at http://www.hhs.gov/ocr/privacy/ (accessed July 24, 2013).

60. Alter J, McKillop P. AIDS and the Right to Know: A Question of Privacy. *Newsweek*, August 18, 1986: 46–47.

61. *Tarasoff v. Regents of the University of California*, 17 Cal. 3d 425 (1976); 131 California Reporter 14 (1976).

62. *Code of Medical Ethics* 2010–2011 Edition. Chicago, IL: American Medical Association, 2010.

CHAPTER 3

The Political and Legal Context of Public Health Ethics

by Ruth Gaare Bernheim and Richard J. Bonnie

Learning Objectives

By the end of this chapter, the reader will be able to:

- describe and distinguish the complementary roles of ethical and legal analyses in public health decision making
- identify the sources of authority for government public health action and the constraints on the use of government authority in public health
- understand the way courts have interpreted and balanced competing legal claims in cases relevant to public health
- examine the way laws can be used as tools to advance public health goals

INTRODUCTION

Throughout human history, societies have undertaken collective activities, often using laws and regulations under authority of the state, to protect the health and safety of its members. The ancient Romans regulated sanitation, for example, and during epidemics in Medieval and Renaissance eras, many European states enacted laws to help prevent and treat infectious diseases.[1] In early English law, conserving the public's health was recognized as one of the core responsibilities of government, and this understanding "came with the colonists to America," according to Tobey, who points out that an act for maritime quarantine was passed by the Massachusetts Bay Colony as early as 1648.[2]

In colonial America, the general authority and duty of the colonies to protect public health was well accepted even before the Revolution, stemming in part from political ideas that the basis of government was an implicit social contract in which the individual and the state were bound by reciprocal obligations, which required government to serve the common good and promote the general welfare (which included public health) in order to fulfill its obligations.[1]

While government's authority and responsibility for protecting the public's health was recognized from the outset in the United States, it was not well defined by early constitutions and statutes. The political and legal context of public health has evolved over time, as new health threats have emerged and as advances in science and technology have created new opportunities for government to intervene to improve population health. The development of modern bacteriology and the related sanitary movement in the late 19th and early 20th centuries, for example, were accompanied by state laws establishing state and local health departments and empowering them to protect and promote health.

Today, government public health practices and policies include and are structured by a wide range of laws from many sources, including constitutions, legislative enactments or statutes, administrative regulations, and the common law (essentially, judge-made law drawing on precedent cases used to decide particular disputes). Governments at every level—federal, state, and local—exert great power and influence in public health by investing public funds in activities ranging from surveillance to public education; empowering public agencies to take preventive action; supporting and coordinating private efforts; and discouraging or constraining behavior thought to be inimical to the public health.

When government public health activities or policies infringe on the liberty interests of individuals or differentially impact particular individuals and stakeholder groups, fundamental and often overlapping political, legal and ethical questions arise. For example, should government's role in public health include regulating and limiting the size of sugared beverages that are sold or the amount of salt added to food? What are the constraints on government authority to intervene in the private lives of individuals? Does government have authority to, for instance, ban smoking in outdoor public spaces such as parks and beaches, or to compel tobacco companies to put anti-smoking graphics on cigarette packages? More generally, what is the appropriate role of government in protecting and promoting public health?

This discussion will provide a brief overview of the political-legal context of public health that is relevant and necessary for undertaking ethical analysis and justification of particular policies and decisions in public health. The goal is to begin addressing the following two questions that are fundamental to discussions of government's role in public health:

1. What is the source and scope of legal authority, if any, and what rules or legal principles constrain the use of this authority?
2. Are there relevant legal and ethical cases or precedents that should be taken into account?

Previous court cases and the opinions written by judges often provide helpful starting points and guidance for ethical, as well as legal, analyses of a public health issue. Thus, this chapter provides excerpts from court rulings to introduce some evolving legal principles—typically anchored in our nation's cultural and moral traditions—that illuminate our political values and public philosophy and inform ethical deliberation, analysis, and justification of policies and decisions in public health.

THE RELATIONSHIP BETWEEN LAW AND ETHICS IN PUBLIC HEALTH

When considering whether to adopt a new public health intervention, such as a tax on sugared beverages to address obesity, public health leaders offer reasons for such interventions, including data about the significance of the problem and the effectiveness of the intervention, and about the benefits and harms and fairness of the interventions. Providing reasons or justifications for particular public health activities and policies takes place within a particular political-legal context that both influences and reflects society's understandings at any point in time about what constitutes the common good, how we think about individual rights and responsibilities, and our notions of collective responsibility and fairness. These ideas lie at the heart of our nation's public philosophy.

Law and ethics have complementary roles in helping public health officials mediate the tensions that exist in our public philosophy and balance public and individual interests in public health practice. For example, there are often deep differences in values among people about whether government should use its authority to intervene on a particular health issue, such as obesity, and about what, if any, intervention is appropriate. Some may believe government should intervene to help communities address obesity, but believe only education, not taxation or regulation, is appropriate. Public health professionals can look to both law and ethics for guidance in addressing different aspects of these questions.

In the most general sense, laws authorize and constrain both public and private action. In relation to public action, laws explicitly establish the foundation for the powers and duties of the government in public health and also set limits on the use of government power to constrain individual liberty. It should be remembered that laws are enacted also to enable private actions as well as constrain them. Ethics, on the other hand, offers a way to identify, understand, and deliberate about the public values that underlie these varied uses of the law or that guide private activity. In addition, ethical perspectives provide guidance about how to specify and assign weights or importance to public values that may be at stake or in tension on a particular issue, so that justification can be offered for a particular course of action, whether taken by state actors or private actors. For example, ethical justifications in support of tobacco control measures have assigned less weight to the rights of smokers to use tobacco products than to the right of third parties to be free from the harms of others' tobacco use.

Ours is a system of limited government in which federal and state judges interpret, apply, and enforce constitutional and legislative constraints on government action. Public values are examined and legal and ethical justifications are offered about what constitutes legitimate use of government authority in two places: (1) in legislatures, which provide public forums for debates about legislation and government activities, and (2) in court proceedings, where parties can provide their arguments about laws or government actions that are in dispute. In some cases, court decisions lead to legislative enactment of new or revised statutes, consistent with judicial rulings. (See **Figure 3.1.**)

For example, court decisions about various state laws on abortion have led to new and revised state laws that regulate abortions within the constitutional parameters set out by the courts. As the cases presented below demonstrate, constitutional law and ethics use similar approaches in addressing competing values or moral claims that arise

FIGURE 3.1 Public Values and the Law

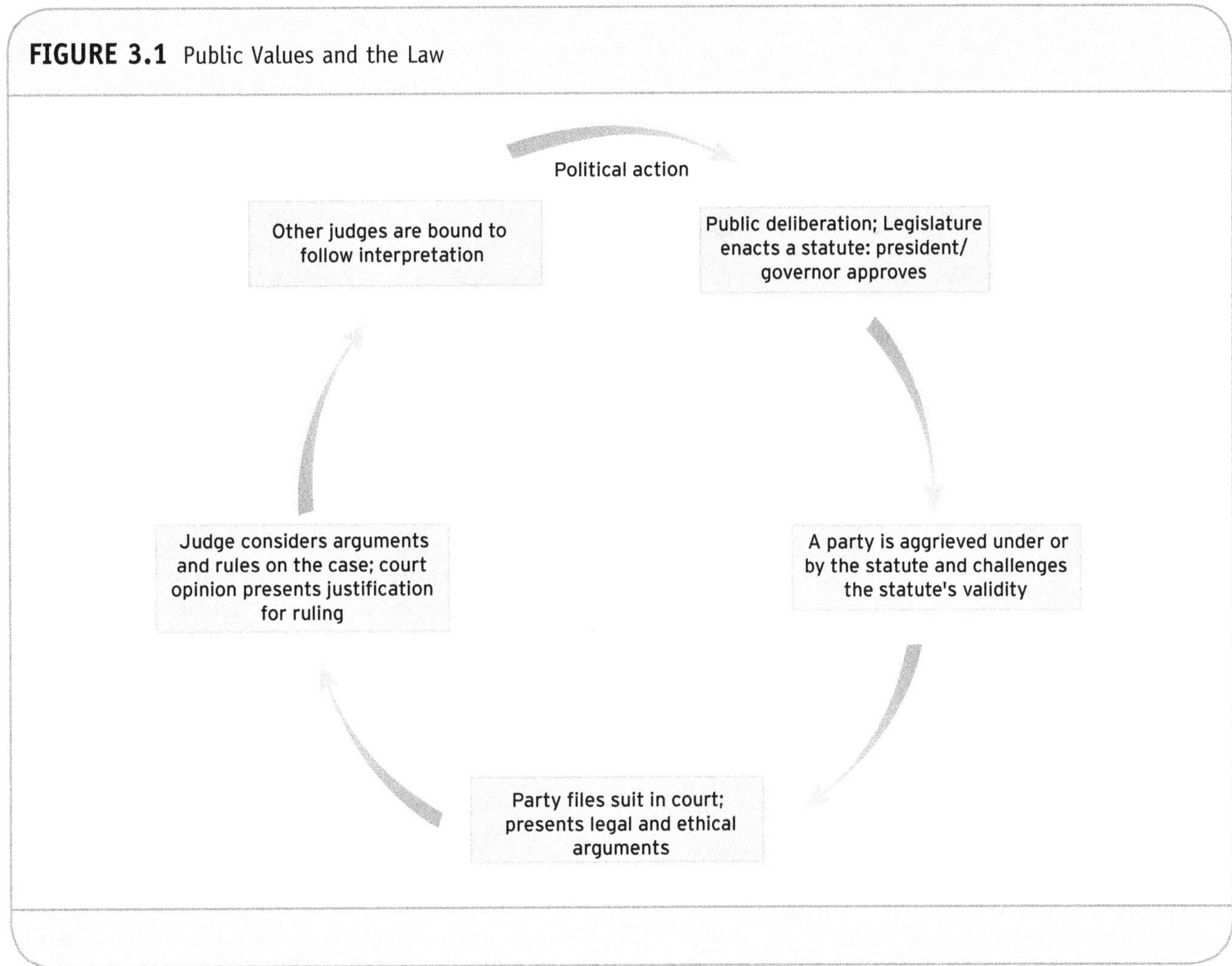

when the government undertakes activities to promote or protect public health. Both assess the need for and particular goals of public health action, weighing and balancing the competing claims about whether government actions and policies are justified, and providing reasons or justifications for decisions. It should be noted that not every use of the law implicates ethical questions. For example, some laws merely set minimum standards for what individuals should do in the interest of health and safety (e.g., stopping at red traffic lights and adhering to posted speed limits). However, other laws may infringe upon important liberties (e.g., immunization requirements) and therefore require more justification informed by both legal principles and ethical considerations.

As formal institutions, courts, legislatures, and executive agencies that exercise authority relating to public health are obliged to adhere to the substantive and procedural requirements that have been set by law. Of course, these legal requirements, which are typically enforceable in courts, do not exist in a social or cultural vacuum; they often crystalize and reflect ethical discourse as well as political considerations and empirical suppositions.

Public health ethics, in contrast, is a less formal process, and draws on moral norms, values, and professional codes. (See **Exhibit 3.1**.) When laws are not determinate or explicitly allow for professional discretion and judgment in public health decision making, or when laws are critiqued and challenged by some because they are thought to no longer express or protect society's values, ethics provides an ongoing systematic approach to assess and provide justifications for what should be done within the boundaries allowed by the law, or alternately how the law should be changed. For example, the laws protecting the confidentiality of persons with reportable diseases were contested in the early years

EXHIBIT 3.1 Centers for Disease Control and Prevention (CDC) Public Health Law Program (PHLP)

- **Law in Public Health:** Provides authority, limitations on state power, incentives and disincentives for behavior, often allows for much professional discretion
- **Ethics in Public Health:** Provides ongoing analysis, deliberation about, and justification for public health action and policy, often when law is indeterminate

Law
- Formal institution
    - Statutes
    - Regulations
    - Court decisions
- Public proceedings with a "reasonable person" standard

Ethics
- Less formal
    - Moral norms, values
    - Professional codes
    - Previous cases
- Publicly justifiable positions based on ethical reasoning

Centers for Disease Control and Prevention (CDC) Public Health Law Program (PHLP), Public Health Law 101, Unit 2 Ethics and the Law, Slide 10. http://www.cdc.gov/phlp/publications/phl_101.html. Last updated date: January 16, 2009. Accessed June 19, 2013.

of the HIV epidemic. Over time, ethical considerations were debated among public and professional stakeholders, and the ethical justifications for different practices for HIV reporting evolved, as did the laws regulating the requirements and procedures for named reporting of HIV-positive individuals to public health authorities. Recent reforms of state laws to recognize civil unions and/or gay marriages also illustrate the way social values and laws continue to evolve over time.

Understanding legal traditions in a particular policy context, and being familiar with the legal framework that governs public health action in that context, are necessary predicates for well-informed ethical judgment by public health officials. Specifically, it is important to understand the source and scope of the power or legal authority conferred on the official in the relevant context. This may require familiarity with the applicable laws and regulations, as well as any relevant precedent legal cases and the embedded values related to the public health issue in question. In many contexts, public health officials will also need to be familiar with superseding limitations or constraints on their authority arising from constitutional provisions (e.g., the First Amendment protection of freedom of speech) or statutory provisions (e.g., the Americans with Disabilities Act). In sum, an understanding of the legal framework is a critical first step in public health decision making and provides a necessary perspective for an ethical analysis of a particular public health action.

Every exercise of public health authority must be traceable to a power conferred by law. This authority is generally established and delineated in statutes, ordinances, and regulations that are passed by legislatures or promulgated by government agencies. Such laws not only set out the authority for government public health activity, but also often provide guidelines about how that government authority should be used. For example, state laws and regulations that authorize public health officials to quarantine individuals or to close a restaurant when there is a risk to the public's health, also generally provide specific criteria, conditions, and procedures that must be followed to guide health officials in the exercise of government authority and set the boundaries for when and how that authority can and cannot be used. Illustrations include laws that require government public health authorities to provide notice to affected parties and to gather and provide evidence about their decisions in court hearings.

In addition to a particular source of authority to act, public health actors must also be aware of extrinsic legal constraints on their authority. For example, the U.S. and state constitutions set limits to government authority by explicitly protecting the rights of individuals, such as the rights to freedom of speech, religion, and association. Public health activities and policies then take place within parameters set by federal and state constitutions, as well as other laws and regulations that may limit the exercise of official power, such as civil rights laws.

Within the prescribed legal boundaries, public health ethics provides a framework for ongoing analysis and deliberation about options for public health action. Ethical analysis then focuses on the following questions: (1) When the law is indeterminate and a number of actions are permissible, which options are ethically justifiable or preferable? (2) In light of underlying legal and ethical principles and considerations, how should the moral claims of different stakeholders

EXHIBIT 3.2 Scenario: Closing Bathhouses and Abatement of a Public Nuisance

Suppose that you are the advisor to the health officer in a medium-size city in upstate New York that is experiencing an increase in syphilis and a rise in HIV infection among a particular population, men who have sex with men. The health officer is concerned that a gay bathhouse in the health district that has both public bath spaces and private stalls provides a venue for activities that facilitate the spread of syphilis and HIV. Given a recent surge in infections in the region, she believes that the bathhouse should be closed and has asked whether a government official has the legal authority to do so—and, if so, whether this would be an ethically justifiable decision.

and the benefits and burdens be weighed and balanced for a specific issue or case in a particular community?

Consider the case scenario in **Exhibit 3.2**, which provides an example of the complementary roles of legal and ethical analyses in public health. Do you believe public health officials should have the authority to close bathhouses? If so, what should they do in this scenario, and why? The section that follows will provide an overview of the source and scope of government public health authority in general, before focusing on the bathhouse scenario in particular.

SOURCE AND DISTRIBUTION OF GOVERNMENT AUTHORITY IN PUBLIC HEALTH

Government authority in public health is shared among different levels of government. In the United States, the authority of the federal government is limited to one of the enumerated powers specified in the U.S. Constitution. As traditionally understood, the Constitution does not confer on the federal government a general power to act to protect public health. Under the U.S. constitutional framework, all powers not specifically delegated to the federal government are reserved for the states; thus, states retain what might be characterized as a "plenary" public health power, while the federal government has only those powers derived from its enumerated powers, such as its power to tax and spend. That said, it must be emphasized that the federal government plays a significant role in ensuring public health, because of the scope of the federal government's power to regulate commerce with foreign nations, among the states, and with the Indian tribes (U.S. Constitution, Article I, Section 8, Clause 3) and its power to tax and spend for the general welfare (U.S. Constitution, Article I, Section 8, Clause 1). In reality, the ever-expanding interpretation of the powers to regulate commerce and to tax and spend provides the federal government with expansive authority and opportunity to engage in many activities to promote public health and safety.

The power to tax and spend for the general welfare, for example, permits the federal government to fund services and activities designed to ensure public health and safety. The taxing power can also be used to regulate the behavior of individuals and other entities, by increasing the cost of behavior it seeks to discourage and by providing tax-related incentives for behavior it seeks to encourage. Tobacco taxes are an example. Indeed, the Supreme Court recently upheld the so-called "individual mandate" to purchase health insurance on the ground that it was a lawful exercise of the power to tax and that taxes are often used to create incentives for desired conduct.[3] The federal spending power also allows Congress to establish federal public health agencies and to allocate public health-specific funds to states and localities for particular programs, including funding that can be contingent on state and local action in order for them to qualify. An example is making a portion of federal highway funds for the states contingent on their adoption of a law setting a minimum age of 21 years for purchasing alcoholic beverages.[4] Organizationally, many public health tasks at the federal level are carried out by the Department of Health and Human Services, including the Public Health Service and the Centers for Disease Control and Prevention (CDC).

Federal agencies also are charged by law to undertake public health functions by regulating goods that flow through interstate commerce; a prime example is the mandate of the Food and Drug Administration (FDA) to protect the quality and safety of the national food supply. A broad interpretation of the commerce clause gives the federal government significant power to regulate local activities that affect interstate commerce, including the cultivation and possession of marijuana for personal medical use.[5] Regulatory functions under the commerce clause are also carried out by the Environmental Protection Agency, the Occupational Safety and Health Administration, and the Consumer Product Safety Commission.

Given the federal government's authority to promote public health by regulating private behavior through its powers to tax and spend and regulate commerce, fundamental questions of legitimacy can arise about the type and level of federal

TABLE 3.1 Sources of U.S. Law

Constitutions	• U.S. Constitution is the source of all legal authority for the federal government • Both state and federal constitutions are sources of legal authority for the states • State constitutions differ in significant ways, producing different styles of government in the states
Statutes	• Statutes are enacted by Congress and state legislatures • Statutes give power to executive branch agencies, such as health departments
Regulations	• Legislatures can give agencies the power to make regulations that have the same force as statutes • Regulations allow agencies to respond to new challenges because they often can be promulgated and amended more quickly than statutes, and can address highly technical aspects of issues • Federal and state laws require agencies to allow the public to participate in rule making

Common Law	• There are three levels of state and federal courts:
	  • Trial courts: make findings of fact based on evidence
	  • Appeals courts: review decisions of trial courts
	  • Supreme courts: reviews decisions of appeals courts to ensure that lower courts' decisions are consistent
	• The state and federal courts determine the guilt of accused criminals, resolve private law disputes between individuals, and review actions of agencies enforcing civil laws such as public health laws

Data from Public Health Law 101. CDC Public Health Law Program. http://www.cdc.gov/phlp/publications/phl_101.html. Accessed June 6, 2013.

involvement in regulating or influencing private behavior. For example, even if the federal government has the authority to do so under the spending power, is it appropriate or prudent for federal agencies to decide what particular family planning services should be supported? Or to make core public health funding for states contingent on the adoption of local ordinances regulating the size of sodas sold in chain restaurants?

While the federal government's power to promote and protect public health is inherently limited by its enumerated powers, the states have sweeping authority to undertake public health activities based on what has traditionally been called the "police power." This is the broad power inherent in a sovereign government to provide for the health, safety, and welfare of its people. The police power was reserved for the state governments when the U.S. federal government was established and thus much public health activity takes place at the state level. The concept of police power—which has its origin in the Latin and Greek words *politia* (Latin: the state, government), *polis* (Greek: the city) and *politeia* (Greek: citizenship, form of government)[6]—represents what is thought to be a core purpose of government, which includes state authority to promote broadly defined social goods.

Through their police powers, state and local governments undertake innumerable public health-related activities for the common good. These range from immunization, quarantine, and investigation of infectious disease outbreaks, to sanitation, nuisance abatement and environmental protection, to the regulation of medical and health professionals and health facilities. All of these activities made significant contributions to the 10 Great Public Health Achievements in the United States, 1900–1999.[7] The top achievements, followed by examples of state and/or local law, include (1) control of infectious diseases (sanitary codes, authorization of disease surveillance, regulation of drinking water); (2) motor vehicle safety (seat belt, child-safety and motorcycle helmet laws; prohibition on alcohol sales to minors; speed limits); (3) fluoridation of drinking water (ordinances authorizing water fluoridation); (4) recognition of tobacco use as a health hazard (excise tax, restrictions on retail sale to minors; clean indoor air laws); and vaccination (state laws requiring school vaccination). Organizationally, states have established and delegated broad authority for public health to state health departments or to local health agencies in cities and counties. The organizational structures of health agencies and the relationships between state and local health agencies vary among the states. For our purposes, the most important point is that every action taken by a state or local public health authority must rest on a specific statutory provision granting the agency the power to do what the agency proposes to do. The first question, particularly for policy innovations in public health, will always be, what is your source of authority to do this? For example, for our bathhouse case scenario, does the public health official have the legal authority to close the bathhouse? And if so, what is the source of that authority?

The concept of dual sovereignty between the state and national governments in our complex federal system creates numerous opportunities for tension and conflict. While states have primary authority for public health, the federal government's power to regulate interstate commerce or to exercise other enumerated powers allows it to regulate activities that the states also have authority to regulate, such as selling tobacco or manufacturing and selling vehicles that emit carbon dioxide. In cases of direct conflict, state laws must yield to the federal requirement under the U.S. Constitution's supremacy clause (Article VI), which states that the U.S. Constitution and the federal laws are the "supreme law of the land." In addition, even in the absence of a direct conflict, the federal government may decide that there should be a uniform national rule for certain areas of commerce, such as regulating nuclear power plants or package labeling requirements for tobacco products, and Congress or a federal agency may decide to "preempt" the field, thereby precluding state and local regulation in that particular field altogether.

Preemption, which generally means that a superior government can block or limit an inferior government's authority to pass laws in an area, also can operate at the level of state and local governments. For the regulation of tobacco products, for example, some state laws limit the authority of local governments to pass more restrictive smoke-free ordinances than the state legislature has adopted. Deeply rooted tensions in our nation's public philosophy are implicit in the frequent debates about which level of government is most appropriate to regulate behavior to achieve public health goals. These tensions were most recently reflected in the momentous litigation regarding the federal government's authority to require individuals to purchase health insurance, ultimately culminating in the Supreme Court's 5–4 decision upholding federal authority in *National Federation of Independent Businesses v. Sibelius* in 2012.[3]

In the context of public health, consider the scope and level of government authority to enact policies encouraging contraception to reduce unwanted pregnancy or to reduce the incidence of sexually transmitted diseases, for instance. Many tools are available to promote these objectives, depending on the target population, including education and increasing access to contraceptive products. As an example, consider the option of free condom distribution in public schools: Which level of government—federal, state, or local (specifically, a local school board)—should exercise the authority to set the policies in this context? And what are the ethical considerations, as well as political factors, that are relevant for such a decision?

Case Study: Bathhouse Scenario

The scenario posed earlier in this chapter about the regulation of bathhouses has confronted public health from the start of the AIDS epidemic in the United States, when public health officials first raised concerns about the potential transmission of infection in gay bathhouses and other commercial sex venues and considered controversial proposals to regulate and close bathhouses. For this scenario, we now turn to the following question: What are the sources and scope of legal authority, if any? One public health approach has been to close bathhouses using the public health's authority to abate public nuisances. Using its police power, a local agency, like a board of health, can identify hazardous or unhealthy conditions and designate them as public nuisances. A public nuisance is an offense that affects the public generally and, in the public health context, poses threats to general health and safety. It potentially covers a wide variety of conditions, such as excessive noise, filth that attracts disease-carrying pests, and contaminants in water. Unlike a private nuisance that usually affects only immediate neighbors, a "public nuisance" affects the entire community. Examples of early public nuisance cases involved a log blocking the road or a factory emitting foul odors. Although certain conditions historically were considered common-law nuisances, most public nuisances today are defined by statute. The local government's authority to "abate" (terminate) a public nuisance is a powerful public health tool. If the condition violates the statute and poses a great risk to the health and safety of the public, the health officer has the authority to summarily eliminate the dangerous condition, including destroying offensive private property, without incurring liability and without a prior hearing.

Does a local government have the authority to close a bathhouse as a public nuisance? The following court case was decided in 1986, after a new regulation was enacted in New York City that authorized health officials to close facilities where high-risk sexual activity took place.

In the St. Mark's ruling, the court deferred to health department's judgment about the significance of the AIDS threat to the public's health and held that the city has the authority to close the bathhouses. The court also rejected additional arguments by St. Mark's and some of its customers that the abatement order violated their constitutional rights. The case suggests that the health department has the authority to close bathhouses, if it presents sufficient supporting evidence about the health threat and risky behavior in the bathhouses to show that there is a reasonable relation between the means and end of the public health action. To say that the agency has authority to close the bathhouses, however, is not to say that it should do so. What are the ethical dimensions of closing the bathhouses? Is closing the bathhouses "necessary"? Are there other options that address health department concerns about potential HIV transmission in the bathhouses? For example, the city could

EXHIBIT 3.3 City of New York et al., Plaintiffs, v. New Saint Mark's Baths et al.[8]

This action by the health authorities of the City of New York is taken against defendant, the New St. Mark's Baths (St. Mark's), as a step to limit the spread of the disease known as AIDS (Acquired Immune Deficiency Syndrome). The parties are in agreement with respect to the deadly character of this disease and the dire threat that its spread, now in epidemic proportions, poses to the health and well-being of the community.... [T]here is no disagreement that the rate of incidence of new cases of AIDS in New York State is approaching 200 a month; effective treatment is wholly lacking, and approximately 50% of all persons diagnosed with AIDS have died. The death rate for this disease increases to nearly 85% two years after diagnosis. The same percentage of AIDS patients suffer from special forms of pneumonia or cancer which are untreatable, and about 30% of these patients show symptoms of brain disease or severe damage to the spinal cord.

... During the five years in which the disease has been identified and studied, 73% of AIDS victims have consisted of sexually active homosexual and bisexual men with multiple partners. AIDS is not easily transmittable through casual body contact or transmission through air, water, or food. Direct blood-to-blood or semen-to-blood contact is necessary to transmit the virus. Cases of AIDS among homosexual and bisexual males are associated with promiscuous sexual contact, anal intercourse and other sexual practices which may result in semen-to-blood or blood-to-blood contact....

Fellatio is also a high risk activity. As stated by the organizer of the AIDS Institute of the New York State Department of Health: "Any direct contact with the semen of an infected person may increase the risk of AIDS transmission. The deposition of semen in areas likely to contain abrasions, open sores, and cuts and concurrent inflammatory processes which could result in the presence of susceptible lymphocytes increases the risk of AIDS transmission. Because the mouth represents such an area (the epithelial tissue in the mouth is more susceptible to injury than the epithelial tissue in the vagina), fellatio presents a high risk for the transmission of AIDS.

On October 25, 1985, the State Public Health Council, with the approval of the ... State Commissioner of Health, adopted an emergency resolution adding a new regulation to the State Sanitary Code. This added regulation specifically authorized local officials, such as the City plaintiffs (City) here, to close any facilities "in which high risk sexual activity takes place." More specifically, the regulation provided: "Prohibited Facilities: No establishment shall make facilities available for the purpose of sexual activities in which facilities high risk sexual activity takes place. Such facilities shall constitute a public nuisance dangerous to the public health."

In 10 NYCRR 24-2.1, the regulation furnished definitions:

"a. 'Establishment' shall mean any place in which entry, membership, goods or services are purchased.

"b. 'High Risk Sexual Activity' shall mean anal intercourse and fellatio."

The Public Health Council based this regulation on the Commissioner's "findings" that: "Establishments including certain bars, clubs and bathhouses which are used as places for engaging in high-risk sexual activities contribute to the propagation and spread of such AIDS-associated retro-viruses. Appropriate public health intervention to discontinue such exposure at such establishments is essential to interrupting the epidemic among the people of the State of New York."

Thereafter, on or about December 9, 1985, the City commenced this action [to close] the New St. Mark's Baths (St. Mark's) as a public nuisance citing the health risks at St. Mark's as defined in the State regulation [and the trial court issued a temporary restraining order.] ... On December 20, 1985, the Public Health Council promulgated the emergency regulation as a permanent regulation. The "findings" of the Public Health Council, as they relate to "high risk sexual activity," were similar to the "findings" of the Council in October. The regulation was approved by the Commissioner of Health and became effective on December 23, 1985.

This action is brought pursuant to the Nuisance Abatement Law. Under that law, the City is empowered to enjoin public nuisances,... including a building, erection, or place (other than certain one- or two-family dwellings) which is a nuisance as defined in Administrative Code ... or a building wherein a criminal nuisance—as defined in Penal Law § 240.45—is occurring. Under Section 240.45 a person is guilty of a criminal nuisance when "(1) by conduct either unlawful in itself or unreasonable under all the circumstances, he knowingly or recklessly creates or maintains a condition which endangers the safety or health of a considerable number of persons; or (2) he knowingly conducts or maintains any premises, place or resort where persons gather for purposes of engaging in unlawful conduct." ...

Under Administrative Code, a public nuisance is defined as follows:

"§ 564-15.0 Definition of nuisance.—The word 'Nuisance' shall be held to embrace public nuisance, as known in common

EXHIBIT 3.3 City of New York et al., Plaintiffs, v. New Saint Mark's Baths et al.[8] (*Continued*)

law or in equity jurisprudence; whatever is dangerous to human life or detrimental to health; whatever building or erection, or part or cellar thereof, is overcrowded with occupants, or is not provided with adequate ingress and egress to and from the same or the apartments thereof, or is not sufficiently supported, ventilated, severed, drained, cleaned or lighted in reference to its intended or actual use; and whatever renders the air or human food or drink, unwholesome. All such nuisances are hereby declared illegal."

The City has submitted ample supporting proof that high risk sexual activity has been taking place at St. Mark's on a continuous and regular basis. Following numerous on-site visits by City inspectors, over 14 separate days, these investigators have submitted affidavits describing 49 acts of high risk sexual activity (consisting of 41 acts of fellatio involving 70 persons and 8 acts of anal intercourse involving 16 persons). This evidence of high risk sexual activity, all occurring either in public areas of St. Mark's or in enclosed cubicles left visible to the observer without intrusion therein, demonstrates the inadequacy of self-regulatory procedures by the St. Mark's attendant staff, and the futility of any less intrusive solution to the problem other than closure.

With a demonstrated death rate from AIDS during the first six months of 1985 of 1,248 plaintiffs and the intervening State officers have demonstrated a compelling State interest in acting to preserve the health of the population. ... to be sure, defendants and the intervening patrons challenge the soundness of the scientific judgments upon which the Health Council regulation is based, citing, inter alia, the observation of the City's former Commissioner of Health in a memorandum dated October 22, 1985 that "closure of bathhouses will contribute little if anything to the control of AIDS." (For a vigorous medical opinion to the contrary from a specialist in this field see letter of Stephen S. Calazza, M.D., dated Jan. 24, 1985.) Defendants particularly assail the regulation's inclusion of fellatio as a high risk sexual activity and argue that enforced use of prophylactic sheaths would be a more appropriate regulatory response. They go further and argue that facilities such as St. Mark's, which attempts to educate its patrons with written materials, signed pledges, and posted notices as to the advisability of safe sexual practices, provide a positive force in combating AIDS, and a valuable communication link between public health authorities and the homosexual community. While these arguments and proposals may have varying degrees of merit, they overlook a fundamental principle of applicable law: "It is not for the courts to determine which scientific view is correct in ruling upon whether the police power has been properly exercised. 'The judicial function is exhausted with the discovery that the relation between means and end is not wholly vain and fanciful, an illusory pretense.' Justification for plaintiffs' application here more than meets that test....

Accordingly, defendants' motion to dismiss the complaint is in all respects denied.

City of New York et al., Plaintiffs, v. New Saint Mark's Baths et al., Defendants
Supreme Court of New York, Special Term, New York County, January 6, 1986

require bathhouses to offer HIV education and/or testing, or mandate condom use, or eliminate private stalls so that risky behavior can be monitored. Are these options more ethically justifiable because they are lesser infringements on individual liberties? What ethical justifications could be offered for the various options?

CONSTRAINTS ON GOVERNMENT AUTHORITY: BALANCING INDIVIDUAL AND PUBLIC INTERESTS

Government public health authority at every level of government is limited by the protection of individual rights and liberty found in the U.S. Constitution, as well as in relevant bills of rights in state constitutions, which are often similar to federal rights.

The defendants in the St. Mark's case also challenged the City's order on the grounds that it violated the constitutional rights of privacy and free association of St. Mark's customers. However, the court held that their rights must give way to the City's compelling interest in protecting the public health. The court also noted that "it is by no means clear that defendants' rights will, in actuality, be adversely affected in a constitutionally recognized sense by closure of St. Mark's" because the constitution's protection for "sexual activity conducted in a private home does not extend to commercial establishments simply because they provide an opportunity for intimate behavior or sexual release...." Nor, the court observed, does closure of the bathhouse "extinguish their opportunities for unrestricted association in establishments which avoid creating a serious risk to the public health."

As for the alleged First Amendment right to freedom of association, the court noted that the impact was tangential in the context of this case "where the nature of the assemblage is not for the advancement of beliefs and ideas but predominantly either for entertainment or gratification."

As in the *St. Mark's* case, courts are frequently called upon to address conflicts that can arise between individual rights on the one hand and state laws or regulations (or health department actions based on them) that protect or promote public health on the other. Many court rulings have an impact on public health, and even when some rulings do not directly relate to a particular public health issue, they often reveal important social and moral consensus and illuminate some of the implicit, widely held beliefs, values, and assumptions in our de facto "public philosophy" that may be relevant for an ethical analysis in public health. Knowledge about laws and their rationale, then, may provide grounding for public health ethical decision making that justifies a higher or different ethical standard than the minimum requirements set by law. Court rulings especially can be a good source for examining the justifications or reasons offered for our beliefs and values regarding the use of government authority and the limits on government actions and also about the legal principles and justifications that have evolved over time. For example, court rulings interpret the U.S. Constitution as allowing, but not requiring, philosophical exemptions for state school immunization requirements, and court opinions provide insight about the ethical tensions and arguments made by different stakeholders when individuals have challenged immunization requirements. An ethical analysis of a public health issue, therefore, can be enriched by an exploration of the broader legal principles and perspectives underlying a public health issue and of the way the courts have weighed and balanced competing claims over time.

The landmark 1905 U.S. Supreme Court case, *Jacobson v. Massachusetts*,[9] is considered a seminal court ruling in public health. It upheld state authority grounded in the police power to protect the public's health by requiring individuals to be vaccinated when the community was threatened by a smallpox epidemic. In the case, Henning Jacobson, a person over 21, refused to be vaccinated, and he challenged the constitutionality of the law on several grounds, including that the law deprived him of his liberty guaranteed under the Fourteenth Amendment of the U.S. Constitution, which provides, in relevant part: "nor shall any state deprive any person of life, liberty or property without due process of law."

The following excerpt from the *Jacobson* court opinion illustrates the way reasons, grounded in important public values, are offered and examined in a court case to justify the use of public health authority and the way the court balances two strong, competing values: the public good and individual liberty.

EXHIBIT 3.4 Jacobson v. Massachusetts[9]

Mr. Justin Harlan delivered the opinion of the Court:

This case involves the validity, under the Constitution of the United States, of certain provisions in the statutes of Massachusetts relating to vaccination.

The Revised Laws of that Commonwealth provide that "the board of health of a city or town if, in its opinion, it is necessary for the public health or safety shall require and enforce the vaccination and revaccination of all the inhabitants thereof and shall provide them with the means of free vaccination. Whoever, being over twenty-one years of age and not under guardianship, refuses or neglects to comply with such requirement shall forfeit five dollars." An exception is made in favor of "children who present a certificate, signed by a registered physician that they are unfit subjects for vaccination."

Proceeding under the above statutes, the Board of Health of the city of Cambridge, Massachusetts, on the twenty-seventh day of February, 1902, adopted the following regulation: "Whereas, smallpox has been prevalent to some extent in the city of Cambridge and still continues to increase; and whereas, it is necessary for the speedy extermination of the disease, that all persons not protected by vaccination should be vaccinated; and whereas, in the opinion of the board, the public health and safety require the vaccination or revaccination of all the inhabitants of Cambridge; be it ordered, that all the inhabitants of the city who have not been successfully vaccinated since March 1, 1897, be vaccinated or revaccinated." Subsequently, the Board adopted an additional regulation empowering a named physician to enforce the vaccination of persons as directed by the Board. . . .

We come, then, to inquire whether any right given, or secured by the Constitution, is invaded by the statute as interpreted by the state court. The defendant insists that his liberty is invaded when the State subjects him to fine or imprisonment for neglecting or refusing to submit to vaccination; that a compulsory vaccination law is unreasonable, arbitrary and oppressive, and, therefore, hostile to the inherent right of every

EXHIBIT 3.4 Jacobson v. Massachusetts[9] (*Continued*)

freeman to care for his own body and health in such way as to him seems best; and that the execution of such a law against one who objects to vaccination, no matter for what reason, is nothing short of an assault upon his person. But the liberty secured by the Constitution of the United States to every person within its jurisdiction does not import an absolute right in each person to be, at all times and in all circumstances, wholly freed from restraint. There are manifold restraints to which every person is necessarily subject for the common good. On any other basis organized society could not exist with safety to its members. Society based on the rule that each one is a law unto himself would soon be confronted with disorder and anarchy. Real liberty for all could not exist under the operation of a principle which recognizes the right of each individual person to use his own, whether in respect of his person or his property, regardless of the injury that may be done to others. This court has more than once recognized it as a fundamental principle that "persons and property are subjected to all kinds of restraints and burdens, in order to secure the general comfort, health, and prosperity of the State. . . ."

Applying these principles to the present case, it is to be observed that the legislature of Massachusetts required the inhabitants of a city or town to be vaccinated only when, in the opinion of the Board of Health, that was necessary for the public health or the public safety. The authority to determine for all what ought to be done in such an emergency must have been lodged somewhere or in some body; and surely it was appropriate for the legislature to refer that question, in the first instance, to a Board of Health, composed of persons residing in the locality affected and appointed, presumably, because of their fitness to determine such questions. To invest such a body with authority over such matters was not an unusual or an unreasonable or arbitrary requirement. Upon the principle of self-defense, of paramount necessity, a community has the right to protect itself against an epidemic of disease which threatens the safety of its members. It is to be observed that when the regulation in question was adopted, smallpox, according to the recitals in the regulation adopted by the Board of Health, was prevalent to some extent in the city of Cambridge and the disease was increasing. If such was the situation—and nothing is asserted or appears in the record to the contrary—if we are to attach any value whatever to the knowledge which, it is safe to affirm, is common to all civilized peoples touching smallpox and the methods most usually employed to eradicate that disease, it cannot be adjudged that the present regulation of the Board of Health was not necessary in order to protect the public health and secure the public safety. Smallpox being prevalent and increasing at Cambridge, the court would usurp the functions of another branch of government if it adjudged, as matter of law, that the mode adopted under the sanction of the State, to protect the people at large, was arbitrary and not justified by the necessities of the case. We say necessities of the case, because it might be that an acknowledged power of a local community to protect itself against an epidemic threatening the safety of all, might be exercised in particular circumstances and in reference to particular persons in such an arbitrary, unreasonable manner, or might go so far beyond what was reasonably required for the safety of the public, as to authorize or compel the courts to interfere for the protection of such persons. . . .

If the mode adopted by the Commonwealth of Massachusetts for the protection of its local communities against smallpox proved to be distressing, inconvenient or objectionable to some—if nothing more could be reasonably affirmed of the statute in question the answer is that it was the duty of the constituted authorities primarily to keep in view the welfare, comfort and safety of the many, and not permit the interests of the many to be subordinated to the wishes or convenience of the few. There is, of course, a sphere within which the individual may assert the supremacy of his own will and rightfully dispute the authority of any human government, especially of any free government existing under a written constitution, to interfere with the exercise of that will. But it is equally true that in every well-ordered society charged with the duty of conserving the safety of its members the rights of the individual in respect of his liberty may at times, under the pressure of great dangers, be subjected to such restraint, to be enforced by reasonable regulations, as the safety of the general public may demand. An American citizen, arriving at an American port on a vessel in which, during the voyage, there had been cases of yellow fever or Asiatic cholera, although apparently free from disease himself, may yet, in some circumstances, be held in quarantine against his will on board of such vessel or in a quarantine station, until it be ascertained by inspection, conducted with due diligence, that the danger of the spread of the disease among the community at large has disappeared. The liberty secured by the Fourteenth Amendment, this court has said, consists, in part, in the right of a person "to live and work where he will," and yet he may be compelled, by force if need be, against his will and without regard to his personal wishes or his pecuniary interests, or even his religious or political convictions, to take his place in the ranks of the army of his country and risk the chance of being shot down in its defense.

(*Continued*)

EXHIBIT 3.4 Jacobson v. Massachusetts[9] (*Continued*)

It is not, therefore, true that the power of the public to guard itself against imminent danger depends in every case involving the control of one's body upon his willingness to submit to reasonable regulations established by the constituted authorities, under the sanction of the State, for the purpose of protecting the public collectively against such danger.

It is said, however, that the statute, as interpreted by the state court, although making an exception in favor of children certified by a registered physician to be unfit subjects for vaccination, makes no exception in the case of adults in like condition. But this cannot be deemed a denial of the equal protection of the laws to adults; for the statute is applicable equally to all in like condition and there are obviously reasons why regulations may be appropriate for adults which could not be safely applied to persons of tender years.

Whatever may be thought of the expediency of this statute, it cannot be affirmed to be, beyond question, in palpable conflict with the Constitution. Nor, in view of the methods employed to stamp out the disease of smallpox, can anyone confidently assert that the means prescribed by the State to that end has no real or substantial relation to the protection of the public health and the public safety. Such an assertion would not be consistent with the experience of this and other countries whose authorities have dealt with the disease of smallpox. And the principle of vaccination as a means to prevent the spread of smallpox has been enforced in many States by statutes making the vaccination of children a condition of their right to enter or remain in public schools. . . .

Jacobson v. Massachusetts 197 U.S. 11 (1905)

The *Jacobson* case illustrates the way courts balance the constitutional protections for individual liberty interests with the use of state police powers to protect the public health. In upholding the vaccination requirement in the *Jacobson* case, the court showed deference to the judgment of public health officials and suggested that it was appropriate for the legislature to refer that question to and invest authority in a Board of Health, composed of persons residing in the locality affected and appointed, presumably, because of their fitness to determine such questions. The court noted that the following conditions were important for the legitimate use of public health power and the infringement of individual liberty: The public health provisions were *necessary*, given the threat of the smallpox epidemic; vaccination was a *reasonable means* to protect the public given the circumstances; and the measure did not cause undue harm to the individual. The court suggested that if Mr. Jacobson had provided evidence that the vaccination would physically or medically harm him, he may have prevailed in court. (For more discussion of the *Jacobson* case, see Chapter 7.)

As in the *Jacobson* case, many public health measures, undertaken with state police powers, can be challenged in courts as an impermissible infringement on individual freedom on a number of Constitutional grounds, such as interference with the freedom of religion, speech, assembly, and protection against unreasonable search and seizure. The idea that individuals should be treated equally under the law and that they should not be denied freedom without due process are of particular importance in public health. The due process clauses in the Fifth (applying to the federal government) and Fourteenth (applying to the states) Amendments of the U.S. Constitution provide broad constraints on the use of government police powers. In the case of *Greene v. Edwards*,[10] for example, the West Virginia Supreme Court established rigorous procedural due-process requirements before persons with infectious disease can be confined, including adequate written notice, access to legal counsel, the right to be present at the hearing, and access to a transcript for appeal. In balancing the need to protect the public's health with the rights of persons who may expose others to infectious disease, the court reasoned that a requirement of fair procedures is justified by the fundamental invasion of an individual's liberty at stake with long-term detention.

Courts also have interpreted due process clauses to include what are called "substantive due process" constraints. These are protections for individuals against arbitrary and capricious government activity. Thus, even if the state holds a hearing before it takes away a person's liberty or property, the law may still be unconstitutional because the government didn't have an adequate substantive justification for limiting the liberty of the citizens. So, for example, a "right to privacy" is not mentioned explicitly in the Constitution, but the Supreme Court has said that such a right is "deeply rooted in our Nation's history and traditions" and that the due process clause limits the scope of power to intrude into a sphere of private life. Jacobson itself is an example of "substantive due process" review by the Supreme Court. Substantive due process protections are controversial because some believe courts are creating rights that are not enumerated in the Constitution. Substantive due process illustrates how courts have used and expanded on the actual language in the Constitution to now protect fundamental social-political values regarding an individual's sphere of privacy and right to be left alone when their actions do not harm others.

Both from an ethical and legal perspective, the concept of a right to privacy is implicit in many public health issues, such as mandatory reporting and treatment, mandatory helmet requirements, etc. On the basis of a right to privacy, the U.S. Supreme Court in *Roe v. Wade*[11] held that the Texas abortion statutes, which prohibited abortions at any stage of pregnancy except to save the life of the mother, were unconstitutional. In the courts opinion, Justice Blackmun noted:

> The Constitution does not explicitly mention any right of privacy. In a line of decisions, however, the Court has recognized that a right of personal privacy, or a guarantee of certain areas or zones of privacy, does exist under the Constitution. In varying contexts, the Court or individual Justices have, indeed, found at least the roots of that right in the First Amendment, in the penumbras of the Bill of Rights, or in the concept of liberty guaranteed by the first section of the Fourteenth Amendment. These (previous court) decisions make it clear that only personal rights that can be deemed 'fundamental' or 'implicit in the concept of ordered liberty' are included in this guarantee of personal privacy. They also make it clear that the right has some extension to activities relating to marriage, procreation, contraception, family relationships, and child rearing and education. This right of privacy, whether it be founded in the Fourteenth Amendment's concept of personal liberty and restrictions upon state action, as we feel it is, or, as the District Court determined, in the Ninth Amendment's reservation of rights to the people, is broad enough to encompass a woman's decision whether or not to terminate her pregnancy.

Citing *Jacobson v. Massachusetts*, among other cases, Justice Blackmun also noted that the woman's right of privacy was not absolute and must be weighed and balanced against important state interests. It should be noted that, since *Roe v. Wade*, the Supreme Court has eschewed the phrase "right of privacy" and has instead characterized the woman's right to choose as a substantive "liberty" interest in making reproductive choices free undue state interference.

Courts continue to address the tensions between civil liberties and state regulation, and in other cases provide further interpretation of the concept of individual liberty protected under the Constitution. For example, in a recent Supreme Court decision in 2003, *Lawrence v. Texas*,[12] which declared the Texas anti-sodomy law unconstitutional, Justice Kennedy began with an explanation of the rights secured by the Constitution: "... Freedom extends beyond spatial bounds. Liberty presumes an autonomy of self that includes freedom of thought, belief, expression, and certain intimate conduct. The instant case involves liberty of the person both in its spatial and more transcendent dimensions." The *Lawrence* case illustrates the evolution and expansion of norms and principles about individual liberty in our public values, and provides an important understanding of the moral context for public health decisions.

Another important limit on government authority, the equal protection clause, prohibits the government from distributing the burdens and benefits of state action arbitrarily or unfairly. It declares a norm of equal treatment of individuals who are similarly situated with respect to the aims of the state action. Under the interpretation of equal protection, while government can differentiate among some people or groups, it generally must do so on rational grounds related to a legitimate government interest. Courts have set more rigorous standards, however, for justifying official actions that use "suspect classifications," such as race, national origin or sex or that affect a "fundamental" interest, such as freedom of speech or religion. For these classifications, government must show that greater need or reasons exist for its different treatment, including a more important government interest at stake and a tighter "fit" between the objective and the classification drawn by the law.

Public health programs often target specific groups, particularly those at high risk, and thus can raise legal and/or ethical concerns regarding fairness and discrimination. For example, a policy that requires homeless people (but not other people) with infectious tuberculosis to be confined until they receive treatment and are no longer infectious creates a classification based on individuals' residence. Another example would be a policy that may have disparate impact on particular groups, such as a policy to target surveillance and screening for a sexually transmitted disease in a particular urban or ethnic population, which could lead to stigmatization of the group. Excerpts from the court opinion in the case *Craig v. Boren*[13] (**Exhibit 3.5**) illustrate how courts reason about equal protection under the law. The case involves a state statute that set different age limits

EXHIBIT 3.5 Craig v. Boren[13]

Mr. Justice Brennan delivered the opinion of the Court.

The interaction of two sections of an Oklahoma statute ... prohibits the sale of 'nonintoxicating' 3.2% beer to males under the age of 21 and to females under the age of 18. The question to be decided is whether such a gender-based differential constitutes a denial to males 18–20 years of age of the equal protection of the laws in violation of the Fourteenth Amendment.

... Before 1972, Oklahoma defined the commencement of civil majority at age 18 for females and age 21 for males. In contrast, females were held criminally responsible as adults at age 18 and males at age 16. After the Court of Appeals for the Tenth Circuit held in 1972, on the authority of Reed v. Reed, 404 U.S. 71 (1971), that the age distinction was unconstitutional for purposes of establishing criminal responsibility as adults, the Oklahoma Legislature fixed age 18 as applicable to both males and females. In 1972, 18 also was established as the age of majority for males and females in civil matters, except that Sections 241 and 245 of the 3.2% beer statute were simultaneously codified to create an exception to the gender-free rule.

Analysis may appropriately begin with the reminder that Reed emphasized that statutory classifications that distinguish between males and females are 'subject to scrutiny under the Equal Protection Clause.' To withstand constitutional challenge, previous cases establish that classifications by gender must serve important governmental objectives and must be substantially related to achievement of those objectives. Thus, in Reed, the objectives of 'reducing the workload on probate courts,' and 'avoiding intrafamily controversy,' were deemed of insufficient importance to sustain use of an overt gender criterion in the appointment of administrators of intestate decedents' estates. Decisions following Reed similarly have rejected administrative ease and convenience as sufficiently important objectives to justify gender-based classification ...

We turn to the question whether, under Reed, the difference between males and females with respect to the purchase of 3.2% beer warrants the differential in age drawn by the Oklahoma statute. We conclude that it does not.

We accept for purposes of discussion (that)... the objective underlying (the statute was)... the enhancement of traffic safety. Clearly, the protection of public health and safety represents an important function of state and local governments. However, ... statistics in our view cannot support the conclusion that the gender-based distinction closely serves to achieve that objective and therefore the distinction cannot under Reed withstand equal protection challenge ...

First, an analysis of arrest statistics for 1973 demonstrated that 18–20-year-old male arrests for "driving under the influence" and "drunkenness" substantially exceeded female arrests for that same age period. Similarly, youths aged 17–21 were found to be overrepresented among those killed or injured in traffic accidents, with males again numerically exceeding females in this regard. Third, a random roadside survey in Oklahoma City revealed that young males were more inclined to drive and drink beer than were their female counterparts. Fourth, Federal Bureau of Investigation nationwide statistics exhibited a notable increase in arrests for "driving under the influence." Finally, statistical evidence gathered in other jurisdictions, particularly Minnesota and Michigan, was offered to corroborate Oklahoma's experience by indicating the pervasiveness of youthful participation in motor vehicle accidents following the imbibing of alcohol. Conceding that "the case is not free from doubt," the District Court nonetheless concluded that this statistical showing substantiated "a rational basis for the legislative judgment underlying the challenged classification.

Even were this statistical evidence accepted as accurate, it nevertheless offers only a weak answer to the equal protection question presented here. The most focused and relevant of the statistical surveys, arrests of 18–20-year-olds for alcohol-related driving offenses, exemplifies the ultimate unpersuasiveness of this evidentiary record. Viewed in terms of the correlation between sex and the actual activity that Oklahoma seeks to regulate driving while under the influence of alcohol the statistics broadly establish that .18% of females and 2% of males in that age group were arrested for that offense. While such a disparity is not trivial in a statistical sense, it hardly can form the basis for employment of a gender line as a classifying device. Certainly if maleness is to serve as a proxy for drinking and driving, a correlation of 2% must be considered an unduly tenuous "fit." Indeed, prior cases have consistently rejected the use of sex as a decisionmaking factor even though the statutes in question certainly rested on far more predictive empirical relationships than this.

There is no reason to belabor this line of analysis. It is unrealistic to expect either members of the judiciary or state officials to be well versed in the rigors of experimental or statistical technique. But this merely illustrates that proving broad sociological propositions by statistics is a dubious business, and one that inevitably is in tension with the normative philosophy that underlies the Equal Protection Clause. Suffice to say that the showing offered by the appellees does not satisfy us that sex represents a legitimate, accurate proxy for the

EXHIBIT 3.5 Craig v. Boren[13] (*Continued*)

regulation of drinking and driving. In fact, when it is further recognized that Oklahoma's statute prohibits only the selling of 3.2% beer to young males and not their drinking the beverage once acquired (even after purchase by their 18–20-year-old female companions), the relationship between gender and traffic safety becomes far too tenuous to satisfy Reed's requirement that the gender-based difference be substantially related to achievement of the statutory objective.

We hold, therefore, that under Reed, Oklahoma's 3.2% beer statute invidiously discriminates against males 18–20 years of age....

In the past, some States have acted upon their notions of the drinking propensities of entire groups in fashioning their alcohol policies. The most typical recipient of this treatment has been the American Indian; indeed, several States established criminal sanctions for the sale of alcohol to an Indian or "half or quarter breed Indian." Other statutes and constitutional provisions proscribed the introduction of alcoholic beverages onto Indian reservations. While Indian-oriented provisions were the most common, state alcohol beverage prohibitions also have been directed at other groups, notably German, Italian, and Catholic immigrants. The repeal of most of these laws signals society's perception of the unfairness and questionable constitutionality of singling out groups to bear the brunt of alcohol regulation. We conclude that the gender-based differential contained in [Oklahoma law] constitutes a denial of the equal protection of the laws to males aged 18–20....

Craig v. Boren 429 U.S. 190 (1976)

for males and females for the purchase of beer. A male, who was then between 18 and 21 years of age and a licensed vendor of 3.2% beer, challenged the statute on the grounds that it constituted invidious discrimination against males 18–20 years of age.

Is there anything ethically problematic about prescribing 21 as the minimum drinking age for everyone? Suppose 18–20-year-olds challenge the constitutionality of the state's minimum drinking age of 21. Would the law survive? Doesn't the data show that 18–20-year-old males are at higher risk for alcohol-related auto crashes than females? Why isn't that enough to justify differential treatment?

DOES GOVERNMENT HAVE A DUTY TO PROTECT HEALTH?

Previous sections of this chapter have explored the significant authority government has in public health, as well as the limitations on the use of that authority when public health activities impinge on individual rights that are protected by the Constitution, for example, under the Fourteenth Amendment due process clause. Another important question, however, is whether the government has an affirmative constitutional duty to protect the public health or, in the language of the Institute of Medicine (IOM) landmark report,[14] a duty "to assure the conditions under which people can be healthy." The answer by standard accounts is no. The federal Constitution, with few exceptions, does not protect "positive rights" (a right to have goods or services provided by the government) and generally imposes no duties on government to provide goods or services, even for the most vulnerable (e.g., clean water, immunization, child protection, prenatal care). Instead, it protects only "negative rights" (i.e., the right to be free from unwarranted government interference with liberty of various types).

DeShaney v. Winnebago County of Department of Social Services,[15] for example, involved a young boy, Joshua DeShaney, who was brutally beaten and permanently injured by his father after the Winnebago County Department of Social Services returned him to the father's custody, despite repeated reports and evidence of suspicious injuries and child abuse. A suit was brought against social workers and other local officials claiming that their failure to act deprived the boy of his liberty in violation of the due process clause of the Fourteenth Amendment to the U.S. Constitution.

In essence, *DeShaney* raises fundamental questions about the nature of the government's obligation to protect its most vulnerable citizens. The Supreme Court essentially says that, under the U.S. Constitution, the tasks of defining and enforcing the government's affirmative obligations are not suitable for courts and are left to the political and moral discourse, where ethical arguments play a major role. The Court also suggests that these questions are best left to the state and the people of Wisconsin. Is the Court right about this? Are political institutions up to the task? Given limited resources for public health and social services in general, state and local

EXHIBIT 3.6 DeShaney v. Winnebago County Dept. of Social Services

Chief Justice Rehnquist delivered the opinion of the Court.

"...The Due Process Clause of the Fourteenth Amendment provides that "[n]o State shall ... deprive any person of life, liberty, or property, without due process of law." Petitioners (contend that the State deprived Joshua of his liberty interest in "free[dom] from ... unjustified intrusions on personal security," by failing to provide him with adequate protection against his father's violence. The claim is one invoking the substantive rather than the procedural component of the Due Process Clause; petitioners do not claim that the State denied Joshua protection without according him appropriate procedural safeguards, but that it was categorically obligated to protect him in these circumstances.

But nothing in the language of the Due Process Clause itself requires the State to protect the life, liberty, and property of its citizens against invasion by private actors. The Clause is phrased as a limitation on the State's power to act, not as a guarantee of certain minimal levels of safety and security. It forbids the State itself to deprive individuals of life, liberty, or property without "due process of law," but its language cannot fairly be extended to impose an affirmative obligation on the State to ensure that those interests do not come to harm through other means. Nor does history support such an expansive reading of the constitutional text. Like its counterpart in the Fifth Amendment, the Due Process Clause of the Fourteenth Amendment was intended to prevent government "from abusing [its] power, or employing it as an instrument of oppression." Its purpose was to protect the people from the State, not to ensure that the State protected them from each other. The Framers were content to leave the extent of governmental obligation in the latter area to the democratic political processes.

Consistent with these principles, our cases have recognized that the Due Process Clauses generally confer no affirmative right to governmental aid, even where such aid may be necessary to secure life, liberty, or property interests of which the government itself may not deprive the individual. As we said [in a previous case]: "Although the liberty protected by the Due Process Clause affords protection against unwarranted government interference ... it does not confer an entitlement to such [governmental aid] as may be necessary to realize all the advantages of that freedom." If the Due Process Clause does not require the State to provide its citizens with particular protective services, it follows that the State cannot be held liable under the Clause for injuries that could have been averted had it chosen to provide them. As a general matter, then, we conclude that a State's failure to protect an individual against private violence simply does not constitute a violation of the Due Process Clause.

Because, as explained above, the State had no constitutional duty to protect Joshua against his father's violence, its failure to do so—though calamitous in hindsight—simply does not constitute a violation of the Due Process Clause.

Judges and lawyers, like other humans, are moved by natural sympathy in a case like this to find a way for Joshua and his mother to receive adequate compensation for the grievous harm inflicted upon them. But before yielding to that impulse, it is well to remember once again that the harm was inflicted not by the State of Wisconsin, but by Joshua's father. The most that can be said of the state functionaries in this case is that they stood by and did nothing when suspicious circumstances dictated a more active role for them. In defense of them it must also be said that had they moved too soon to take custody of the son away from the father, they would likely have been met with charges of improperly intruding into the parent-child relationship, charges based on the same Due Process Clause that forms the basis for the present charge of failure to provide adequate protection.

The people of Wisconsin may well prefer a system of liability which would place upon the State and its officials the responsibility for failure to act in situations such as the present one. They may create such a system, if they do not have it already, by changing the tort law of the State in accordance with the regular lawmaking process. But they should not have it thrust upon them by this Court's expansion of the due process clause of the Fourteenth Amendment.

DeShaney v. Winnebago County Dept. of Social Services, 489 U.S. 189 (1989)

health officials often are required to set priorities and make decisions about the allocation of scarce public resources. Does ethical analysis provide a more robust approach for examining options and addressing resource allocation than legal remedies?

LAW AS A TOOL FOR IMPROVING PUBLIC HEALTH

Legal principles and rules establish the framework for government action by defining and locating authority in political institutions, defining and enforcing individual rights and other limits or constraints on that authority, and, on rare occasions, imposing legally enforceable duties on public officials to protect the health and well-being of the people. Now we turn to the instrumental functions of law a "tool" for public health action.

It is helpful to keep two broad functions of law in mind. In many contexts, a central aim of legal rules and procedures is to ensure that particular disputes are resolved justly and fairly according to law. In criminal law, for example, the aim is to ensure that the defendants are convicted only if proven guilty beyond a reasonable doubt, and also to ensure that their punishment is proportionate to the seriousness of their wrongdoing. Similarly, in tort cases, an important aim is to ensure that people or companies who wrongfully cause injury compensate their victims. Aside from reaching just results in individual cases, however, the rules of criminal law and tort law are also designed to deter and prevent criminal offenses and careless behavior. These preventive and instrumental functions of law are most important to public health, including prohibitions or requirements that discourage or inhibit unsafe or unhealthy behavior, promote or facilitate safe or healthy behavior or otherwise create conditions conducive to public health, safety and welfare.

A recurrent question in public health policy is what legal tools or policy levers can be most useful from a preventive point of view and what limits our society places, or should place, on the use of these particular instruments. **Exhibit 3.7** provides a functional taxonomy of legal tools for achieving public health goals based on the target of the intervention (e.g., collecting information and monitoring, regulating or restricting communications, regulating dangerous places, modifying individual behavior, etc.) In the context of modifying individual behavior, Figure 3.1 offers a typology based on the mechanism for affecting decision making that is being deployed (informing or otherwise shaping the informational environment, persuading, creating incentives or disincentives, restricting choices, coercing or requiring action, and compulsion or control). Ethical and legal constraints on the use of these tools are highly contextual, and subsequent chapters of this book will explore those constraints in several particular contexts.

The use of coercion (e.g., penalizing someone for not wearing seatbelts) is often controversial in public health, particularly when the prohibited behavior does not harm or create a risk of harming someone else. Threatening to take away a person's rights also amounts to coercion. Compulsory vaccination as a condition of public school attendance is "coercive" because students have a right under the laws of every state to attend public schools. Proposals to require adolescent girls to receive the HPV vaccine have been controversial on a variety of grounds, including whether less restrictive measures would be sufficient, whether they will encourage sexual activity, whether they violate parental control over the upbringing of their children, and whether requiring the vaccination only for girls is discriminatory. (See further discussion about immunization policy in Chapter 7.)

No one would doubt that government has authority to discourage and deter HIV-positive individuals from engaging in risky behavior that could lead to HIV transmission, but what legal tools are appropriate? Should having sexual intercourse with someone without disclosing one's HIV status be a crime? In 2001, 26 states had at least one law criminalizing HIV exposure, and between 1986–2001 there were 316 reported cases of prosecution of persons in the U.S. for knowing or willful exposure or transmission of HIV.[16] While some suggest that criminal laws may have beneficial symbolic or normative value in deterring risky behavior, others raise concerns about the challenge of fair and effective enforcement, given poor dissemination of information about the laws and

EXHIBIT 3.7 Legal Tools to Reduce Disease or Injury

1. Assembling information through mandated or leveraged reporting and collection of information from otherwise private records
2. Control of dangerous persons (quarantine or isolation; monitoring)
3. Control of dangerous places (abatement of nuisance; quarantine)
4. Regulation of natural environment
5. Regulation of "built" environment
6. Regulation of commercial products
   - Control of dangerous products
   - Facilitating access to risk-reducing products
7. Regulation of communication
   - Require communication of information, messages
   - Restrict communication of information, messages
8. Regulation of individual behavior (e.g., prohibiting dangerous or unhealthy conduct or requiring safe or healthy conduct)
9. Use of media to promote "healthy" behaviors
10. Provision of preventive services and education/information or requiring others to provide them

* Whenever used in all of the above contexts, "regulation" may include screening, hazard abatement, creation of incentives or disincentives, and standard-setting.

about the illegal nature of the conduct, and the need for highly intrusive monitoring to detect violations. The use of criminal law also could have unintended consequences, such as the discouragement of HIV testing, since some may fear exposure to criminal sanctions. On the other hand, indirect regulation of unhealthy behavior and products through civil litigation to collect monetary damages for harms or loss, for example, may be more ethically justifiable in some circumstances. However, in this context, one might well doubt that the threat of civil liability for transmitting the disease to one's unknowing sexual partner will be likely to have much deterrent effect.

Of course, civil litigation against manufacturers of dangerous products by injured victims or even by the state or federal governments for their own costs in treating product-related disease and injury can be a useful tool of product regulation as a supplement to direct regulatory action. Although this type of product liability litigation brought by government is controversial, it has led to many benefits for public health efforts in tobacco control. The Master Settlement Agreement between tobacco companies and 46 states and the District of Columbia, which had brought a lawsuit against tobacco companies, for example, resulted in the tobacco industry providing approximately $206 billion in revenue over a 25-year period for anti-smoking campaigns, and included numerous other financial and regulatory outcomes that supported tobacco prevention.[17] Even when tobacco-related revenues generated by the Master Settlement Agreement and by cigarette excise taxes increased, however, the amount actually appropriated by state and federal governments for tobacco control remained low and below that required to fund best practices recommended by the CDC, illustrating the importance also of building public and legislative support to prioritize spending on tobacco prevention and control programs. (See **Figure 3.2.**)

FIGURE 3.2 Total State Tobacco-related Revenues and State and Federal Tobacco Control Appropriations Compared with CDC Best Practices for Comprehensive Tobacco Control Recommendations for Tobacco Control Funding—United States, 1998–2010

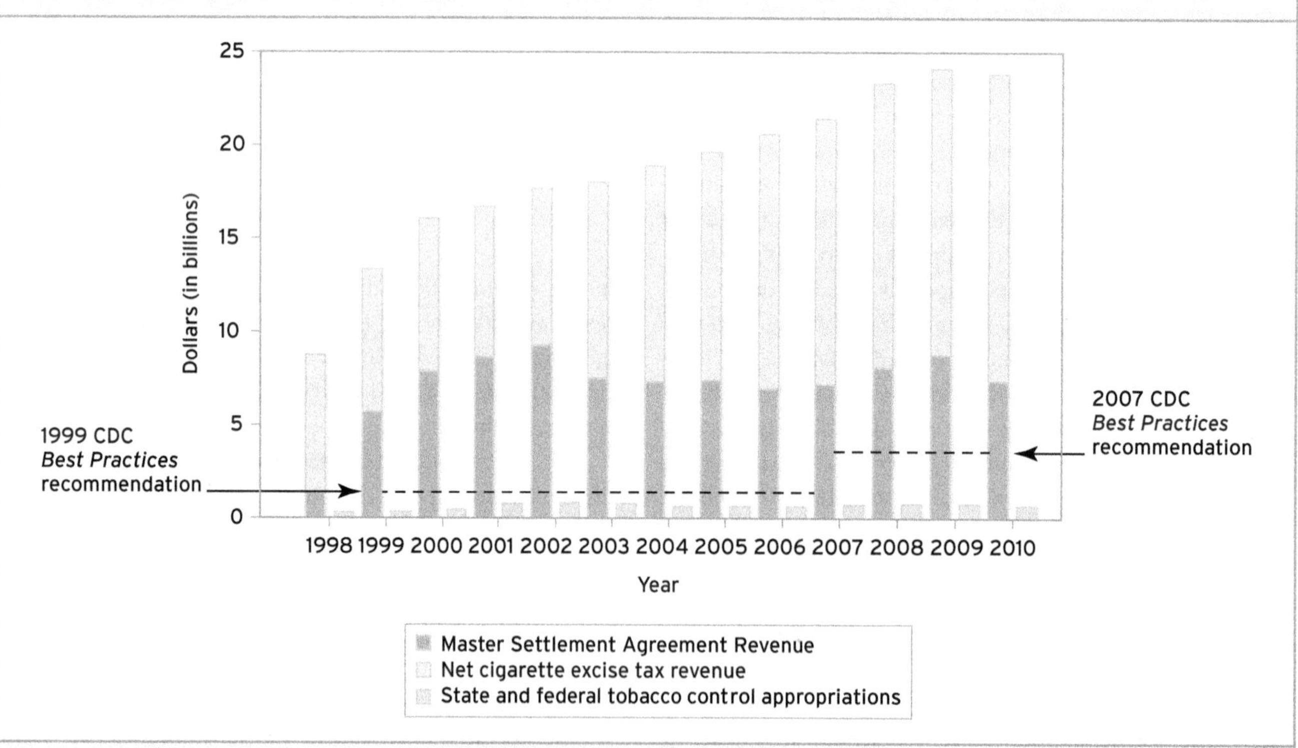

Reproduced from: State Tobacco Revenues Compared with Tobacco Control Appropriations—United States, 1998–2010. MMWR 61(20);370–374 May 25, 2012 http://www.cdc.gov/mmwr/preview/mmwrhtml/mm6120a3.htm?s_cid=%20mm6120a3.htm_w, (retrieved 4/14/13)

Other laws increasingly are promulgated as mechanisms to regulate individual behavior and shift the social norms in the desired direction. Some examples include zoning laws requiring that more land be set aside for parks to promote exercise, or laws that tax tobacco or other unhealthy products as a way of deterring their use. Health promotion through environmental regulation of this type is, in general, ethically justified because it produces public health benefit while still allowing for individual choice. Health impact assessments of laws and policies are providing new methods to measure the benefits, harms, and costs of laws and regulations on public health, and the evidence provides justification for public health action.

Some public health interventions, however, although constitutional, are still politically and ethically controversial, given the widely varying norms, beliefs, and values in society that often come into conflict when these tools are proposed or implemented. Laws that require helmets when riding motorcycles have been upheld by the courts as constitutional, but nonetheless often require ethical justification to address the ethical tensions and garner the political support needed so that the statutes are enacted in state legislatures. Implementation of publicly acceptable laws and policies, therefore, requires an understanding of the competing moral claims of the various stakeholders and developing justifications for laws and policies that resonate ethically with the public at any given time.

PUBLIC DELIBERATION AND LEADERSHIP

The story of tobacco control illustrates the importance of offering justifications that can shift public understanding and public ethical discourse over time. In the wake of the Surgeon General's 1964[18] report on the dangers of tobacco smoking, strong claims of paternalism (and the "right to be foolish") were mounted against proposals to use tools of public health policy to reduce tobacco use. For two decades, the locus of tobacco control was at the local level, where grassroots campaigns were launched for smoke-free laws. However, during the 1980s and 1990s national leaders in public health science, public health advocacy, and public policy orchestrated a gradual shift in public opinion regarding the ethical basis of tobacco restrictions. As summarized by the IOM's 2007 report, *Ending the Tobacco Problem*:[19]

> Until the late 1980s, the operating assumptions of tobacco policy in the United States were rooted in the society's general preference for individual liberty and freedom of choice, especially in matters that affect individual health. Thus, although it has been widely understood for many years that smoking poses serious health risks, the prevailing assumption was that the weighing of the benefits and the health risks of consumer products, including tobacco products, is up to the consumer and that government efforts to force people to make healthy choices would amount to an unacceptable form of paternalism. The underlying intuition is that people are and ought to be free to make their own choices and are responsible for the consequences of their choices. This perspective was also reflected in the unbroken line of jury verdicts and judicial decisions refusing to hold tobacco companies liable for smoking-induced disease and death among informed consumers.
>
> The first major change in tobacco policy was consistent with the antipaternalism principle and with traditional economic theory. The nonsmokers' rights movement, which took root in California in the late 1970s, called attention to the fact that some of the costs of smoking are borne by third parties and urged lawmakers to adopt bans on smoking in public buildings and workplaces. The antismoking movement received a major boost when the U.S. Environmental Protection Agency classified environmental tobacco smoke as a carcinogen in 1992. Although the tobacco industry disputed the nature and the extent of the risks associated with exposure to side stream smoke and continues to do so, the evidence documented suggesting the considerable health dangers of environmental tobacco smoke has been definitively summarized by the Surgeon General, and the moral legitimacy of smoking restrictions in enclosed public places is now taken for granted.
>
> In the late 1980s, the weaknesses in the libertarian point of view began to seep into public understanding and to transform the policy debate about tobacco. This profound change in the political dynamic occurred as a result of three intertwined developments.
>
> The first important development was a profound change in public understanding as the addictive nature of nicotine became scientifically established. The simultaneous proliferation of nicotine replacement treatments (NRTs) and other cessation tools, along with evidence of their effectiveness, helped to reinforce public

understanding of the grip of nicotine addiction and the need for stronger measures to help people quit. This development also began to erode the anti-paternalism objection against efforts to reduce consumption directly on the grounds that many people who have become hooked would like to quit.

The second convergent development was a concerted focus on the problem of smoking initiation. It became clear that almost all adult smokers began smoking as teenagers and that prevention of the initiation of smoking needed to be a core aim of tobacco policy. (Although it is not the only aim, prevention of smoking initiation is essential if the nation is to achieve a long-term permanent reduction in prevalence.) Understanding of nicotine addiction as a "pediatric disease" also strengthened the ethical case for aggressive efforts to reduce smoking initiation by teenagers, even if the measures also had spillover effects on adult smokers. Reports by the Surgeon General and the Institute of Medicine in 1994 established the scientific foundation for a youth-oriented policy initiative (eventually spearheaded by Food and Drug Administration Commissioner David Kessler in 1995) and also galvanized public opinion against the tobacco industry for targeting young people.

Third, the state Medicaid lawsuits and other tobacco litigation led to revelations of industry deception and duplicity and confirmed the industry's role in fostering and perpetuating tobacco use. These disclosures weakened the force of the antipaternalism principle as a constraint on tobacco policy and eroded the supposition that smokers have freely assumed the risks of smoking and are responsible for the often fatal consequences. Instead of being a champion of individual freedom and consumer sovereignty, the tobacco industry is now more often seen as a vector of disease and death, bringing public understanding into alignment with the premises of the public health community.[19 (p. 146)]

Reprinted with permission from the National Academies Press, IOM (Institute of Medicine). 2007. Ending the tobacco problem: A blue-print for the nation. Washington, DC: The National Academies Press.

In sum, over the last two decades of the 20th century, the operating assumptions of tobacco policy in the United States and elsewhere in the world changed dramatically in part because of the fundamental realizations that (1) tobacco use is grounded in addiction to nicotine and (2) nicotine addiction typically begins before smokers become adults. Most smokers start smoking and become addicted while they are adolescents; and most addicted adult smokers want to quit, try to quit, and would rather be nonsmokers. The deeper public understanding of tobacco addiction was nurtured and sustained by the nation's public health leadership and transformed the ethical and political context of tobacco policy-making. A widespread popular consensus in favor of aggressive policy initiatives emerged, leading to enactment of the comprehensive Family Smoking Prevention and Tobacco Control Act in 2009.[20] This groundbreaking law gives the Food and Drug Administration (FDA) the authority to regulate the manufacture, distribution, and marketing of tobacco products to protect public health.

The shift in popular sentiment has also been accompanied by support across most of the political spectrum for a variety of aggressive measures of tobacco control, including stronger package warnings, higher cigarette excise taxes, point of sale advertising restrictions, and tighter public smoking bans. However, the challenge of reducing tobacco use so that it is "no longer a public health problem" remains a daunting one, especially in certain regions of the country and among less educated and economically disadvantaged populations. (See further discussion of advertising restrictions in Chapter 9.)

As public health science provides more and better data about effective public health interventions, public health leaders have responsibility to continually advocate for ethically responsive policies and to develop the rhetorical strategies needed to win public support for them. Tobacco control, for example, is one of the "winnable battles" that the CDC has prioritized for two reasons: first, because of tobacco's large-scale impact on health—CDC reports that tobacco use, which varies widely by state/region and disproportionately affects disadvantaged populations, is responsible for more than 430,000 deaths each year[21]—and second, because of there are evidence-based tactics and approaches that are known to be effective in addressing tobacco use.

These include legal strategies, such as excise tax increases, smoke-free laws and policies, and advertising restrictions (see **Figures 3.3** and **3.4**), which remain controversial in legislative and political forums. For example, despite compelling evidence about the effect of cigarette price increases on cigarette sales, state adoption of higher excise tax rates varies greatly. Public health leaders have important opportunities in public forums to shape the public's understanding about

FIGURE 3.3 When Cigarette Prices Increase, Cigarette Sales Decrease

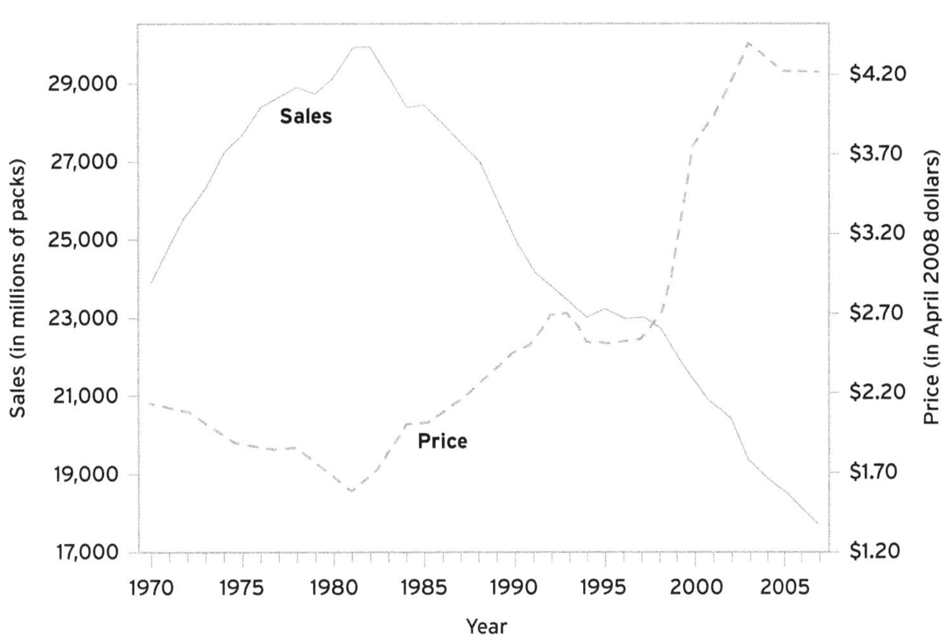

Reproduced from CDC Winable Battles Website Accessed 3/25/13; http://ww.cdc.gov/winnablebattles/tobacco/index.html Source: ImpacTeen Chartbook: Cigarette Smoking Prevalence and Policies in the 50 States

FIGURE 3.4 Comprehensive Smoke-free Indoor Air Laws Have been Enacted in 25 States and the District of Columbia

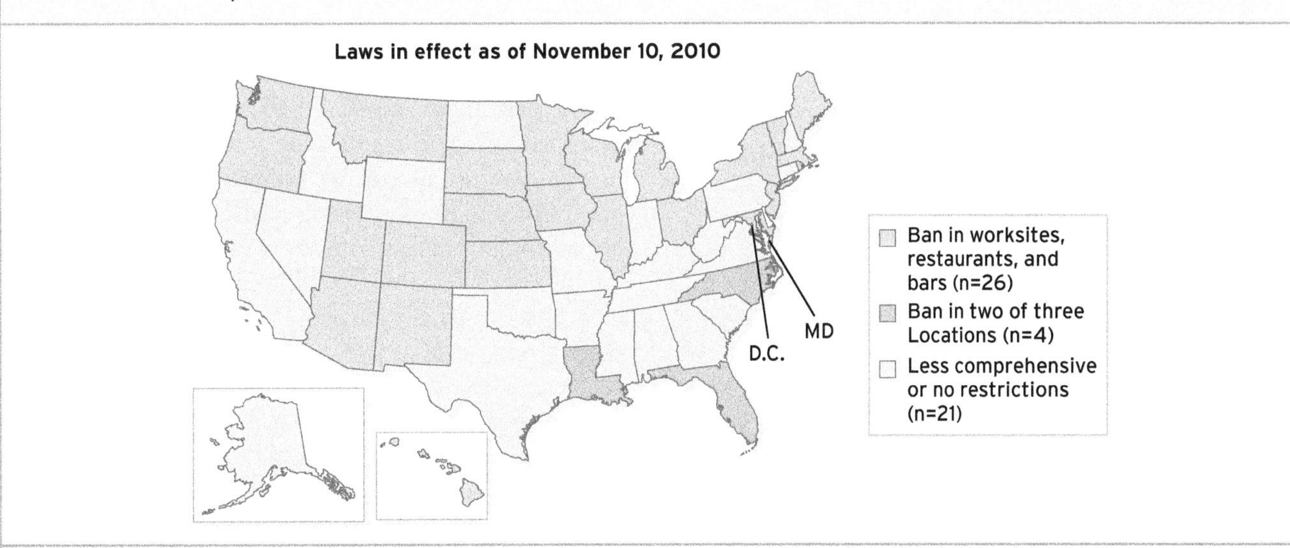

Data from CDC, Office on Smoking and Health, State Tobacco Activities Tracking and Evaluation (STATE) System.

the legitimacy of these laws and regulations by offering justifications for them that are grounded in scientific evidence, public values, and ethical considerations.

One intriguing new strategy to consider is the latest frontier in "smoke-free" laws—proposals to ban smoking in open-air public areas. Laws and other policy tools that aim to reduce access to tobacco and to deter its use through high prices and other disincentives also have the added virtue of declaring and manifesting social disapproval of—and "denormalizing"—the behavior. Is using the law or the resources of the state to express disapproval of smoking in itself a violation of public values embedded in our tradition, such as anti-paternalism sentiments? Is making it less convenient to buy cigarettes or to smoke them? Ostracizing smokers? What if companies refuse to hire people who smoke? Should the state allow discrimination against smokers? Is stigmatization a permissible tool of public health? If stigmatization and shaming do contribute to a decrease in tobacco use or tobacco initiation, is it justifiable to use such strategies?

The IOM report, *Ending the Tobacco Problem*,[19] endorsed the use of smoking restriction laws, pointing out that clean air laws "have done more to reduce tobacco consumption than any other intervention that cigarette price increases." It stated that smoking restrictions serve three purposes: (1) they protect nonsmokers from the health effects and the noxious odors of secondhand smoke; (2) they help smokers quit, cut down on their smoking, and avoid relapses; and (3) they reinforce a nonsmoking social norm. Among others, the report made the following recommendations:

- Recommendation 4: States and localities should enact complete bans on smoking in all nonresidential indoor locations, including workplaces, malls, restaurants, and bars. States should not preempt local governments from enacting bans more restrictive than the state ban.
- Recommendation 10: States should not preempt local governments from restricting smoking in outdoor public spaces, such as parks and beaches.

The IOM report described smoking in outdoor spaces as "the last frontier in the progressive restriction of smoking" and suggested these restrictions would be controversial because some doubted they can be defended on the basis of environmental tobacco smoke exposure by nonsmokers and therefore contend that banning outdoor smoking is unambiguously paternalistic.

Why did the IOM refrain from endorsing adoption of open-air public smoking bans? Why did it urge that the issue be addressed at the local level and not at the national or state level? A few locales are adopting or considering outdoor smoking bans,[22] despite claims that such bans are paternalistic and not ethically justifiable. Consider the following scenario, and in particular the broader questions it raises about the role of law in a liberal democracy and about the ethical justifications for laws, such as smoking restrictions in outdoor spaces, which restrict individual choices. (An exercise on smoke-free policies in outdoor public spaces is presented at the end of this chapter.)

The recent history of tobacco policy, like the evolution of the initial public policy response to HIV/AIDS in the 1980s, demonstrates how prudent public health leadership, together with effective education and advocacy, can promote public understanding and help mold a public consensus on the need to address important public health challenges. In the context of tobacco, effective leadership emerged initially in national health advocacy organizations (such as the American Cancer Society), then in cities and counties where clean-air advocacy led to ground-breaking local ordinances, later among state attorneys general in class action litigation against the tobacco industry based on novel legal theories, and finally among politicians and public health office-holders in Washington. This sequence of creative and committed leadership gradually transformed public discourse and all but erased anti-paternalism objections to aggressive tobacco regulation. State tobacco control programs now provide a backbone for prevention activities, including public smoking bans, excise taxes, and youth access restrictions. In 2009, after almost five decades of debate and deliberation, Congress embraced a major regulatory intervention.

A similar transformation may be underway in accelerating policy initiatives aiming to reverse the striking increase in the nation's average body mass index, especially among children. However, despite the growing chorus of concern among public health leaders, the general public remains skeptical about the acceptability of aggressive measures to alter the nation's eating habits, especially regulation of high calorie foods.

Creative use of existing authority can be a key component of a transformative agenda, as the Medicaid reimbursement litigation initiated by the state Attorneys General turned out to be. However, pushing the envelope can also set back the cause if it galvanizes vociferous political opposition or provokes a successful legal challenge. In the context of tobacco control, FDA Commissioner David Kessler's innovative effort to regulate cigarettes as nicotine delivery devices under the Food, Drug and Cosmetic Act in 1996 was eventually invalidated by the Supreme Court in 2000. New York City's Mayor Michael Bloomberg has been a pathbreaking activist in many domains of public health, including tobacco prevention and gun control, but his signature effort to break new ground in obesity prevention—the 16-ounce

Sugary Drinks Portion Cap Rule—was stuck down decisively by the New York courts. That case, *New York Statewide Coalition of Hispanic Chambers of Commerce v. New York City Department of Mental Health and Hygiene*,[36] represents a fitting counterpoint to the 1986 decision in *Saint Marks Bath* upholding New York City's creative use of the power to abate public nuisances with which this chapter began. It is a fitting reminder that the first question to be asked in public health innovation is whether the public health agency has legal authority to do what it proposes to do.

In May 2012, Mayor Bloomberg announced the Portion Cap Rule proposing to require food service establishments to cap at 16 ounces the size of cups and containers used to sell and serve sugary beverages. The Board of Health received 38,000 written comments about the proposal, 80% of which supported the Rule—but 6,000 of the commenting organizations and individuals opposed the Rule. In addition, a petition opposing the Rule, signed by more than 90,000 people, was submitted by a coalition of individuals, businesses, and community organizations. After the Board adopted the Rule in September 2012, a lawsuit was immediately filed. A New York City trial judge quickly enjoined to rule on the grounds that it exceeded the City's lawfully delegated authority. This decision was affirmed unanimously by an appellate court in July 2013. The unprecedented and highly controversial Portion Cap Rule never went into effect.

New York City Charter § 556 authorizes the New York City Department of Health and Mental Hygiene (DOHMH), an administrative agency in the executive branch of the City government, to regulate and supervise all matters affecting health in the City, including conditions hazardous to life and health, to regulate, among other things, the City's food and drug supply of the City, and to enforce the New York City Health Code. The Board of Health promulgated the Portion Cap Rule to amend Article 81 of the Health Code that sets forth the rules governing "food service establishments."

What is noteworthy about these enabling provisions in the City Charter is how broad they are. It was certainly plausible for the City to argue that this broad authority to regulate "all matters affecting the health of the City," together with specific authority to regulate food service establishments, authorizes the Board of Health to adopt regulations designed to reduce excessive sugar consumption, especially by children. But the New York appellate court pointed out that if the power were as expansive as the City claimed, the enabling legislation would have virtually no limits at all and would amount to an unconstitutional delegation of legislative authority to an executive agency, violating a fundamental tenet of the constitutional structure—"separation of powers" between legislative and executive branches of government. The court therefore read the New York City Charter language ("all matters affecting the health of the City") more narrowly to authorize only regulations "designed to protect the public from inherently harmful and inimical" threats to health, including "the power to supervise and regulate the safety of water and food supplies as well the control of diseases." The court explained:

> "If soda consumption represented such health hazard, then the [Rule] would be exactly the kind of interstitial rule-making intended by the legislature ... The Board of Health, however, does not claim that soda consumption can be classified as such a health hazard. Rather, the hazard arises from the consumption of sugary soda 'in excess quantity.' The risks of obesity and developing diabetes and other illnesses are greater in those who drink soda to excess than in those who drink it in moderation or not at all. Thus, since soda consumption cannot be classified as a health hazard, per se, the Board of Health's action in curtailing its consumption was not the kind of interstitial rulemaking intended by the legislature."

Further, the court reasoned, a hallmark of proper delegation of authority to administrative agencies is the need for special expertise and competence, and no special scientific expertise is needed in the context of drafting the Portion Cap Rule: The regulation had carve-outs for alcoholic beverages, milk shakes, fruit smoothies, mixed coffee drinks, mochas, lattes, and 100% juice drinks; and it would have applied to restaurants, delis, fast-food franchises, movie theatres, stadiums, and street carts, but not to grocery stores, convenience stores, corner markets, and gas stations. Thus, the agency's decisions about the scope and application of the Rule were essentially value judgments balancing the uncertain health gains achieved by setting the cap in a particular business context against the competing concerns about the impact of the ban on commercial activity and employment.

In sum, the Board of Health was writing on a clean slate rather than fleshing out and implementing a previously made legislative judgment or policy. The City Council is the proper forum for public deliberation about the competing societal values at stake and for deciding the extent to which the sale and service of sugary drinks should be curtailed in the interest of public health.

Do you agree with the court's decision? The Board of Health undertook an extensive effort to elicit public opinion.

Was its deliberative process faulty? Why shouldn't the elected Mayor or the lawfully appointed members of the Board of Health make this decision? Recall the *Saint Mark's Bath* case discussed earlier in the chapter, where the New York Court of Appeals upheld the Board of Health's authority to close the City's bath houses. Sexual behavior is not inherently harmful. How are the two cases different?

In striking down Mayor Bloomberg's Portion Cap Rule, the appellate court ended its opinion with the following observation:

> "[W]e must emphasize that nothing in this decision is intended to circumscribe [the agency's] legitimate powers. Nor is this decision intended to express an opinion on the wisdom of the soda consumption restrictions, provided that they are enacted by the government body with the authority to do so. Within the limits described above, health authorities may make rules and regulations for the protection of the public health and have great latitude and discretion in performing their duty to safeguard the public health."

The court draws a clear distinction between the "legal" question presented in the case (the Board's "authority" to enact the policy) and the wisdom of the policy (whether the intervention is justified). Is the distinction clearly and persuasively drawn in this case?

Case Study: Smoke-Free Policies in Outdoor Public Spaces[a]

Comprehensive smoke-free policies have become commonplace in the United States. Recently, some jurisdictions have taken action to extend these policies prohibiting smoking to include some outdoor spaces, such as parks and beaches. Several health justifications have been offered in support of these policies. First, as described in a 2006 report by the U.S. Surgeon General, there is no risk-free level of second-hand smoke exposure.[23] Even brief exposures to second-hand smoke can cause adverse health effects, particularly among vulnerable populations, triggering asthma attacks in children and adverse events for individuals with heart disease.[24] Some evidence suggests second-hand smoke levels in outdoor spaces can be substantial under certain conditions, in which factors such as wind direction and close proximity can yield concentrations that rival those of indoor areas.[25] In addition to reducing the health impact of second-hand smoke, prohibiting smoking in outdoor spaces such as parks might have other benefits. Some studies have shown that children are influenced by adult smoking behaviors, suggesting that if children do not view smoking in public places such as parks, they may be less likely to grow up to become smokers themselves. Finally, the smoke-free policy may have a positive environmental impact, reducing the litter produced by discarded cigarette butts and the risk of cigarette-related fires—as well as the associated labor and other costs incurred by municipalities in litter removal and other maintenance.[24]

In addition, these smoking bans also serve to promote health by increasing restrictions on the practice of smoking itself. By further restricting the permissibility of smoking, these smoke-free policies can be viewed as part of a broader anti-tobacco strategy aimed at changing social norms associated with smoking and tobacco use.[26,27] Such policies are consistent with a decades-long anti-tobacco strategy that has sought to "de-normalize" smoking from being an everyday, accepted—even glamorous—practice to one that is increasingly viewed as an undesirable behavior.[28,29] Finally, smoke-free policies may also provide motivation for tobacco users to quit smoking.[30] By reducing opportunities to smoke, these policies may support more individuals to begin cessation—and more to be successful at doing so. As nearly 70% of current U.S. adult smokers report that they want to quit completely, policies to support successful cessation have considerable potential to reduce smoking-related morbidity and mortality.[31]

Some objections to smoke-free policies have been made. First, opponents assert that the evidence base for the harm caused by second-hand smoke in outdoor spaces is not sufficiently strong to prohibit smoking in these areas. Studies which have measured the effects of second-hand smoke may not be comparable to the typical exposure in a park or other outdoor space.[32] If the health impacts of second-hand smoke to bystanders in these outdoor settings are low, the primary force of extending smoke-free policies to outdoor spaces may be in reducing the harms to smokers themselves, which invokes consideration of the appropriate extent of paternalism to promote public health.[33,34] Further, opponents question whether indirect or behavioral harms, such as the risk to children for modeling smoking behavior, are sufficient justifications for restricting smoking.[35]

Scenario: Outdoor Smoking Ban

An outdoor smoke-free policy has recently been proposed by your community's Board of Health. The policy would apply

[a] Disclaimer: The following case study draws on material developed by the Centers for Disease Control and Prevention Public Health Ethics Program and is used with the permission of that program. It is solely an educational exercise and does not necessarily reflect the position of Centers for Disease Control and Prevention on this issue.

to all public parks and beaches. The Board has called you, the local health department director, to testify at the upcoming hearing on the potential policy. How would you, as the local health department director, evaluate whether and how the policy should be enacted?

CONCLUSIONS

Legal and ethical principles and analyses offer complementary and often overlapping perspectives about government's legitimate role and activities in public health. Understanding the source and scope of legal authority, as well as the specific laws and regulations related to a particular public health issue in question, provides important background information for undertaking an ethical analysis of public health options. Laws not only set the boundaries of what constitutes legitimate government action, they also make explicit the moral baseline and minimal expectations for government action. When laws are indeterminate and allow the use of discretion about whether and how to use government authority in public health or when there is an option to pass a new law as a tool to improve public health, ethical considerations can offer important guidance and justification for making decisions and policies. In addition, previous court rulings can provide a rich source of knowledge not only about whether a public health law or intervention is constitutional, but also about the deeply held public values at stake on a particular issue and the ways both to balance those values when they are in tension and to justify decisions.

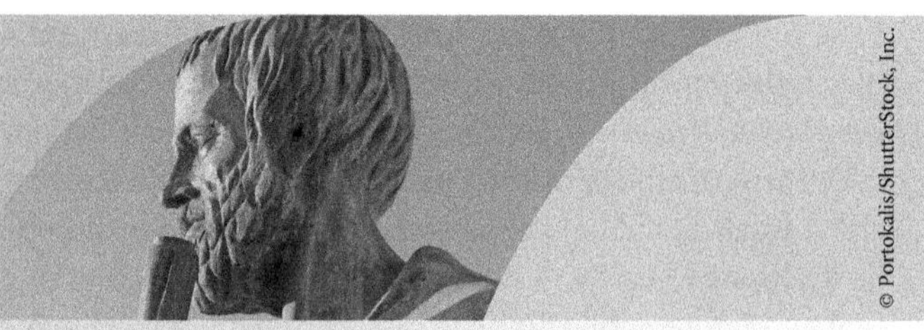

Discussion Questions

1. What are some of the important public values and principles embedded in our public philosophy and legal tradition?
2. The amendments in the Bill of Rights include the freedom of religion, speech, press, and assembly (First Amendment); the right to keep and bear arms (Second Amendment); the freedom from unreasonable searches and seizure (Fourth Amendment); and the right to due process, equal protection, and just compensation for private property taken for public use (Fifth Amendment). What public health activities might be constrained or limited by one of these amendments?
3. What recommendations, based on the history of tobacco control presented in this chapter, would you make to public health professionals who wanted to address the obesity epidemic? From a policy perspective, what would be the differences between tobacco and obesity?
4. A number of the court decisions presented in this chapter based some of their conclusions on scientific and/or medical data. What did the court decisions suggest was the role of the courts regarding data and evidence? In comparison, what then might be the roles of state legislatures and departments of health?
5. For the case scenario on banning outdoor smoking, what are the ethical arguments for and against such a ban? Using the Framework for Ethical Analysis presented in Chapter 1, what would be your position on whether the ban should be adopted?

REFERENCES

1. Parmet W. Health care and the constitution: Public health and the role of the state in the framing era. *Hastings Constitutional Law Quarterly* 1993;20:267–335.

2. Tobey JA. Public health and the police power. *New York University Law Review 1927;*. 4:*126*–133.

3. *National Federation of Independent Business et al. v. Sebelius, Secretary of Health and Human Services et al.* Certiorari to the United States Court of Appeals for the Eleventh Circuit. No. 11–393. Argued March 26, 27, 28, 2012—Decided June 28, 2012.

4. *South Dakota v. Dole*, 483 U.S. 203 (1987).

5. *Gonzales v. Raich*, 545 U.S. 1, 125 S.Ct. 2195, 162 L.Ed.2d 1 (2005).

6. Gostin L. *Public Health Law Power, Duty, Restraint.* Berkeley and Los Angeles, CA: University of California Press, 2000: 48.

7. Centers for Disease Control and Prevention (CDC). Ten great public health achievements—United States, 1900–1999. *Morbidity and Mortality Weekly Report*, 1999;48(12):241–243. Available at http://www.cdc.gov/mmwr/preview/mmwrhtml/00056796.htm (accessed July 27, 2013).

8. *City of New York et al., Plaintiffs, v. New Saint Mark's Baths et al., Defendants.* Supreme Court of New York, Special Term, New York County, January 6, 1986.

9. *Jacobson v. Massachusetts* 197 U.S. 11 (1905).

10. *Greene v. Edwards*, 263 S.E.2D 661 (1980).

11. *Roe v. Wade*, 410 U.S. 113 (1973).

12. *Lawrence v. Texas*, 539 U.S. 558 (2003).

13. *Craig v. Boren*, 429 U.S. 190 (1976).

14. Institute of Medicine. *The Future of Public Health.* Washington DC: National Academies Press, 1988. Available at http://iom.edu/Reports/1988/The-Future-of-Public-Health.aspx (accessed July 27, 2013).

15. *DeShaney v. Winnebago County Dept. of Social Services,* 489 U.S. 189 (1989).

16. Goodman RA, Hoffman RE, Lopez W, Matthews GW, Rothstein MA, Foster KL (eds). *Law in Public Health Practice.* New York, NY: Oxford University Press, 2007:157.

17. Centers for Disease Control and Prevention (CDC). Comprehensive smoke-free laws—50 largest U.S. cities, 2000 and 2012. *Morbidity and Mortality Weekly Report*, 2012;61(45):914–917. Available at: http://www.cdc.gov/tobacco/data_statistics/mmwrs/byyear/2012/mm6120a3/intro.htm (accessed July 27, 2013).

18. Office of the U.S. Surgeon General. *Smoking and Health: Report of the Advisory Committee to the Surgeon General of the Public Health Service.* United States Public Health Service, Office of the Surgeon General, 1964. Retrieved from http://profiles.nlm.nih.gov/ps/retrieve/ResourceMetadata/NNBBMQ (accessed July 27, 2013).

19. Institute of Medicine. *Ending the Tobacco Problem: A Blue-Print for the Nation.* Washington, DC: The National Academies Press, 2007.

20. Family Smoking Prevention and Tobacco Control Act, Public Law 111 31, June 22, 2009. Retrieved from www.gpo.gov/fdsys/pkg/PLAW-111publ31/pdf/PLAW-111publ31.pdf

21. Centers for Disease Control. Winnable Battles. Retrieved from http://www.cdc.gov/winnablebattles/tobacco/index.html (accessed July 27, 2013).

22. Slade D. Charleston approves outdoor smoking ban for streets and sidewalks in the hospital district. *The Post and Courier* (2013, January 9). Retrieved from http://www.postandcourier.com/article/20130109/PC16/130109371/charleston-approves-outdoor-smoking-ban-for-streets-and-sidewalks-in-the-hospital-district (accessed July 27, 2013).

23. Office of the U.S. Surgeon General. *The Health Consequences of Involuntary Exposure to Tobacco Smoke: A Report of the Surgeon General.* Atlanta: U.S. Department of Health and Human Services, Centers for Disease Control and Prevention, Coordinating Center for Health Promotion, National Center for Chronic Disease Prevention and Health Promotion, Office on Smoking and Health, 2006.

24. Bloch M, Shopland D. Outdoor smoking bans: More than meets the eye. *Tobacco Control* 2000;9:99.

25. Kleipeis N, Ott W, Switzer P. Real-time measurement of outdoor tobacco smoke particles. *Journal of Air and Waste Management Association*, 2007;57:522–534.

26. Bayer R, Stuber J. Tobacco control, stigma, and public health: Rethinking the relations. *American Journal of Public Health*, 2006;96(1):47–50.

27. Bayer R, Colgrove J. Science, politics, and ideology in the campaign against environmental tobacco smoke. *American Journal of Public Health*, 2002;92(6):949–954.

28. Brandt A. Blow some my way: Passive smoking, risk, and American culture. In: Lock S, Reynolds L, Tansey E, (eds). *Ashes to Ashes: The History of Smoking and Health.* Amsterdam, The Netherlands: Rodolpi BV, 1998:164–191.

29. Francis J, Abramsohn E, Park H. Policy-driven tobacco control. *Tobacco Control*, 1998;19(Suppl 1):16–20.

30. Hopkins D, Razi S, Leeks K, et al. Smokefree policies to reduce tobacco use: A systematic review. *American Journal of Preventive Medicine*, 2010;38(2S):S275–S289.

31. Centers for Disease Control and Prevention. Quitting smoking among adults—United States, 2001–2010. *Morbidity and Mortality Weekly Report*, 2011;60(44):1513–1519.

32. Chapman S. Should smoking in outdoor spaces be banned? *British Medical Journal*, 2008;337:a2804.

33. Rabin R. Tobacco control strategies: Past efficacy and future promise. *Loyola Los Angeles Law Review,* 2008;41:1721–1768.

34. Colgrove J, Bayer R, Bachynnski K. Nowhere left to hide? The banishment of smoking from public spaces. *New England Journal of Medicine*, 2011;364:2375–2377.

35. Blanke D, Cork K. Exploring the limits of smoking regulation. *William Mitchell Law Review*, 2007;34(4):1587–1593.

36. *Matter of New York Statewide Coalition of Hispanic Chambers of Commerce v. New York City Dept. of Health & Mental Hygiene*, 2013 NY Slip Op 05505, 2013 WL 3880139, New York Appellate Division, First Department, decided July 30, 2013.

CHAPTER 4

Public Health Perspectives

by Ruth Gaare Bernheim

Learning Objectives

By the end of this chapter, the reader will be able to:

- understand key concepts in public health, such as population health goals, prevention, determinants of health, and health equity
- identify the types and use of evidence in public health practice
- describe and assess a range of public health interventions that can be undertaken to achieve "healthy communities" and stakeholder engagement

INTRODUCTION

Charged with broad responsibilities to protect and promote the health and general welfare, government public health officials today are confronted with wide-ranging challenges as they aim to ***protect*** the public from infectious disease threats, ***prevent*** chronic diseases and injury, and ***promote*** healthy lifestyles and healthy environments. While the availability of clean water, safe foods, and other improvements in living standards accounted for the 20 years of life expectancy gained in the first half of the 20th century,[1] public health leaders suggest that additional major gains will require complex, multi-tiered efforts that focus on social, economic, and environmental factors that impact health. Multiple stakeholders, from school superintendents and urban planners to physicians and corporate wellness counselors, must aim to improve socioeconomic conditions; change social norms; and integrate preventive clinical interventions, such as smoking cessation counseling, with medical care.

To address cardiovascular disease (CVD), for example, healthcare providers currently treat risk factors such as hypertension and high cholesterol on an individual basis through medication and screening. "But even assuming perfect treatment, this approach fails to prevent almost half of the disease burden caused by elevated blood pressure,"[1 (p. 591)] points out Dr. Thomas Friedan, director of the Centers for Disease Control and Prevention (CDC). He calls for additional public health interventions that also change the environment, for example, by providing greater access to healthier foods with reduced sodium or trans fat and by improving community design to increase physical activity. To accomplish this, public health leaders endorse a Health in All Policies (HiAP) approach, which highlights the importance of identifying and addressing government policies and programs in nonhealth sectors, such as housing, agriculture, labor, and transportation, that have an impact on population health and health equity.[2]

Given the limited resources available for public health activities, however, challenging ethical questions arise about the scope and priorities of government public health activity. How should health officials and communities make decisions about which particular public health goals to pursue and what means or interventions they should use to achieve them? For example, if a particular community's mortality rates for both cardiovascular and cancer are higher, and its childhood immunization rate lower, than the state and national averages, how should it focus its efforts, given limited resources?

This chapter explores some perspectives in the field of public health that are relevant to an ethical inquiry about setting goals and priorities, given public health's broad mandate. A case study on CVD will illustrate the wide range of interventions in public health practice and the ethical dimensions of making choices from among the many options available, particularly when resources are limited.

IMPROVING POPULATION HEALTH

Public health is both a social and political undertaking, as we have noted elsewhere, and thus involves scientific analyses, as well as the art of communicating knowledge to the public and building the community collaborations and support needed to improve population health. Constraints on public health activity also are social and political and include not only the lack of economic resources (public health competes with other social goods, such as education, for public funding), but also social norms and health literacy. For example, some might oppose particular public health activities because they "believe that the health burden is low, the intervention is too costly or is likely to be ineffective, and therefore the expected benefits don't warrant the costs."[3]

Others may have philosophical concerns about public health goals, such as apprehension that pursuing a particular goal may lead to a slippery slope that significantly undermines individual interests, "such as perceived loss of personal autonomy or the belief that these actions will undermine self-reliance or individual choice."[3] And still others might challenge whether particular actions fall within the appropriate role or scope of government public health activity, such as public health advocacy for zoning laws that prohibit particular food establishments in certain neighborhoods as a way to address obesity. One commentator, for example, points out the potentially boundless scope of public health, now that data show correlations between health and individual behaviors, and health and social conditions such as poverty, illiteracy, and homelessness.[4]

Such controversies about public health's activities are not new and have been fueled, in part, by "the anti-authoritarian ethos that is a historically prominent feature of U.S. politics and civic culture," according to Ronald Bayer.[5 (p. 1099)] He and others call for an explicit acknowledgement of the ethical and political tensions embedded in public health and a public debate about our public health choices. Bayer states: "Across the spectrum of threats to the public health—from infectious diseases to chronic disorders—are inherent tensions between the good of the collective and the individual. To acknowledge this tension is not to foreordain the answer to the question 'How far should the state go?'; rather, it is to insist that we are fully cognizant of difficult trade-offs when we make policy determinations."[5 (p. 1102)]

Understanding different aspects of public health's role—protection, prevention, and promotion—can provide a general starting point for addressing some of the philosophical tensions that arise when translating science into practice and offering justifications for public health interventions (**Figure 4.1**). Public health efforts that aim to protect the public against infectious disease outbreaks, for example, are generally well accepted by the public, eliciting less political controversy or ethical tension, in particular because of the increased risk of direct physical harm to others in the population. Factors that can further support government actions are the severity, probability, and imminence of the risk or harms to the health and safety of others. Protective strategies to prevent injuries, such as child safety features in consumer products and requirements for airbags in motor vehicles, as

FIGURE 4.1 Public Health Role

Public health role	Protection	Prevention	Promotion
Mandate for government action	Higher	→	Lower
Tension among public values, particularly for liberty-limiting interventions	Lower	→	Higher
Intervention focus	Infectious disease Injury Chronic disease Healthy communities		

well as environmental health interventions such as removal of lead from paints and gasoline, also are widely accepted as within government's appropriate mandate because they are understood by the public as ways to reduce social costs, are cost effective, and achieve public goals that individuals acting alone could not.

Public health activities aimed at addressing chronic disease conditions and creating healthy living conditions, however, often elicit greater controversy because these efforts seek behavioral, social, and economic changes that some in the public believe inappropriately or unnecessarily curtail liberty and/or property interests or impose excessive costs on businesses. Health promotion efforts aimed at creating healthy communities, for example, through changes to land use design or zoning to increase physical activity, are considered by some to be primarily social and political decisions and not within public health's realm of responsibilities. For initiatives aimed at promoting health and creating healthy communities, therefore, government public health often must undertake public engagement and public communication, using rhetorical strategies that imaginatively emphasize our *individual* and *collective* interests in ensuring social and environmental conditions conducive to health. Unlike with communicable disease outbreaks for which there is an identifiable agent to eliminate or contain, typically evoking military metaphors, activities aimed at promoting healthy communities often evoke metaphors about caring and stewardship, which can seem less urgent and compelling to the public in our liberal democracy.

Another challenge in launching health promotion activities in particular can be the insufficiency of data. The evidence about the causes and threat to the "public's" health of chronic diseases, for example, is often complex, given the multiple, indirect, and long-term factors, sometimes called pathways, that contribute to the development of chronic disease morbidity and mortality. In addition it is difficult to set composite measures that document community health outcomes. For example, there "is no coordinated, standard set of true measures of a community's health—not aggregated information about the health of individuals residing in a community, but rather measures of green space, availability of healthy foods, land use and zoning practices that are supportive of health, safety, social capital, and social cohesion."[6]

Evidence-Based and Value-Based Approaches

One approach to garner support for chronic disease prevention and to promote healthy communities is to set particular goals, based on data about the population health burdens and evidence demonstrating the benefits of specific interventions. For example, the Centers for Disease Control and Prevention (CDC) identified goals by focusing on Winnable Battles, which "are public health priorities with large-scale impact on health and with known, effective strategies to address them."[7] Current Winnable Battles, such as nutrition, physical activity and obesity, and tobacco have been chosen because of the magnitude of their impact on population health, because there are evidence-based interventions that exist to address them, and because intensive focus could have an impact in a short time period.

Another complementary strategy in public health is to build public understanding and consensus in the gap (see **Figure 4.2.**), as persuasive data emerges demonstrating the public health impact of a behavior or condition, in order to galvanize the necessary support for effective community interventions. A successful example was the use of federal funding as leverage to induce states to raise the minimum purchase age for alcohol when it was shown that lowering the "drinking age" was associated with substantial increases in alcohol-related auto crashes among teen drivers. However, public health often must compete with other public values and moral claims of different stakeholders in the political forum, when offering ethical justification for health goals and priorities.

Oliver points out that politics plays a significant role in agenda setting in public health. Political factors include not only documentation about the severity of a health problem, but also the public's understanding about who bears responsibility for the health problem, as well as the public's perceptions about the population affected. Oliver states; "When public health problems are stratified by income, age, race, gender, geographic location, or other markers, one group's problems may not be treated the same as another's. Instead, the popularity of affected individuals, occupational or social groups, or industry will influence the likelihood and nature of governmental action."[8 (p. 200)]

Public narratives about the causes of health-related problems and about the affected populations often include fundamental questions of fairness and personal autonomy that should be discussed and resolved in the political forum. For example, Oliver suggests that "if a significant proportion of individuals with solid jobs and incomes are perceived to be uninsured by choice, or overweight individuals are perceived to reject healthier diets and opportunities for exercise that they know are in their best interest, the conflicting public images diminish pressure for governmental solutions to these problems, however serious they are."[8 (p. 200)] Thus examining the moral perspectives of different stakeholders and the

FIGURE 4.2 Moral Considerations in Expediting Knowledge to Action

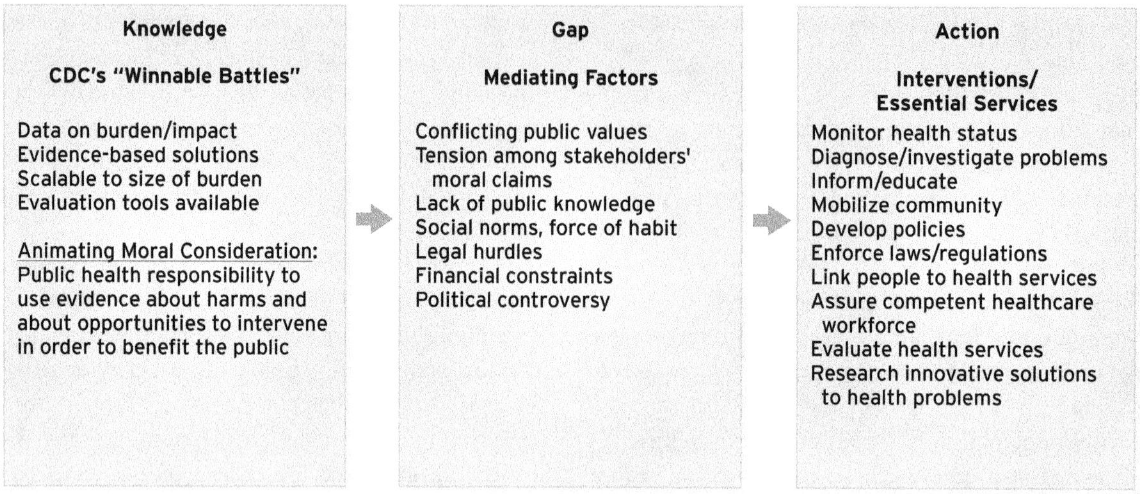

Knowledge	Gap	Action
CDC's "Winnable Battles"	**Mediating Factors**	**Interventions/ Essential Services**
Data on burden/impact Evidence-based solutions Scalable to size of burden Evaluation tools available Animating Moral Consideration: Public health responsibility to use evidence about harms and about opportunities to intervene in order to benefit the public	Conflicting public values Tension among stakeholders' moral claims Lack of public knowledge Social norms, force of habit Legal hurdles Financial constraints Political controversy	Monitor health status Diagnose/investigate problems Inform/educate Mobilize community Develop policies Enforce laws/regulations Link people to health services Assure competent healthcare workforce Evaluate health services Research innovative solutions to health problems

Modified from: the Centers for Disease Control and Prevention "The Public Health System and the 10 Essential Public Health Services": http://www.cdc.gov/nphpsp/essentialservices.html

culture and history of particular communities, including the public narratives and metaphors at play, provides important information for public health leaders and community partners when they deliberate about the ethical dimensions of various options.

We propose that the starting point of our ethical analyses, then, is to identify the gravity of the public health problems or needs (e.g., what are the harms to be prevented or mitigated), and to clarify the public health goal/s (what is the good to be produced), before considering the means or strategies to achieve them. Since public health goals often require long-term, sustained commitments, setting goals involves making difficult trade-offs, based on the data available, and attending to the particular cultural and social perspectives of the community. For example, setting a goal to reduce HIV transmission by providing clean needles to drug users or to reduce teenage pregnancy by providing condoms in high schools involves assessing evidence about the social, cultural, and political context of a particular community.

Public health decision making in the public forum, then, must be evidence-based and value-based. It is properly characterized as both *science* and *art* in that it involves using information from many sources, professional experience, and a wide variety of stakeholder perspectives, as well as knowledge about "which information is important to a particular stakeholder at the right time."[9] Evidence-based public health engages the community in the assessment of the problem and creation of goals. Brownson et al explain that, in contrast to a math problem, "significant decisions in public health must balance science and art because rational, evidence-based decision making often involves choosing one alternative from among a set of rational choices."[9]

At the national level, the Healthy People initiative provides an example of a goal-setting process. First launched in 1979, it sets specific, quantified targets every 10 years to guide prevention efforts across the country. (See **Table 4.1** to view overarching goals.)

TABLE 4.1 *Healthy People 2020* Overarching Goals

Attain high-quality, longer lives free of preventable disease, disability, injury, and premature death.
Achieve health equity, eliminate disparities, and improve the health of all groups.
Create social and physical environments that promote good health for all.
Promote quality of life, healthy development, and healthy behaviors across all life stages.

Reproduced from the U.S. Department of Health and Human Services. Healthypeople.gov

To set goals and more specific objectives for each goal, the Healthy People initiative engages in an ever-widening stakeholder process that includes government and non-government agencies at the national, state, and local levels, as well as professional, academic, and community stakeholders. *Healthy People 2020* contains 42 topic areas with nearly 600 objectives and 1,200 measures, as well as 12 leading health indicators that are used for national tracking and assessing progress at national, state, and community levels (**Table 4.2**).[10]

From the start of the *Healthy People* initiative, the science and data available to guide decision makers about the choice of potential goals, objectives, and interventions for many health problems were limited. Thus, "(s)etting priorities for a manageable and credible set of objectives required considerable professional and scientific judgment. … These judgments, in turn, required some weighing of ethical, equity, and political considerations," according to Green and Fielding.[11]

Another national initiative, the National Prevention Strategy, created a road map with the goal of increasing "the number of Americans who are healthy at every state of life" by engaging the leaders of 17 federal agencies in the National Prevention Council.[12] The federal agencies included the departments of Agricultures, Education, Transportation, Labor, Homeland Security, Interior, Defense, Housing and Urban Development, and Justice. In announcing the comprehensive prevention plan in 2011, Department of Health and Human Services (HHS) Secretary Kathleen Sebelius noted that the National Prevention Strategy, "which was called for under the Affordable Care Act, will helps us transform our healthcare system away from a focus on sickness and disease to a focus on prevention and wellness."[13] The Strategy calls for actions by public and private partners on its seven priorities: tobacco free living, preventing drug abuse and excessive alcohol use, healthy eating, active living, injury and violence free living, reproductive and sexual health, and mental and emotional well-being. Its four strategic directions include Clinical and Community Preventive Services, which emphasizes the need for the integration of prevention-focused medical care and community efforts, as well as Empowered People, Elimination of Health Disparities, and Healthy & Safe Community Environments (see **Figure 4.3**). At the national level, then, setting health goals includes the assessment of the available data and the perspectives of political and professional leaders and community stakeholders.

TABLE 4.2 *Healthy People 2020*

Leading Health Indicators	Examples
Access to Health Services	Persons with medical insurance
Clinical Preventive Services	Adults with hypertension whose blood pressure is under control
Environmental Quality	Air Quality Index exceeding 100
Injury and Violence	Homicides
Maternal, Infant, and Child Health	Infant deaths
Mental Health	Suicides
Nutrition, Physical Activity, and Obesity	Adults who are obese
Oral Health	Persons aged 2 years and older who used the oral healthcare system in past 12 months
Reproductive and Sexual Health	Persons living with HIV who know their serostatus
Social Determinants	Students who graduate with a regular diploma 4 years after starting 9th grade
Substance Abuse	Adults engaging in binge drinking during the past 30 days
Tobacco	Adults who are current cigarette smokers

Reproduced from the U.S. Department of Health and Human Services. Healthypeople.gov

Setting Goals in State and Local Public Health

Public health agencies at every level of government are confronted with similar challenges of setting goals and choosing among strategies when data and resources are limited. How should public health agencies make these decisions in state and local public health practice? We will explore this question, as well as provide a snapshot of the wide variety of public health interventions undertaken in communities today, through the scenario that follows.

Case Study: Addressing Heart Disease

A state's health department receives a five-year $50 million grant from a private foundation to launch a new cardiovascular disease (CVD) health initiative to address the high rate of CVD in the state. The health department has solicited and received 11 proposals (listed below) for new programs from

FIGURE 4.3 National Prevention Strategy

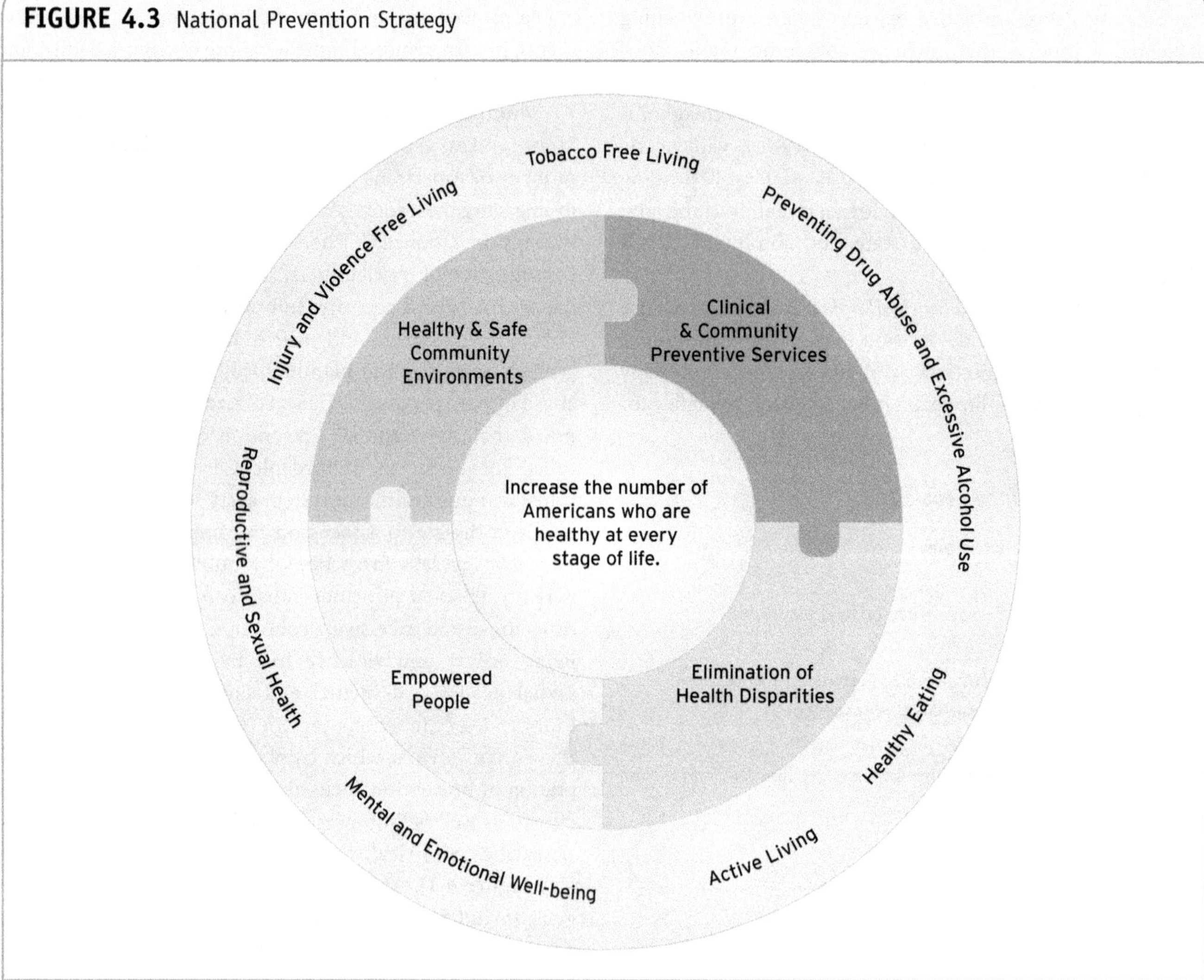

Modified from: National Prevention Council, National Prevention Strategy, Washington, DC: U.S. Department of Health and Human Services, Office of the Surgeon General, 2011. http://www.surgeongeneral.gov/initiatives/prevention/strategy/report.pdf

local health districts around the state and from state agencies. The health department convened an advisory committee of three physicians and three nurses recommended by the state professional societies to assess and prioritize the proposals, drawing on the information provided below about CVD from local and national sources.

Background

Heart disease is the leading cause of death in the state, accounting for approximately 40% of deaths in the previous year. The state ranks in the top five states in the country for stroke deaths. Strokes also are the leading cause of serious, long-term disability in the state. In the previous year, the state had more than 200,000 hospitalizations attributed to heart disease and stroke, with total direct and indirect costs for CVD estimated at $2.5 billion. According to the Behavioral Risk Factor Surveillance System (BRFSS), survey results show that adults in the state have the following risk factors for heart disease and stroke: 24% had high blood pressure; 30% had high blood cholesterol; 14.5% had diabetes; 19.5% were current smokers; and 53% were overweight or obese. Approximately 77% had one or more of these five risk factors.

Two groups in particular have been identified for potential targeted interventions: African American and rural indigent. Thirty percent of state residents are African American, and they carry a disproportionate burden of cardiovascular-related deaths and hospitalizations. African Americans in the state have a stroke rate that is 50% higher than the national average and have a shorter life expectancy than other state residents. Being overweight contributes to 32% of heart disease deaths annually, and 70% of African Americans in the state are overweight or obese. The prevalence of other risk factors among African Americans in the state are: current smokers, 27%; sedentary lifestyle, 62%; high blood pressure, 36%; diabetes, 13%; and high cholesterol, 38%. The rural poor in the state have limited access to medical services. More than half of the rural counties are classified as medically underserved. African Americans are more likely to live in the state's rural areas. One rural, predominantly African-American region in particular has the highest poverty levels and highest CVD rates and is known as the "stroke belt" region of the state.

Previous state CVD funding for local and state data collection and planning has identified the need for health education, community-level interventions, and medical care throughout the state, and highlighted the interplay of environmental and economic conditions that are correlated with CVD in the state. Focus groups of different community stakeholders have identified the following barriers that prevent individuals from adopting or changing behaviors to reduce their CVD risk: few community programs provide education, facilities, and screening to identify CVD risk factors; worksites do not support healthy behaviors; and grocery stores and restaurants in many communities do not offer healthy choices.

The Community Guide Recommendations for CVD[14]

Three recommendations for CVD interventions are supported by evidence, according to the national Community Preventive Services Task Force, which is administered and supported by the Centers for Disease Control and Prevention. The recommendations, provided in The Community Guide, are based on previous research that has been compiled in systematic reviews to learn what works to promote public health on a particular topic, such as CVD. The Community Preventive Services Task Force uses the results of systematic reviews to issue evidence-based recommendations and findings to the public health community. In contrast to research findings from a single study, a systematic review, involves a formal process to identify all relevant research studies on a topic, assess their quality, and summarize the evidence. The following are the only three evidence-based recommendations on CVD:

- *Clinical decision-support systems (CDSS)*: computer-based information systems designed to assist healthcare providers in implementing clinical guidelines at the point of care. CDSS use patient data to provide tailored patient assessments and evidence-based treatment recommendations for healthcare providers to consider. Patient information is entered manually or automatically through an electronic health record (EHR) system. CDSS for cardiovascular disease prevention (CVD) include such interventions as: reminders for overdue CVD preventive services including screening risk factors such as high blood pressure, diabetes, and high cholesterol; recommendations for health behavior changes to discuss with patients such as quitting smoking, increasing physical activity, and reducing excessive salt intake; and alerts when indicators for CVD risk factors are not at goal.
- *Reducing out-of-pocket costs for cardiovascular disease preventive services for patients with high blood pressure and high cholesterol*: program and policy changes that make cardiovascular disease preventive services more affordable. These services include medications, behavioral counseling (e.g., nutrition counseling) and behavioral support (e.g., community-based weight management programs, gym membership). ROPC is coordinated through the healthcare system and preventive services may be delivered in clinical or nonclinical settings (e.g., worksite, community).
- *Team-based care to improve blood pressure control*: a health systems-level organizational intervention that incorporates a multidisciplinary team to improve the quality of hypertension care for patients. Each team includes the patient, the patient's primary care provider, and other professionals such as nurses, pharmacists, dietitians, social workers, and community health workers. Team members provide process support and share responsibilities of hypertension care to complement the activities of the primary care provider. These responsibilities include medication management; patient follow-up; and adherence and self-management support. Team-based care interventions typically include activities to facilitate communication and coordination of care support among various team members and actively engage patients by providing them with education about hypertension medication, adherence support (for medication and other treatments), and tools and resources for self-management (including health behavior change).

The *Healthy People 2020* goal as it relates to heart disease and stroke is to "improve cardiovascular health and quality of life through prevention, detection, and treatment of risk factors for heart attack and stroke; early identification and treatment of heart attacks and strokes; and prevention of repeat cardiovascular events."[15] The report lists the leading modifiable (controllable) risk factors for heart disease and stroke as high blood pressure, high cholesterol, cigarette smoking, diabetes, poor diet and physical inactivity, overweight and obesity. The *Healthy People 2020* report points out that cardiovascular health is significantly influenced by the physical, social, and political environment, including maternal and child health; access to educational opportunities; availability of healthy foods, physical education, and extracurricular activities in schools; opportunities for physical activity, including access to safe and walkable communities; access to healthy foods; quality of working conditions and worksite health; availability of community support and resources, and access to affordable, quality health care.

In addition, *Healthy People 2020* reports the following challenges: "No national system exists to collect data on how often cardiovascular events occur or recur, or how often they result in death. Similarly, there is inadequate tracking of quality indicators across the continuum of care, from risk factor prevention through treatment of acute events to post-hospitalization and rehabilitation. New measures and tools are needed to monitor improvement in cardiovascular health over the next decade."[15]

Proposals for Advisory Committee Review

The 11 proposals submitted to the state are roughly equal in cost ($2 million for each of 5 years), and thus only five of the following proposals can be funded. Before assessing and ranking the proposals and providing justification for its choices, the advisory committee has been asked to address some preliminary questions: What are the appropriate public health goals in this context? What criteria should the committee use to evaluate the proposals? For example, number of people reached through the intervention? Number of people in high-risk categories reached? Evidence of program effectiveness in producing a particular outcome, e.g., lowered blood pressure rates, for a particular population, in the short-term or of cost-effectiveness in achieving a goal over a sustained time-period? Should the level of community participation or engagement in the proposed intervention be a criterion for ranking? And if so, how would "community" be defined? Should others be invited to join the advisory committee, and if so, who? The Advisory Committee also is invited to make recommendations to the state health department about goals or interventions not included in the proposals listed below.

1. **Statewide social marketing campaign** in the media and in partnership with schools and youth and adult organizations to provide messages about a "heart-healthy" diet. One major focus is a low-fat milk campaign throughout the state involving media, taste tests, and school contests. Another is a campaign to limit intake of sugared beverages to address obesity.
2. **Stroke awareness and preparedness program** that promotes public and professional awareness of the warning signs of stroke, of the importance of treating and controlling high blood pressure to prevent stroke, and of the importance of calling for emergency transport to a hospital upon experiencing symptoms. Program includes training 1,200 emergency medical services technicians and paramedics throughout the state on stroke, as well as providing more emergency services to underserved geographical areas.
3. **Community centers and blood pressure control program** that offers training for health practitioners and peer counselors at community centers throughout the state. This training focuses on developing programs to monitor community members' blood pressure and providing ongoing educational and counseling programs on healthy lifestyles through peer counselor outreach and home visits.
4. **Teacher workshops** for middle school and high school teachers throughout the state that focus on programmatic and curricular development about helping students avoid behaviors that put them at risk for heart disease and stroke later in their lives. Workshops include training on how to help students become "empowered" health decision makers.
5. **Screening program for "stroke belt" residents** that provides screening (every week) for high cholesterol and high blood pressure at grocery stores in the stroke belt region and grocery stores in other neighborhoods with residents at "high risk." The program also will include a nutrition education program that focuses on changing the "cultural" propensity in the communities to consume certain foods that are particularly unhealthy.
6. **Physical activity intervention** to provide community venues for physical activity and health promotion by renovating three community health centers in the rural "stroke belt" counties. Safe playgrounds, basketball courts, and track with dusk-to-dawn lighting will be made available in a central location in each county, as well as nutrition education classes and fitness programs that include aerobics training and certification for community members.

7. **Community wellness program** that develops a network of African-American women in community churches throughout the "stroke belt" counties. The program seeks to improve individual and community health by developing a social support network and building social capital in the community. Church members will be trained and paid to organize and work in a "health ministry" that partners with local churches, leaders, businesses, community groups, and families to focus the community on a heart healthy lifestyle. Emphasis will be put on educational and awareness campaigns that can facilitate community action on social and environmental changes, such as healthy neighborhood land development, enforcement of youth tobacco restrictions, and meetings with business such as grocery stores about heart healthy business practices.
8. **Statewide worksite wellness program** that hires worksite wellness coordinators in different regions throughout the state to work with businesses in the region on worksite wellness programs that focus on CVD. Initial projects would include providing preventive health screening programs at worksites and working with companies to develop physical fitness incentives, tobacco reduction programs for employees, etc.
9. **Medical treatment for the least-served communities**, a program in which the three least-served communities in the stroke belt region would be visited weekly by a "traveling" medical clinic that primarily provides screening and treatment for CVD. Efforts would include setting up an initial appointment for patients with primary care physicians in the area who agreed to take referrals from the traveling clinic.
10. **Community gardens for the stroke belt region**, including development of community sites throughout the region where community members contribute time and work together, along with funded staff, to plant, grow, and prepare healthy food for themselves and for local consumption. The program includes nutrition education and cooking lessons.
11. **Campaigns to raise awareness** of unhealthy food, particularly fast food, and to advocate and build grass-root support for zoning laws that prohibit fast-food outlets in geographical zip codes with higher CVD burdens.

The next sections provide a brief introduction to some public health perspectives that can provide background for assessing and deliberating about goals and justifications for choosing among the various public health strategies. We will invite readers to consider the questions raised in the scenario again at the end of the chapter, drawing on the ideas raised in the next sections.

POPULATION PREVENTION

At the core of public health is a focus on population health and prevention, which is a broader and different scope than the healthcare delivery system's primary emphasis on clinical interventions for individuals and, in particular, for those already sick or identified as high risk. The primary science of public health is epidemiology, which focuses on the distribution, causes, and determinants of health and disease in populations. It is a problem-solving method "to get to the root of health problems in a community, whether the problem is a measles outbreak on a small college campus or a global influenza pandemic, an increase in homicide in a single community, a national surge in violence, or a localized or widespread rise in cancer."[16] Numerous measures are used in public health to assess population health and to set goals (**Table 4.3**), and the choice of measures and goals has ethical implications.

Identifying whether the goal of an intervention is a population health goal, in contrast to a clinical one, for example, can have an impact on an ethical analysis. Verweij and Dawson illustrate with the example of a hepatitis B vaccination initiative for high-risk groups in the Netherlands. The ethical question was whether "it was necessary to offer all participants post-vaccination blood tests, in order to see if they showed a sufficient immune response to the vaccine."[17] The rationale was that if participants had a low immune response, they then could be offered extra vaccinations. If the goal of the initiative was a preventive medical goal to provide protection to particular high-risk individuals, then it could be argued that it was more ethically justified to offer the post-vaccine tests if there was evidence that not all of those vaccinated acquired immunity. However, if the goal of the immunization program was to reduce the transmission of hepatitis B in a population, then there would not be as strong a justification to do follow-up testing, since a few individuals with insufficient immunity would not have a major population impact.

A population perspective recognizes that individual medical care is only one of numerous determinants of health, and that others, such as behavioral, social, and environmental factors, are significant determinants of health and present great opportunities to focus preventive measures across communities and populations to achieve health gains. Rose's seminal 1985 article, "Sick Individuals and Sick Populations," points out the difference in etiology, for example, between why some *individuals* have hypertension and why some

TABLE 4.3 *Healthy People 2020* Measures of General Health

• *Life expectancy (with international comparison)*: summary mortality measure defined as the average number of years a population of a certain age would be expected to live. *Healthy People 2020* monitors life expectancy at birth and at age 65.
• *Healthy life expectancy*: average number of healthy years a person can expect to live, allowing for easy comparisons across populations and over long periods of time. *Healthy People 2020* tracks expected years of life in good or better health; of life free of limitation of activity, of life free of selected chronic disease.
• *Years of potential life lost (YPLL) (with international comparison)*: summary measure of premature mortality (early death), i.e., the total number of years not lived by people who die before reaching a given age, e.g., in the United States, the age limit is often placed at 75.
• *Physically and mentally unhealthy days*: a measure of the number of days that individuals rated their physical or mental health as not good in the previous 30 days.
• *Self-assessed health status*: a measure of how an individual perceives his or her health—rating it as excellent, very good, good, fair, or poor.
• *Limitation of activity*: a measure of the long-term reduction in a person's ability to do his or her usual activities. Since 1997, in the National Health Interview Survey, limitation of activity has been assessed by asking people about such limitations as: activities of daily living (such as bathing/showering, dressing, eating, getting in and out of bed, walking, using the toilet) and instrumental activities of daily living (such as using the telephone, doing light housework, doing heavy housework, preparing meals, shopping for personal items, managing money).
• *Chronic disease prevalence*: the proportion of a population with chronic diseases, which cause 7 out of 10 deaths in U.S. each year. Heart disease, cancer, and stroke alone cause more than 50% of all deaths each year. In 2008, 107 million Americans—almost 1 out of every 2 adults age 18 or older—had at least 1 of 6 reported chronic illnesses: Cardiovascular disease, arthritis, diabetes, asthma, cancer, and chronic obstructive pulmonary disease (COPD).

Data from the U.S. Department of Health and Human Services. 10-Year Agenda, retrieved 5/11/13 http://www.healthypeople.gov/2020/about/GenHealthAbout.aspx

populations have more hypertension than others, and on that basis he distinguishes two types of prevention.[18]

The first is the "high-risk" strategy used in medicine to target individuals for interventions that reduce their risk. An example would be identifying and treating patients with elevated blood pressure who are at risk for stroke because of elevated blood pressure and who can be treated. While Rose points out some advantages of this approach, such as subject and physician motivation, he describes a number of disadvantages including the limitations of screening, e.g., it is often used more frequently by those with the least risk of disease, it can identify "borderline" individuals for whom there is no appropriate treatment to reduce risk, and does not change the underlying causes of disease.[18]

In contrast, the population strategy advocated by Rose attempts to change the risk of disease in the entire population, for example, through environmental interventions such as policies to reduce salt intake or through changing society's behavioral and social norms regarding exercise. Rose calls such an approach to prevention "radical" since its goals are "to remove the underlying causes that make the disease common" in a population and to shift the entire distribution of risk in a population to lower levels. As examples, he points out that changing the social norms in a population from smoking to "nonsmoking" and from unhealthy to healthy diets could eliminate the need for targeted education to change individual behavior. "Much more powerful as motivators for health education are the social rewards of enhanced self-esteem and social approval," he states.[18]

Rose's perspective also suggests that an individual's risk is related to the population in which he or she lives, although individuals often are unaware of an association. Rose acknowledges that the population strategy for prevention has drawbacks, however, citing the Prevention Paradox, which means population prevention measures often bring little benefit, particularly little immediate benefit, to any one individual. Thus, population strategies such as required immunization policies often elicit resistance and challenge by those who raise moral arguments based on respecting autonomous choices. Population strategies also encounter motivation problems with physicians since "(g)rateful patients are few in preventive medicine, where success is marked by a nonevent."[18]

Implications of Population-Wide Approaches

While shifting the entire distribution of risk in a population to lower levels through population-wide strategies may lead to the greatest gains in population health, this approach might also obscure the disparities that continue to exist in the distribution of risk among subgroups in the population after implementing population-wide preventive measures. Considerations of justice may argue for targeting smaller subpopulations or individuals who are most at risk, particularly if they have much greater risk and need than those with health measures at the population mean. Zulman et al also suggest that since new multivariable prediction tools have made it easier to identify high-risk individuals in recent years, the optimal prevention policy will often use both high-risk and population-wide strategies. In comparing preventive approaches, they highlight the impact of costs and limited resources as considerations for policymakers. "For example," they point out, "an affordable population-based intervention that offers short-term improvements in quality of life (such as a diet or exercise program that makes people feel better within a short time) will theoretically almost always be preferable to a targeted approach."[19] On the other hand, they note that cheap population strategies that result in just a small health impact across the population would be less justifiable than a targeted intervention for high-risk individuals that had great impact for the few.

Rose also sketches a general principle for allocating the burden of proof regarding the utility of an intervention when a decision is being made about whether to implement it across the population: Whenever we know that an existing "exposure" in the population is "causing" a health problem, he argues, we can generally presume that steps taken to reduce that exposure are "safe," whereas steps taken to counteract the effects of exposure with a new product or activity (such as a vaccine) should be proven to be safe before being implemented. He justifies this principle with appeals to avoiding harm and utility: "In mass prevention, each individual has usually only a small expectation of benefit, and this small benefit can easily be outweighed by a small risk."[18] Rose cites the example of a WHO trial of a cholesterol-lowering drug that "seems to have killed more than it saved, even though the fatal complication rate was only about 1/1000/year."[18] Rose contrasts two approaches to population prevention: (1) restoring a normal baseline in the population by removing an abnormal exposure, such as air pollution or tobacco use and (2) introducing a new protective intervention, such as drugs or jogging, that does not change the underlying exposure (which should be proven safe before implementation).[18]

Rose's analysis offers considerable insight and calls attention to the need to take precautions before using an intervention that carries its own uncertain risks. However, the distinction between reducing and counteracting the unhealthy or hazardous exposure is not as clean as he suggests. On the one hand, removing a hazardous product or condition may not produce a net gain in population health. Making the environment appear to be safer alters risk perceptions and may lead people to underestimate the risks of possible substitutes or to adapt their behavior in a way that erodes or offsets the predicted benefits of the intervention. Reducing exposure to "high-tar" cigarettes led to increased use of "low tar" alternatives that probably resulted in a net increase in population harm due to reduced quitting by smokers who incorrectly perceived the "low tar" cigarettes as safer.

On the other hand, proving the safety of population-based countermeasure in advance is a challenge since, as noted by Zulman et al, even educational campaigns are "rarely without some disutility, be it in the form of lost time or the intrusiveness or cost of lifestyle change. Even resentment of public health officials may sometimes need to be considered."[19] Based on their research, they caution that population strategies can potentially lead to many people experiencing small disutility (that adds up to much population disutility), while few in the population receive the benefits. Thus, difficult trade-offs must be weighed; they conclude: "... population-based prevention strategies may be appropriate when the risk for a disease is widely dispersed in the population and the proposed intervention is very safe and cheap. Furthermore, the appeal of a population-based approach increases when it is more costly and difficult to identify and intervene on high-risk individuals."[19]

Determinants and Pathways

Over the last 50 years, research has documented the interconnectedness of many biological, behavioral, and social-environmental factors that contribute to human health, and public health has developed models to showcase different approaches to prevention, given the evidence about these complex factors (**Table 4.4**).

The Institute of Medicine's (IOM) 2002 report, *The Future of the Public's Health*,[20] notes that public health has long had an ecological approach with the agent-host-environment triad as a model, which illustrated that health often was the result of complex interactions among all three factors. New models developed in the last decades, however, specify more determinants of health, as described in the IOM report: "Most models of health determinants identify macro-level conditions and policies (social, economic, cultural, and environmental) as potent forces in shaping mid-level (working conditions, housing) and proximate (behavioral, biological) determinants of health. Macro-level or upstream determinants (such as policies and societal norms) and micro-level determinants (such as sex or the virulence of a disease agent) interact along complex and dynamic pathways

TABLE 4.4 Determinants of Health and Examples

Social determinants: Gender, socioeconomic status, employment status, educational attainment, food security status, availability of housing and transportation, racism, and health system access and quality
Behavioral determinants: Patterns of overweight/obesity and exercise; use of illicit drugs, tobacco, or alcohol
Environmental determinants: Lead exposure, asthma triggers, workplace safety factors, unsafe or polluted living conditions
Biological and genetic determinants: Family history of heart disease and inherited conditions such as hemophilia or cystic fibrosis

Data from: National Partnership for Action to End Health Disparities. *National Stakeholder Strategy for Achieving Health Equity*. Rockville, MD: U.S. Department of Health & Human Services, Office of Minority Health. 2011 retrieved 5/11/13 from http://www.minorityhealth.hhs.gov/npa/files/Plans/NSS/NSSExecSum.pdf

to produce health at a population level."[20] Implicit in these models also is the understanding that the determinants of both individual and population health are always interacting and changing over time, so that public health approaches also must continually adapt. Citing the obesity epidemic as an example, Teutsch and Fielding emphasize that the "complexity of many contemporary health problems requires multiple avenues of attack."[21]

One avenue or approach is public health's focus on changing behavioral and lifestyle factors that contribute to poor health. As early as 1990, McGinnis and Foege showed that more than 50% of deaths were the result of behaviors such as tobacco use, alcohol consumption, and poor diets.[22] Further analyses by Mokdad et al a few years later highlighted the difference between the immediate causes of death most often listed on death certificates from 1990 to 2000 (heart disease, cancer, and stroke) and what they suggest are the actual or underlying causes of death.[23] In the United States in 2000, according to Mokdad et al, the most common actual causes of death were tobacco (435,000), poor diet and physical inactivity (400,000), alcohol consumption (85,000), microbial agents (e.g., influenza and pneumonia, 75,000), toxic agents (e.g., pollutants and asbestos, 55,000), motor vehicle accidents (43,000), firearms (29,000), sexual behavior (20,000), and illicit use of drugs (17,000).[23]

For some, a focus on the actual causes as represented by Mokdad et al raises ethical concerns about the appropriate reach of public health behavioral interventions. Such interventions often extend the meaning of concepts such as "epidemic" from infectious outbreaks to widespread conditions such as obesity. This is done to justify public health action by labeling individual behavior itself as a public health problem requiring societal attention. Given the moral considerations of respecting autonomous choices of individuals and our public values that favor the protection of individual preferences, some might ask, Why is public health implicated by the poor diets and sedentary lifestyles of individuals? Is public intervention justified by data documenting the effect of individual behaviors on overall population health measures, or the cost to society of treating diseases that are eventually caused by these behaviors? Might not the private purchase of insurance allow a person to internalize these costs, so that individuals essentially can bring their behavior back into a "private" sphere? Others raise concerns that encouraging and emphasizing behavioral and ecological approaches to population health could lead to a "tyranny of health" that becomes part of our secular morality. For example, Conrad claims that the "pursuit of wellness is inherently a moral pursuit, the achievement of a sense of virtue."[24] Fitzgerald raises concerns about the "dark side" of focusing on health lifestyles and cautions against developing a "a zealotry about health, in which we take ourselves too seriously and believe that we know enough to dictate human behavior, penalize people for disagreeing with us, and even deny people charity, empathy, and understanding because they act in a way of which we disapprove."[25] Embracing a notion of health as the ability to cope with disease effectively, rather than obtaining complete freedom from disease, Fitzgerald suggests that the more society directs "individual behavior, the less autonomous, and therefore the less healthy, the individual may become."[25] Given these concerns, public health officials should be prepared when implementing behavioral or lifestyle interventions to provide data on the burden of disease, and specify and justify particular goals, in ways that acknowledge the impact, however minor, on autonomous individual choices.

Ecological Approaches and Health Inequalities

While public health has long recognized the impact of the environment on human health, early interventions focused most often on the physical environment. Addressing ecological-level influences, public health is now expanding its focus to many aspects of the environment, including the social, economic, natural, and built environment, as well as to the important role of social determinants of health, such as socioeconomic status, racial and ethnic disparities, social networks and support, and work conditions (**Table 4.5**).

TABLE 4.5 *Healthy People 2020:* A "Place-Based" Framework for Social Determinants

Economic Stability	• Poverty • Employment Status • Access to Employment • Housing Stability (e.g., homelessness, foreclosure)
Education	• High School Graduation Rates • School Policies that Support Health Promotion • School Environments that are Safe and Conducive to Learning • Enrollment in Higher Education
Social and Community Context	• Family Structure • Social Cohesion • Perceptions of Discrimination and Equity • Civic Participation • Incarceration/ Institutionalization
Health and Health Care	• Access to Health Services—including clinical and preventive care • Access to Primary Care—including community-based health promotion and wellness programs • Health Technology
Neighborhood and Built Environment	• Quality of Housing • Crime and Violence • Environmental Conditions • Access to Healthy Foods

Reproduced from the U.S. Department of Health and Human Services. Healthypeople.gov

New research in the last 20 years demonstrates that "place matters" in complex ways. In 2001 researchers established, for example, that the risk of cardiovascular disease was impacted by the neighborhood of residence, even after controlling for such factors as income and education.[26] Strong epidemiological evidence documents the many and varied ways socioeconomic status (SES) impacts health, with heart disease providing a strong example of the association between SES and mortality.[20 (p. 58)]

Highlighting the uneven distribution of social determinants, Daniels emphasizes the impact on health of "the cumulative experience of social conditions across the life course. In other words, by the time a sixty-year-old patient presents to the emergency room with a heart attack to receive medical treatment, that encounter represents the result of bodily insults that accumulated over a lifetime."[27] He calls for intersectoral efforts to improve primary social conditions, such as education and workplace environments, as a way to improve health and reduce health inequalities. Others maintain that improvements in social conditions also are important considerations for respecting the autonomous choices and self-determination of individuals. Extensive research now shows how behavioral choices are influenced and constrained by the environment. Efforts to change behaviors to prevent obesity are prime examples, because of the cultural and social factors that shape eating, exercise, etc. Sufficient social resources to make choices "real" are required, because as Faden and Powers maintain, "... a self-determining life is not merely the ability to shape a life for oneself, but the ability to be self-directing under social conditions that make possible the realization of a sufficient level of well-being in all of its core dimensions."[28]

The central idea of the ecological, multi-level framework, according to the 2002 IOM report, is "that characteristics of places—neighborhoods, schools, work sites, and even nations—carry with them health risks for the individuals who live in those environments."[20] Since the health risk "conferred" by these places is beyond what the individuals carry themselves, this model suggests that aspects of places, such as economic inequality and social capital, have an impact on population health and health disparities. For example, noting that the IOM's report, *Unequal Treatment,*[29] reported that racial and ethnic health disparities existed in the population even after controlling for social and demographic factors, insurance status, and clinical need, Bleich et al. point out that the "remaining disparities were attributed to factors such as discrimination and the healthcare system and the regulatory climate in which it operates."[30] Although research has documented health disparities for more than 30 years and initiatives like *Healthy People 2020* (see **Table 4.1**) have made health equity a national goal, health disparities continue to exist, and in some cases are even widening. For example, "disparities among racial/ethnic populations increased for heart disease deaths (1999–2006), chronic obstructive pulmonary disease deaths (1990–1998), and chronic lower respiratory disease deaths (1999–2006)."[11]

Setting public health goals to reduce health inequalities, then, can be justified through appeals to both social justice and efficiency. (See **Exhibit 4.1** for relevant definitions related to disparities.)

EXHIBIT 4.1 Definitions Related to Health Disparities

Health equity: The attainment of the highest level of health for all people. Achieving health equity requires valuing everyone equally with focused and ongoing societal efforts to address avoidable inequalities, historical and contemporary injustices, and the elimination of health and healthcare disparities.

Health inequality: The difference in health status or in the distribution of health determinants between different population groups.

Health disparity: A particular type of *health difference* that is closely linked with social or economic disadvantage. Health disparities adversely affect groups of people who have systematically experienced greater social and/or economic obstacles to health and/or a clean environment based on their racial or ethnic group; religion; socioeconomic status; gender; age; mental health; cognitive, sensory, or physical disability; sexual orientation; geographic location; or other characteristics historically linked to discrimination or exclusion.

Courtesy of DHHS/Office of Minority Health.

Woolf et al maintain that since health differences exist for those with low incomes and some minority groups, targeting public health interventions on those populations and their living conditions are likely "to yield proportionately greater public health benefit."[31] Others justify targeted interventions based on the costs to society, which a 2009 study that included both direct costs (i.e., medical spending) and indirect costs (i.e., lower productivity and premature mortality) found to be $1.24 trillion between 2003 and 2006.[30]

Public health, then, aims in general to improve population health through preventive strategies and efforts to reduce health risk. Health risks, which vary among subpopulations, are related to complex upstream social and economic factors "that both surpass and powerfully interact with 'downstream' elements such as individual behaviors, biological traits, and access to healthcare services."[20 (p. 71)] More research is needed, however, about the mechanisms underlying behavioral and socioeconomic risk factors and about the contextual factors that affect the success of interventions in improving population health and health equity in particular communities.

EVIDENCE IN PUBLIC HEALTH PRACTICE

Public health draws on a wide variety of evidence for decision making, including quantitative data, program evaluation, and qualitative data, which are obtained in numerous ways such as through surveillance, clinical and laboratory reporting systems, large national surveys, observation, focus groups, and traditional research. Jacobs et al explain: "Public health evidence often derives from cross-sectional studies and quasi-experimental studies, rather than the so-called 'gold standard' of randomized controlled trials often used in clinical medicine. Study designs in public health sometimes lack a comparison group, and the interpretation of study results may have to account for multiple caveats. Public health interventions are seldom a single intervention and often involve large-scale environmental changes that address the needs and balance the preferences of large, often diverse, groups of people."[32]

A recent national study recommended transforming the current statistics and information system to greatly enhance coordination and integration of data collection and analysis across public and private sectors, based on its finding that "at all levels of American life—including local, state, and national—decision makers lack sufficient information to make important choices about the health of their communities." The study strongly endorsed an ecological health model for public health and noted the particular challenge of acquiring population data for assessing the upstream determinants of health, such as "defining socioeconomic environments and elucidating the complex and interrelated pathways between many determinants and health outcomes of interest." In addition, many upstream determinants are risk factors for and have wide-ranging effects on multiple diseases. Given the co-occurrence of many lifestyle-related chronic conditions, measurement and analyses is further complicated because, for example, "higher levels of educational attainment are strongly linked with better health outcomes, but there are multiple confounding influences, including neighborhood conditions, early life experiences, and race and ethnicity."[6 (p. 27)]

In practice, public health professionals use a number of methods to identify public health burdens and set goals, including surveillance, national surveys, collecting information through outbreak investigations, community needs assessments, all of which often include professional discretion and ethical dimensions. For example, the threshold of when to act on a health issue or decline to act can be set in a variety of ways, such as statistical, intuitive, or mandated (for example, by the acceptance of funding), and for all of these, ethical factors may arise, such as whether the confidentiality of affected parties or particular groups in the community can be adequately protected when action is taken. Even analyzing data, which involves setting a statistical threshold that signifies the existence of a problem (is the problem significant when $P < 0.05$? Or $P < 0.001$? Or perhaps $P < 0.10$?) and presenting data in written or oral reports both involve interpretation and framing risk factors and other demographic information that can stigmatize groups and affect the levels of trust in affected communities.

Economic evaluation is another type of evidence that can be used in public health, although its use in practice is often limited because of a lack of reliable data about the effectiveness of interventions and related population outcomes. Methods such as cost-effectiveness analysis provide ways to compare the relative costs and health gains for different interventions by using a common outcome measure, such as number of deaths or cases of disease prevented, or number of life-years or quality-adjusted life-years (QALY) saved. However, Grosse et al point out that "valuing different types of outcomes is an inherently subjective, value-laden process in which economic methods need to be combined with broad stakeholder input and deliberation."[33]

The use of cost-effectiveness results requires interpretation about the calculation of benefits and costs. For example, the decision about what threshold to use for a condition such as hypertension or diabetes can have a significant impact on measures of benefits, such as an increased life expectancy or quality of life associated with early diagnosis of a condition if the threshold for a disease is lowered.[34] What gets counted as a cost, for instance, often includes only those items that are relatively easy to measure. Grosse et al cite the example of a cost-effectiveness analysis for kidney dialysis, which excluded from the assessment of cost the unpaid time for caregivers during home dialysis, thus making home dialysis look more cost effective.[33]

In addition, comparing two interventions by using QALYs gained as the effectiveness measure can advantage interventions for younger and/or healthier people, who have longer life expectancies. "Some argue that shifting from valuing whole lives to any form of life-years unfairly discriminates against older people, who may value the remainder of their lives as highly as do younger people. Similar arguments can be put forward for people with life expectancies shortened by their socioeconomic status or preexisting health conditions or disabilities."[35 (p. 135)]

Since cost-effectiveness analysis is used most often to assess different medical treatments, and the costs depend on medication expenditures, in some studies prevention has been shown to actually increase spending. For hypertension, as an example, an analysis has shown that "the accumulated costs of treating hypertension are nonetheless greater than the savings, because many people, not all of whom would ever suffer heart disease or stroke, must take medication for many years."[36 (p. 45)]

Of most importance in using cost-effectiveness assessments in public health decision making is understanding the context of the decision, however. In contrast to clinical studies where the values of particular groups of patients can be included in the assessment, in public health settings, "community values (i.e., the aggregated and averaged judgments of a representative sample of individuals in the general population) regarding the relative desirability of different states of health should be used."[26] Whose values count, however, and what is counted in the costs and outcomes are complex questions. For community-based prevention efforts, for example, cost-effectiveness analysis "does not include—and has not developed methodologies to measure—the effects of an intervention on community well-being or community process and does not usually take into consideration the differences among communities."[26 (p. 101)]

Given the moral claims and different perspectives of numerous stakeholders in each community, it could be argued that economic evaluation, such as cost-effectiveness studies, might be done from the perspective of each stakeholder group that is affected by a public health intervention, as well from a composite community perspective, to ensure deliberation can include a comparison not only of the cost-effectiveness of different interventions, but also a comparison of analyses as viewed by different stakeholder groups with different values and assessments of costs and benefits. (See Chapter 2 for a discussion of the ethical dimensions of measuring costs and benefits.)

Particularly for the analyses of community interventions, the question of "Whose values?" is key to assessing the evidence about the effectiveness of interventions. A recent IOM report emphasizes the importance of and differences among a community stakeholders: "A program may have a very different value depending on whether the perspective is that of the federal budget, of a specific employer, of specific segments of society or a particular community or of society in general. For example, the success of tobacco control is partly due to smoking restrictions in such places as workplaces, restaurants, and airplanes. To a nonsmoker with a generally positive view of regulation, such restrictions are valuable. To others, such as business owners who fear losing customers, such restrictions can be seen as harmful."[26 (p. 20)]

Another example cited in the report is the use of needle-exchange programs to accomplish a goal that all stakeholders in the community support, reducing the transmission of HIV. Stakeholder groups in communities, however, often value the trade-offs differently, with public health professionals valuing the benefits of needle-exchange program based on research data showing effectiveness in reducing HIV transmission, while others view the programs as facilitating or implicitly accepting illegal drug use in the community.[26]

Thus, for community-based prevention efforts, an IOM report calls for a new framework for assessing evidence about the value and benefits of interventions that includes three elements:

1. Benefits and harms should include not only impact on individual health, but also on community well-being and community process. Measuring the investment of individuals in their community's well-being, and their engagement in the process of making decisions about how to live and what their environment should be like provides legitimacy for health decisions—an added value that contributes to health outcomes.
2. Benefits and harms, based on the community's valuation, should be compared with the resources used.
3. Differences among communities should be specified, because "communities vary so much in their characteristics, the causal links between interventions and valued outcomes may be different for different communities."[26 (p. 113)]

HEALTHY COMMUNITIES: COLLABORATIONS, STAKEHOLDERS, AND SYSTEMS

The recent Institute of Medicine (IOM) report, *The Future of the Public Health in the 21st Century*,[20] emphasized that public health's broad mission is to ensure healthy communities, which requires the engagement of and interactions among many sectors in the community such as governmental public health, the healthcare delivery system, businesses, academia, and media to name just a few. IOM uses the term community "to mean any group of people who share geographic space, interests, goals or history. It includes the built environment, social networks, and the organizations and institutions that sustain the individual and collective life of the community."[26 (p. 15)]

Healthy communities or "healthful environments" have common characteristics that include other sectors of the community as well, such as strong school systems, good public safety, and neighborhoods with parks, all of which contribute to health and to the common good in different ways. Thus, some public health leaders call for public health to shift its emphasis from biomedical approaches to an intersectoral agenda and policies that harkens back to the social hygiene movement in the 19th century. "To achieve our national health objectives, the biomedical reductionist approach and continued rapid expansion of the biomedical industry need to give way to a new paradigm favoring interventions that have multiple, broad, beneficial impacts," state Teutsch and Fielding,[37] who use the example of childhood education to demonstrate the potential to improve both health and other quality of life measures at the same time. They conclude that the field of public health needs to move away from a model based on categorical funding of disease-specific interventions "to emphasize changes in the greatest determinants of health: our social and physical environments."[37a]

Public engagement and relationship-building, it might be argued, are the bedrock of public health practice. The IOM report highlights the importance of relationships built on common goals: "All partners who can contribute to action as a public health system should be encouraged to assess their roles and responsibilities, consider changes, and devise ways to better collaborate with other partners. They can transform the way they 'do business' to better act to achieve a healthy population on their own and position themselves to be part of an effective partnership in assuring the health of the population."[20]

Thus, attention to the ethical dimensions of day-to-day public health practice should be integrated into the health department's provision of essential services (see the list of Public Health Essential Services in **Figure 4.2**) which is presented earlier in the chapter. For example, state and local public health departments increasingly use metrics or standards, established by the Public Health Accreditation Board (PHAB), to demonstrate their services and outcomes to the community, and the Public Health Code of Ethics provides a complementary tool to create "ethically-sensitive" measures. **Table 4.6** presents a crosswalk between a public health essential service (mobilize community partners ...) that public health departments have responsibility to provide in column 1; the PHAB standard that delineates specific ways for public health departments to actually provide the service in column 2; relevant ethical principles drawn from the Public Health Code of Ethics that offers ethical perspectives in column 3; and questions to help set metrics in column 4 that integrate ethical considerations into day-to-day practice.

The crosswalk attempts to show ways to integrate ethical considerations into practice, by asking, what would constitute meaningful community engagement as informed by the

[a] Teutsch S, Fielding JE (2013) "Rediscovering the Core of Public Health," Frontiers in Public Health Services and Systems Research: Vol. 2: No. 3, Article 1.

TABLE 4.6 Using Ethical Principles to Highlight Metrics for Community Engagement

Essential Services	PHAB Standard	Ethical Principles	Metrics: Examples
Essential Service—Mobilize community partnerships to identify and solve health problems.	Domain 4. Engage with the community to identify and address health problems. Standard 4.1. Engage with the public health system and the community in identifying and addressing health problems through collaborative processes. Standard 4.2. Promote the community's understanding of and support for policies and strategies that will improve the public's health.	Principle 3. Public health policies, programs, and priorities should be developed and evaluated through processes that ensure an opportunity for input from community members. Principle 6. Public health institutions should provide communities with the information that they have that is needed for decisions on polices or programs and should obtain the community's consent for their implementation. Principle 12. Public health institutions and their employees should engage in collaborations and affiliations in ways that build the public's trust and the institution's effectiveness.	1. How is the "community" identified and involved? 2. In what ways are the values of the community elucidated and affirmed in the definition of the health problem; generation of solutions; implementation of the solution; and dissemination of the results? 3. Is the context of the local community (for example, history, availability of key stakeholders, inclusion of underrepresented groups) reflected in the type and structure of the engagement techniques? 4. What is the public's level of trust after engagement (as measured for example in an evaluation of the attitudes of engaged participants or by actions taken to address stakeholder concerns?

Reproduced from: Bernheim RG, Stefanak M, Brandenburg T, Pannone A, Melnick A. (2013) Public Health Accreditation and Metrics for Ethics, J Public Health Manag Pract., Jan-Feb;19(1):4–8.

ethical principles in the Code? According to public health leaders,[38]

> "In public health, public engagement is essential for developing and maintaining the social connections and relationships between public health professionals and the community—and as captured in the Code, community engagement is a way of obtaining the community's consent. The Code recognizes that society's trust in the authority of the public health profession is premised on public health professionals' consistent and transparent conduct aligned with commonly held community values. Thus, meaningful community engagement depends on the particular context and is as much art as science. ... Seeking community consent for a particular issue, for example, would involve determining what a specific community would believe to be respectful and appropriate communication and participation, based on community values. The objectives, level of expertise, and available evidence for engagement, therefore, are situation dependent. Other relevant aspects of engagement include type of communication (e.g., whether the communication is one way or two way), intention (e.g., education, input, consensus), participants (citizens, community representatives, leaders, experts), structure (formal or informal), and outcome (e.g., whether there is a specific decision or choice to be made). Experts also suggest that when developing

> community engagement activities, one should assess the range of 'problem-solving activities' in which a particular community might be involved, including problem definition, generation of solutions, implementation of the chosen solution, and dissemination of results. Ethical principles in the Code and ethics metrics based on them, therefore, can provide a frame of reference for public health officials when they assess what kind of activities would constitute meaningful community engagement."[38b]

For example, community-based public health activity often focuses on primary and secondary prevention (**Table 4.7**) and requires intersectoral action that engages "actors from a variety of relevant sectors in the planning, implementation, and governance of interventions."[26 (p. 25)]

A public health strategy to address obesity illustrates the need for sweeping changes in the community, such as in the dietary standards and physical activity norms. Efforts to do this may require the coordinated, simultaneous activity of a wide variety of actors: elected officials who approve zoning regulations and the creation of new parks or bike paths; parent groups and school boards that approve nutritional requirements for school menus; corporations who endorse community wellness goals; public transportation officials who approve new bus routes; private restaurants that offer healthy choices on their menus, etc.[26]

How should the community be engaged? There is new emphasis on the role of community organizing and system change as an approach for improving community health, which shifts responsibilities from individual institutions and the health department to inter-organizational coordination, collaboration among partners, and the pooling of community resources and efforts.[39] In describing the creation of "active living communities," using as an example the safe streets and safe routes to school legislation in Hawaii, Moore and Maddock suggest that mounting transformative change at the community level involves viewing the community as a complex system with the public health practitioner acting as a "super connector."[40] "The main goal of a systems approach is to understand the relationship between the actors, information and concepts in the system, and the communication and flow of knowledge between those points. Tools like network analysis and surveys of policy makers can be important in documenting the success of our efforts."[40] Thus, for a systems approach to creating healthy communities, community consent may involve the use of new forms of social media and communication flow among key stakeholder groups and organizations from different sectors, as well as eliciting their commitment to help implement strategies to undertake social change. As Oliver points out: "To the extent that Americans support collective action in the pursuit of public health or any other social good, they exhibit a strong preference for voluntary organization and participation."[8 (p. 196)]

TABLE 4.7 Three Levels of Prevention

Primary Prevention: aims to prevent disease from occurring. Example: encourage people to protect themselves from the sun's ultraviolet rays
Secondary Prevention: detects or identifies disease after it has occurred but before the person notices anything is wrong or has symptoms. Example: screen for suspicious skin growths
Tertiary Prevention: targets the person who already has symptoms of the disease to slow or halt the disease process and provide better care to those with disease. Example: provide better treatments for melanoma.

Data from: CDC Excite Training, retrieved 5/11/13 http://www.cdc.gov/excite/skincancer/mod13.htm

CONCLUSIONS

Addressing cardiovascular disease from a public health perspective, as presented in the case scenario presented earlier in this chapter, illustrates the opportunity for transformative, system-level changes in the community, based on public health's population perspectives, evidence-based practices, (**Table 4.8**), and community-engaged approaches.

TABLE 4.8 Evidence-Based Public Health

Engaging the community in assessment and decision making
Using data and information systems systematically
Making decisions on the basis of the best available peer-reviewed evidence (both quantitative and qualitative)
Applying program planning frameworks (often based in health behavior theory)
Conducting sound evaluation
Disseminating what is learned

Data from: Jacobs JA, Jones E, Gabella BA, Spring B, Brownson RC. Tools for Implementing an Evidence-Based Approach in Public Health Practice. Prev Chronic Dis 2012;9:110324.

[b] Reproduced from Bernheim RG, Stefanak M, Brandenburg T, Pannone A, Melnick A. (2013) Public Health Accreditation and Metrics for Ethics, Journal of Public Health Management and Practice, Jan-Feb;19(1):4–8.

At the end of the chapter, we suggest now that you reconsider questions raised by the scenario. What assessment criteria and justifications might now be offered in support of the five proposals you chose earlier, taking into account the perspectives from public health presented in this chapter and in light of public health moral considerations or principles from the code of ethics? How might the Advisory Committee use the questions for community engagement metrics in Table 4.6?

This chapter describes public health's ecologic (determinants-of-health, population-based) model, which aims to create healthy communities and to complement the biomedical, clinical care approach of medicine. The goal for cardiovascular disease strategies might be to create a "heart-healthy community" by providing selective interventions to targeted individuals or groups that ensure basic needs, such as access to essential services that include medical care and screening as a priority to address disparities. A "heart-healthy" community also might provide universal, population-wide interventions to build social support and social capital through, for example, widespread marketing campaigns to change social norms. These choices have significant ethical dimensions that can be useful in setting goals and choosing interventions. For some of the CVD interventions described in this chapter's scenario, evidence about effectiveness is lacking, so that the population benefits of interventions (utility) are difficult to assess. The scenario illustrates the importance for public health to evaluate the outcomes of their activities and contribute to a much-needed body of knowledge about evidence-based CVD best practices in the community. The scenario also illustrates a shift to integrate healthcare delivery, including primary care, and public health to improve population health.

Public health goals, benefits, and burdens are broad concepts and require specification in particular contexts, given the range of values, cultural interpretations, and socioeconomic conditions that bear on the meaning and use of health data and evidence. Thus, the documentation of benefits and harms includes not only the collection of data through the use of scientific methods such as epidemiology and cost-effectiveness analysis, but also the incorporation of social information, based on community values, and the moral claims of varying stakeholders, about how data should be collected, interpreted, and assessed.

Even decisions about the collection of data are increasingly recognized to require the engagement of the public. Decision making in public health, particularly for setting goals and assessing health burdens in the public realm, inevitably requires interpreting public health data, reaching judgments about its social and political significance, formulating proposals for action, and developing rhetorical strategies for building support for them. Public health decision makers always need to be sensitive to perpetual questions of political legitimacy, such as who has the authority to make decisions; what is the appropriate role of government agencies; at what level of government—federal, state, or local—should action be taken; and what stakeholders should be appropriately involved in the process.

For some public health problems, such as infectious disease control and reducing environmental hazards to health and safety, the public generally understands and accepts both the role of government and its goals. As public health embraces an increasingly muscular approach toward chronic disease prevention, expanding its focus to goals that involve changing individual behavior and creating a healthy social environment, public health activities often encounter ethical and political tensions and require attention to community values and the need for public justification. Providing population data is helpful and sometimes necessary, but often insufficient. Community engagement in and consultation about the creation and use of evidence ensure that both public health decision makers and community stakeholders can act with (1) *understanding* of the fundamental values and tensions entailed by setting public health goals and priorities and designing and implementing public health initiatives, (2) *respect* for diverse interests of individuals and groups, including the collective interest in a healthy community and the public good, and (3) *political responsibility* within the parameters of legitimate political institutions and deliberative processes. Modern public health, which is at once evidence-based and value-based, is inescapably—and properly—grounded in the political process.

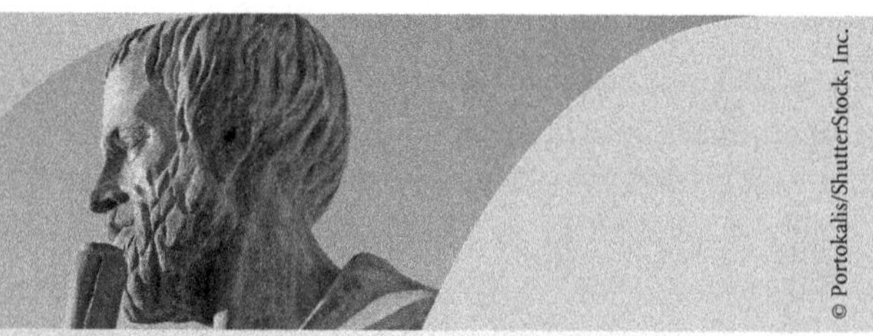

© Portokalis/ShutterStock, Inc.

Discussion Questions

1. It is customary to use the term "epidemic" to characterize the recent weight increase in the United States, thereby appropriating concepts associated with the spread of infectious disease—a classic public health concern. Do you think it is appropriate to characterize the increase in American's collective body mass index as an "epidemic"? Is this a useful label?
2. A sudden increase in the incidence of infectious disease implicates the public health by threatening to spread throughout the population. Why is the *public* health implicated by poor diets and sedentary lifestyles of individual Americans? Does calling these behaviors public concerns tug against the idea that people are entitled to make their own choices about how to live their lives based on their own values and preferences?
3. From a population perspective, the goal, according to Rose, is "to move the distribution," and he suggests that changing social norms would be needed to reduce exposure to risks associated with certain behaviors. Is changing social norms to reduce "behavioral causes" of disease analogous to improved sanitation?
4. Given the ecological approach to health that focuses on behavioral and social determinants of disease and injury, what, if any, are the boundaries of public health or limits on public health's scope?

REFERENCES

1. Frieden T. A framework for public health action: The health impact pyramid. *American Journal of Public Health*, 2010;100(4):590–595.

2. Association of State and Territorial Health Officials. Available at: http://www.astho.org/Programs/HiAP/ (accessed August 24, 2013).

3. Frieden T. Government's role in protecting health and safety. *The New England Journal of Medicine*, 2013;368:1857–1859.

4. Hall M. The scope and limits of public health law. *Perspectives in Biology and Medicine*, 2003;46: S199–S209.

5. Bayer R. The continuing tensions between individual rights and public health. *EMBO Reports*, 2007;8(12), 1099–1103.

6. Institute of Medicine. *For the Public's Health: The Role of Measurement in Action and Accountability*. Washington, DC: The National Academies Press, 2010:5.

7. Centers for Disease Control & Prevention. Winnable Battles. Available at http://www.cdc.gov/about/resources/pdf/WBGeneralFAQs.pdf (accessed May 10, 2013).

8. Oliver TR. The politics of public health policy. *Annual Review of Public Health*, 2006;27:195–233.

9. Brownson R, Fielding J, Maylahn M. Evidence-based public health: A fundamental concept for public health practice. *Annual Review of Public Health*, 2009;30:175–201.

10. U.S. Department of Health and Human Services. *Healthy People 2020*. Available at http://www.healthypeople.gov/2020/default.aspx (accessed May 13, 2013).

11. Green LW, Fielding J. The U.S. Healthy People initiative: Its genesis and its sustainability. *Annual Review of Public Health*, 2011;32:451–470

12. U.S. Department of Health and Human Services. Available at http://www.surgeongeneral.gov/initiatives/prevention/strategy/index.html (accessed August 27, 2013).

13. U.S. Department of Health & Human Services. Available at http://www.hhs.gov/news/press/2011pres/06/20110616a.html (accessed August 26, 2013).

14. U.S. Department of Health and Human Services. *The Guide to Community Preventive Services*. Available at http://www.thecommunityguide.org/cvd/index.html (accessed May 19, 2013).

15. Centers for Disease Control & Prevention. Heart Disease. Available at http://www.cdc.gov/heartdisease/cdc_addresses.htm (accessed May 19, 2013).

16. Centers for Disease Control & Prevention, Office of Surveillance, Epidemiology, and Laboratory Services. Excite website. Available at http://www.cdc.gov/excite/about.htm (accessed July 30, 2013).

17. Verweij M, Dawson A. The meaning of 'public' in "public health.' In Dawson A, Verweij M (eds). *Ethics, Prevention, and Public Health*. Oxford, UK: Oxford University Press, 2007:28.

18. Rose G. Sick individuals and sick populations. *International Journal of Epidemiology*, 1985;14:32–38.

19. Zulman D, Vijan S, Omenn G, Hayward R. The relative merits of population-based and targeted prevention strategies. *The Milbak Quarterly* 2008;86:557–580.

20. Institute of Medicine. *The Future of the Public's Health in the 21st Century*. Washington, DC: The National Academies Press, 2002.

21. Teutsch SM, Fielding JE. Rediscovering the core of public health. *Annual Review of Public Health*, 2013;34:287–299.

22. McGinnis JM, Foege WH. The immediate vs. the important. *JAMA* 2004;291:1263.

23. Mokdad AH, Marks JS, Stroup D, Gerberding JL. Actual causes of death in the United States, 2000. *JAMA*, 2004;91:1238–1245.

24. Conrad P. Wellness as virtue: morality and the pursuit of health. *Culture, Medicine & Psychiatry*, 1994;18:385–401.

25. Fitzgerald F. The tyranny of health. *The New England Journal of Medicine*, 1994;331(3):196–198.

26. Institute of Medicine. *An Integrated Framework for Assessing the Value of Community-Based Prevention*. Washington, DC: The National Academies Press, 2012.

27. Daniels N, Kennedy B, Kawachi I. Justice, Health, and Health Policy. In: Danis M, Clancy CM, Churchill LR (eds). *Ethical Dimensions of Health Policy*. New York: Oxford University Press, 2002;19–51.

28. Powers M, Faden R, Saghai Y. Liberty, Mill, and the framework of public health ethics. *Public Health Ethics*, 2012;5(1):6–15.

29. Institute of Medicine. *Unequal Treatment: What Health Care System Administrators Need to Know about Racial and Ethnic Disparities in Healthcare*. Washington, DC: The National Academies Press, 2002.

30. Bleich S, Jarlenski M, Bell C, LaVeist T. Health inequalities: Trends, progress, and policy. *Annual Review of Public Health*, 2012;33:7–40.

31. Woolf SH, Dekker MM, Byrne FR, Miller WD. Citizen-centered health promotion. *American Journal of Preventive Medicine*, 2011;40;1 (Suppl 1):S38–S47.

32. Jacobs JA, Jones E, Gabella BA, Spring B, Brownson R. Tools for implementing an evidence-based approach in public health practice. *Preventing Chronic Disease*, 2012;9:110324. Available at http://dx.doi.org/10.5888/pcd9.110324 (accessed July 30, 2013).

33. Grosse SD, Teutsch SM, Haddix AC. Lessons from cost-effectiveness research for United States public health policy. *Annual Review of Public Health* 2007;28:365–391.

34. Kaplan RM, Ong M. Rationale and public health implications of changing CHD risk factor definitions. *Annual Review of Public Health* 2007;28:321–344.

35. Institute of Medicine. *Valuing Health for Regulatory Cost-Effectiveness Analysis*. Washington, DC: The National Academies Press, 2006.

36. Russell LB. Preventing chronic disease: an important investment, but don't count on cost savings. *Health Affairs (Millwood)*, 2009;28(1):42–45.

37. Teutsch S, Fielding JE. Rediscovering the core of public health. *Frontiers in Public Health Services and Systems Research*, 2013;2(3): Article 1. Available at http://uknowledge.uky.edu/cgi/viewcontent.cgi?article=1047&context=frontiersinphssr (accessed July 30, 2013).

38. Bernheim RG, Stefanak M, Brandenburg T, Pannone A, Melnick A. Public health accreditation and metrics for ethics. *Journal of Public Health Management Practice*, 2013;19(1):4–8.

39. Woulfe J, Oliver TR, Zahner SJ, Siemering KQ. Multisector partnerships in population health improvement. *Preventing Chronic Disease* 2010;7(6):A119. Available at http://www.cdc.gov/pcd/issues/2010/nov/10_0104.htm (accessed July 30, 2013).

40. Moore JB, Maddock JA. The role of the public health practitioner in creating active living communities. *Journal of Public Health Management Practice*, 2012;18(5):397–398.

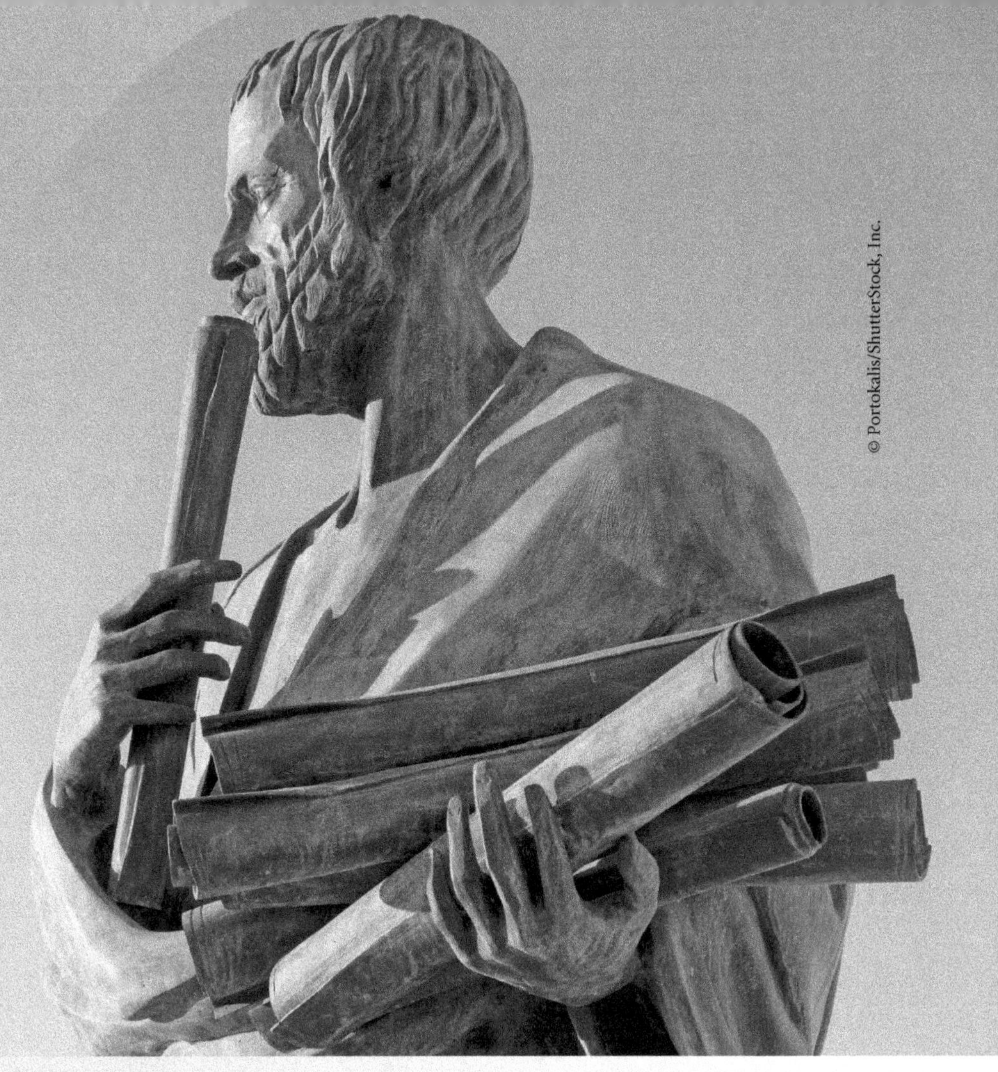

© Portokalis/ShutterStock, Inc.

PART II

Tools and Interventions in Public Health

CHAPTER 5

Surveillance and Public Health Data: The Foundation and Eyes of Public Health

by James F. Childress

Learning Objectives

By the end of this chapter, the reader will be able to

- Define public health surveillance and sketch its major features and aims
- Distinguish active and passive surveillance
- Understand the different ethical issues raised by anonymous or anonymized data, on the one hand, and personally identified or identifiable data, on the other
- Use the norms of privacy and confidentiality in assessing different surveillance practices
- Identify the major similarities and differences between surveillance in public health practice and surveillance in public health research
- Understand the different issues raised by surveillance in controlling infectious diseases versus controlling non-communicable chronic conditions, as in the New York City diabetes control program

INTRODUCTION

During the 2012 Summer Olympics in London, public health officials operated a wide-ranging health surveillance system, based on rapid identification and containment of any pathogen emerging in the population. The United Kingdom's Health Protection Agency (HPA) "developed what is being billed as 'the world's largest health surveillance system.' By rapidly meshing many different streams of information pouring in from hospitals, general practitioners, clinics, infirmaries, and healthcare hotlines across the U.K., the HPA has developed a way to measure and monitor the public health in near- real-time, ensuring that any pathogen outbreak is quickly identified, diagnosed, and contained before the whole of London comes down with the sniffles—or worse."[1] Whatever its scale, surveillance has played a key role in public health policy and practice for a long time, particularly in regard to infectious diseases; the U.K.'s Olympics surveillance concentrated on agents that could spread from person to person or from animals, plants, or food to humans.

This chapter will examine public health surveillance: its definition, major features, dominant aims, and challenges, as well as its indispensable role in public health policies and practices, and the ethical issues it raises. The data generated by this important tool enable effective public health actions, but, insofar as the surveillance obtains personally identifiable information, there are concerns about threats to individual privacy and to the confidentiality of health-related information as well as about the lack of, or presence of only attenuated, individual consent.[2] These concerns become more urgent as public health surveillance continues to expand its scope in order to better address naturally emerging infectious diseases and bioterrorist threats—as well as looking beyond infectious diseases to target noncommunicable, chronic diseases, such as diabetes. Each state has legal authority to conduct public health surveillance, and this legal foundation, we have argued, includes ethical values as well. However, that legal authority is often indeterminate rather than prescriptive. The law often authorizes public health officials to act without determining which actions they must undertake. Moreover, legal authority does not indicate whether a particular policy, practice, or action is ethically justified. Apart from simply saying "It's the law," Lee and colleagues ask the important question that is the focus of this chapter: "How can the public health system ethically defend the *collection* of personally identifiable, private health information without patient consent for the purposes of public health practice?" (italics added).[2] And, we might add, "How can the public health system defend *various uses* of these data?"

PUBLIC HEALTH SURVEILLANCE: ITS NATURE AND GOALS

What Is Public Health Surveillance?

There are numerous definitions of public health surveillance. Following is one used by the Centers for Disease Control and Prevention (CDC)[3 (p. 4)]:

> Public health surveillance is a series of ongoing systematic activities, including collection, analysis, and interpretation of health-related data essential to planning, implementing, and evaluating public health practice closely integrated to the dissemination of data to those who need to know and linked to prevention and control. Public health surveillance is predicated on the need to address a defined public health problem or question and aimed at the use of data to guide efforts to protect and promote population health.

This definition helpfully characterizes public health surveillance as "a series of ongoing systematic activities" that include collecting, analyzing, and interpreting health-related data, which are deemed to be "essential to planning, implementing, and evaluating public health practice." Then it explicitly connects these activities with two further activities: (1) the dissemination of data to those in public health policy or practice who need that information for the judgments and decisions they must make, and (2) "prevention and control" as two major public health endeavors. These activities preclude any simplistic misinterpretation of surveillance in public health as an *end* in itself. It is rather a *tool* for developing appropriate public health policies and practices, goals and interventions.

Types of Public Health Surveillance

The practice of public health surveillance has undergone a remarkable evolution in the United States. As Buehler[4] observes,

> Public health surveillance in the United States has evolved from monitoring infectious diseases to tracking the occurrence of many noninfectious conditions, such as injuries, birth defects, chronic conditions, mental illness, illicit drug use, environmental, and occupational exposures to health risks. In 2001, the intentional dissemination of *Bacillus anthracis* spores and subsequent cases of anthrax in the United States provided an impetus for automating surveillance to enable early detection, rapid characterization, and timely continuous monitoring of urgent public health threats.
>
> As the topics of surveillance have evolved, so have the methods of surveillance, spurred by rapid advances in information technology. With the impending mass adoption of electronic health records, procedures for conducting surveillance are taking another turn, and new opportunities for strengthening surveillance capacities are emerging. Electronic health records offer an opportunity to improve links between health-care providers and public health departments, making surveillance more effective and timely, although fulfilling that promise poses substantial challenges.

What distinguishes public health surveillance from other types of surveillance, such as criminal surveillance, military surveillance, and so forth? The distinction has to do with the *purpose* for which the information and data are being collected. Surveillance is an activity that can be undertaken for various purposes—some good, some bad, some indifferent. As we will see in the course of this chapter, it is important in an ethical assessment of public health surveillance to be very specific about its purposes. It is not enough to say that the proposed surveillance is for the purpose of public health. Instead, the specific public health goals in collecting and using the data need attention in the process of ethical assessment.

Among the important distinctions in ethically analyzing and assessing public health surveillance is the distinction between anonymous (or anonymized) data and personally identified (or identifiable) data. Even though anonymous data obviously derive from persons, they do not compromise individual privacy and, furthermore, usually cannot create risks, such as stigmatization, for those persons. Similar points hold for anonymized data, where identifiers have been removed, if we assume that the data are protected, that any links are secure, and the like. The main ethical issues in public health surveillance concern personally identified or identifiable information.

Epidemiological data can often be anonymous. Much epidemiological work based on public health surveillance does not require personal identifiers; it focuses on patterns related to diseases or health conditions, particularly risk factors and demographic characteristics. Determining these patterns often is sufficient for public health practice. However, a public health surveillance system will sometimes need individuals' names or other personal identifiers for effective action—for instance, to be able to alert individuals about their risks after having been exposed to a person with tuberculosis. Name-based reporting is mandated for some conditions.

To take another example: for a food-borne disease, such as the deadly *E. coli* outbreak in Europe in 2010, it is important to know the names and activities of the individuals infected. Those infected with the *E. coli*, if alive, could be interviewed to learn exactly where they ate, what they consumed, and so forth, so that public health officials could attempt to track down the source of the infection to prevent further cases. For similar reasons, it is also important to have name-based reporting for diseases such as meningitis or gonorrhea that are transmitted person-to-person in order to determine when the infection occurred, the infected person's contacts, and the like. In such cases, important public health actions need to be undertaken to protect others, such as vaccination for meningitis or treatment of gonorrhea in sexual contacts. Where direct individual follow-up and interventions are not available—for either the person infected or his/her contacts—personally identified information is less important.[5 (p. 14)]

Another distinction is between active and passive surveillance.[6] In *passive* surveillance—i.e., passive from the standpoint of public health agencies—healthcare providers or laboratories submit information about diseases, syndromes, etc., often as required by law. In *active* surveillance, public health officials contact healthcare providers or laboratories for such information. Most public health surveillance systems in the U.S. are passive at least from the perspective of state and local health departments; the reporting is certainly active from the standpoint of the healthcare providers and laboratories who provide information and data. The advantage of active surveillance by public health officials is that it tends to be more comprehensive and its data tend to be more complete; the disadvantage is that it requires more resources than passive surveillance. Active surveillance is sometimes used not only to ensure more complete data but also to follow-up on passive reports, to establish that the passive reports are representative, and to address particularly important problems.[6] Some interpretations of active surveillance encompass even more active case-finding—for instance, house-to-house search for individuals suffering from an Ebola outbreak in an African country, or follow-up with a sexual contact of a person identified with a sexually transmitted disease in the U.S.[5 (p. 12)] (We will spend more time on these last types of active surveillance in the chapter on case identification.)

This distinction between passive and active surveillance becomes less important as public health moves to systems that acquire data from linked medical records, without the initiative and actions of healthcare providers or laboratories, beyond their usual record keeping. The distinction is also relatively unimportant when the government mandates that all or some healthcare providers or laboratories report information. This we already have for infectious diseases, as is evident in the National Notifiable Disease Surveillance System for tracking what's happening in diseases from the states. Below we will consider the further and increased expansion of surveillance into noncommunicable diseases such as diabetes.

We should also note another use of the terms active and passive surveillance, now directed at the individuals who are the source of the information. Consider, for instance, surveillance of individuals' reactions to vaccinations. In active surveillance, healthcare providers actively follow those who are vaccinated by asking, at set intervals, direct, specific questions about any reactions. They can then follow-up initial responses to obtain more information and determine with greater reliability the nature and significance of those reactions. By contrast, in passive surveillance individuals may self-report at any time they believe they have a negative reaction to report, and then healthcare providers can follow-up. As previously suggested, the advantage of active surveillance, over passive surveillance, is that the data will probably be more complete, less susceptible to selection bias, and more readily available.[7 (p. 139)]

Who Is Involved in Public Health Surveillance?

In the U.S., the primary responsibility for public health surveillance, especially in the form of disease surveillance, falls on state health departments. However, they represent only a fraction of the agents involved in public health surveillance, all of whose cooperation is essential for effective surveillance. The responsibility is thus a shared one (see **Table 5.1**).[8]

Surveillance: Necessary but Insufficient for Effective Public Health

The tool of surveillance is commonly hailed as the key to public health policy and practice. Tracking the population's health is variously described as "an essential component of effective public health practice"[9] or the "cornerstone"[10 (p. 14)] or "foundation"[11] of public health practice. Some even say that surveillance is where public health starts. "In public health," said David Satcher, MD (U.S. Surgeon General, 1998–2002), "we can't do anything without surveillance. That's where public health begins."[11] These various claims

TABLE 5.1 Agents in Public Health Surveillance

Agents
Hundreds of thousands of healthcare providers (physicians, nurses, etc.) and healthcare institutions, such as hospitals and clinics
59 state and territorial health departments
> 3,000 local health departments (county, city, and tribal)
> 180,000 public and private laboratories
Public health officials in federal agencies and departments (Health and Human Services [HHS], which includes the Centers for Disease Control & Prevention [CDC] and the Food & Drug Administration [FDA]; U.S. Department of Agriculture [USDA]; Department of Defense [DOD]; and Department of Homeland Security [DHS])
World Health Organization [WHO]: Coordination of international surveillance

Data from: Government Accountability Office, *Emerging Infectious Diseases: Review of State and Federal Disease Surveillance Efforts*. Washington, DC: Government Accountability Office, September 2004, pp. 8–11.

point to the necessity of information and data to identify, gauge, and quantify public health problems, set specific public health goals, and determine effective public health interventions. In short, as Thacker and colleagues write, "public health surveillance is the foundation for decision making in public health and empowers decision makers to lead and manage more effectively by providing timely, useful evidence."[11] In view of these claims, it should not be surprising that we examine surveillance in the first chapter of the second part of this book devoted to tools and interventions.

The role and function of public health surveillance is often expressed in the metaphor of "eyes," or less commonly the metaphor of "radar."[12] For instance, a very important book on disease surveillance in the U.S. is entitled *Searching Eyes: Privacy, the State, and Disease Surveillance in America.*[13] Surveillance enables public health officials to acquire the information and data they need in order to understand and respond to health problems in the population. To switch to the other metaphor, radar—in its most dramatic (but not only) form, public health surveillance functions like an early alert system to warn of an approaching storm or enemy that could threaten a community's health. This early warning system enables preparation for effective actions.

The last observation indicates why, even though surveillance is essential for public health, it is not sufficient. By itself, information does not affect public health—it does not protect the public, prevent ill health, or promote health. It affects public health only if it is used as a basis for action. In the graphic language of Hermann Biggs, an influential figure in 19th century public health, the collection of information about diseases is not undertaken "in order to keep clerks or adding machines busy."[13 (p. 5)] William H. Foege, director of the CDC from 1977–1983, made a similar point: "The reason for collecting, analyzing, and disseminating information on a disease is to control that disease. Collection and analysis should not be allowed to consume resources if action does not follow."[14 (p. 47)]

This means that part of the justification for undertaking public health surveillance must be the anticipated actions that will follow, their precise nature to be determined by the characterization and extent of the public health problem to be addressed and the appropriate goals and means given the definition of the problem. Hence, it is important to attend to the probable uses of the information and data in the ethical analysis and assessment of public health surveillance. The overall goal is to protect the public health, to prevent health problems, and to promote health. This is what distinguishes public health surveillance from some other forms of surveillance, for instance, for security, but the ethical justification requires attention to more specific public health goals.

In short, justifying public health surveillance depends on the proposed uses of the data generated and how effective, cost-effective, and ethically defensible those uses are. To repeat the main point: the data by themselves will not protect or promote public health—only actions based on those data can do that. As a tool, surveillance can be used to develop effective public health interventions. Many of these possible interventions that data generated by surveillance can warrant are discussed elsewhere in relation to particular public health needs. For now, it's sufficient to say that in certain contexts, depending on the health problem, appropriate actions could include education, vaccination, partner notification, quarantine and isolation, or case management, such as directly observed therapy for tuberculosis.

Here we will just refer to major types of uses of public health surveillance data, with some illustrations, before addressing specifics. These indicate the range, but they do not include all the possible uses in any specificity.

For the first—and perhaps most common and obvious—use of public health surveillance, an excellent example comes from the early detection of severe acute respiratory syndrome (SARS) in 2002–2003. As Rein notes, this early detection was made possible by surveillance, and it

TABLE 5.2 Major Types of Uses of Public Health Surveillance

1. Recognize cases or clusters of cases that require interventions for preventing transmission or reducing morbidity and mortality
2. Assess the impact of health events on public health or identify and track trends
3. Establish the need for resources and interventions and allocation of resources in planning
4. Monitor interventions and prevention and control programs
5. Identify populations or geographical areas at high-risk for purposes of targeted interventions and analytic studies
6. Develop hypotheses for studies of risk factors

Data from: Garcia-Abreu A, Halperin W, Daniel I. *Public Health Surveillance Toolkit: A Guide for Busy Task Managers*. Washington, DC: The World Bank, 2002, p. 20.

contributed significantly to the prevention of a global outbreak that could have been devastating if not catastrophic.[15] The second use is evident in the regular reports by the CDC that help public health officials and others track trends in the incidence of diseases and their effects. An example of the third use is identifying correlative risk factors for disease acquisition or progression—for instance, surveillance data on the early cases of AIDS enabled public health officials to determine that the cause of AIDS was an infectious agent (subsequently identified as HIV) transmitted through bodily fluids such as blood and semen. As a result, it was possible to develop preventive programs that helped to reduce the spread of HIV and save numerous lives.[15] Continuing surveillance of HIV/AIDS has also been used in the fourth way identified above, while the fifth use—evaluating the effectiveness and impact of interventions, policies, and public health strategies—is evident in the National Immunization Survey, which monitors vaccination rates and enables officials to evaluate programs to increase those rates.[15] (See our chapter on immunization.)

Regarding the sixth use—supporting research inquiries and scientific hypothesis generation—Rein calls attention to the expansion of the National Mesothelioma Virtual Registry as a possible way to enable scientists to better understand the etiology of this deadly lung cancer so they can develop more effective treatments for disease.[15] As we will see below, surveillance is not research, but the distinction between them is not always clear.

Health Security, Securitization, and Surveillance

Until the last 15 years or so, public health and national security tended to be viewed as separate. To be sure, worries have long existed about infections crossing national boundaries, and historical experience has confirmed the legitimacy of those worries—for instance, in 19th century encounters with cholera and other infectious agents. In part as a result of several dramatic events, including the mailing of weaponized anthrax spores through the U.S. postal system in 2001, coupled with heightened anxiety in the U.S. about terrorist threats following the 9/11 attacks, the dangers of biological, chemical, and other weapons used against a population became even more patent.[16] Added to this was the increased sense of danger from existent and emerging infectious agents rapidly spreading from one country to another as a result of globalization, with its widespread and rapid travel. In such a context, the notion of "health security" became more common, along with the associated notion of "securitization" of public health. This perspective not only reflects the perceived connection between the war against disease (e.g., infectious diseases) and the war against external enemies (e.g., terrorists), but also the recognition that serious threats to public health, whatever their source, threaten society politically, economically, and in other ways.

This perspective has had an impact, even when the language is absent, on the approach to public health within the U.S. (and within other countries) as well as in international discourse and agreements, particularly regarding the threat of biological and other forms of terrorist activity. When public health is considered a problem of health security, and when the war against disease is connected with the war against human enemies, surveillance becomes even more important. One result may be that it has become easier to accept and justify public health surveillance without close attention to the relevant ethical considerations, to which we now turn.[17]

ETHICAL CONSIDERATIONS IN PUBLIC HEALTH SURVEILLANCE

Surveillance is clearly an important and indispensable means in protecting and promoting public health—it provides the essential information for defining problems and designing and implementing effective interventions. In principle, surveillance is an ethically justifiable means. Whether it is actually justifiable in particular circumstances will depend on specific public health purposes as well as on other conditions. (We should emphasize that this chapter concentrates on surveillance information from and about humans; a significant part of surveillance in public health focuses on animals and plants—for instance, monitoring mosquito populations for the Eastern equine encephalitis and West Nile viruses in order to alert the public about precautionary measures and to undertake spraying and other activities, if necessary, to reduce the risks.)

The metaphors for public health surveillance we discussed earlier—"eyes" and "radar"—and other metaphors such as "a finger on the pulse of the health of the community"[2 (p. 38)] suggest that individuals' privacy is compromised at least to some extent in public health surveillance. A person has privacy if others do not access the person in certain ways—for instance, through touching, observing, listening, etc. *Privacy* presupposes limited access, whether by others' choices, indifference, or respect for personal rights. A *right to privacy* is an individual's justifiable claim against others that they not violate his or her privacy; it can be a legal and/or a moral claim. Privacy can take a variety of forms, but we are here focusing mainly on informational privacy; that is, limited access to information about individuals. In clinical care or research, the collection of information about individuals generally presupposes their consent, which may be express or tacit, general or specific, etc. Rarely, however, do individuals consent to the collection, analysis, use, storage, and transfer of personal information for public health purposes. The first ethical question—about the justifiability of collecting information without consent—can be distinguished from, though it is not unconnected with, questions about subsequent uses and risks of misuses of the collected information. The risks are mainly psychosocial in nature—embarrassment, stigmatization, difficulties in employment, and the like.

Neither the legal nor the ethical right to privacy is absolute. At most, they set a presumption against using personal identifiers in the collection and use of information; they establish a priority for the collection and use of anonymous or anonymized information whenever possible. Determining whether and when collecting information with personal identifiers through public health surveillance is ethically warranted will depend, in the first instance, on the legitimacy of the specific public health goal. As we have suggested, it is not sufficient to appeal to the broad goals of protecting or promoting public health or reducing social and economic burdens; it is essential to carefully examine the specific goal(s). Then, in line with our ethical framework, which will be further illustrated in cases in this chapter, it is important to determine whether the proposed surveillance is likely to realize the goal(s) being sought and whether the infringement of privacy rights is necessary, proportionate, and the least intrusive means consistent with realizing the goal(s). Another question is whether adequate security measures have been developed and implemented to protect individuals' personal information; such measures can help to minimize the negative effects of overriding the right to privacy by reducing the risks of misuses of personal information.

Similar points also apply to the confidentiality of personal information. *Confidentiality*, in many ways, is a subset of personal privacy, but it is distinctive because it presupposes relationships and a pledge or promise, whether explicit or implicit, to protect personal information generated in a relationship—for example, within health care—from disclosure without the source individual's (or surrogate's) permission. In the context of public health surveillance, healthcare professionals often have a legal and an ethical duty to report information to public health officials. This information need not always have personal identifiers—for instance, where the goal is to follow the spread of influenza in a region—but sometimes, as we previously observed, personal identifiers are essential for public health officials to be able to undertake effective interventions, such as notifying sexual contacts of HIV status or determining the sources of an outbreak of foodborne illness. Here we are focusing primarily on information with personal identifiers. Anonymous or anonymized information does not constitute an infringement of privacy and thus is to be preferred if the public health goal can be pursued without personal identifiers.

One way to avoid some of the ethical problems surrounding privacy and confidentiality would be to obtain individuals' voluntary and informed consent, as is common in clinical practice and research. However, in confidential relations between healthcare providers and patients, requiring individuals' specific, explicit consent for the collection and sharing of information would entail the cooperation of overburdened healthcare professionals, consume additional time, reduce the timeliness and completeness of the information, and so forth.[18]

However much the "stewardship" metaphor illuminates public health as a whole, it is certainly helpful in thinking about public health responsibilities in certain contexts. Surveillance is a good example. As Buehler stresses,

> Despite these changes in scope and methods, the fundamental premise of public health surveillance remains constant. It should provide information to the public health community regarding the health of the populations served. Stewards of public health surveillance have a

> responsibility to ensure that the information is used to advance public health and to safeguard the confidentiality of persons who are represented in the data.[4]

This stewardship metaphor fits well with another important ethical consideration that we emphasize here and elsewhere: public engagement. Public engagement includes providing information to the public and justifying surveillance activities in light of public values. However, in its ideal form, it is more than a one-way activity, with public health officials providing information and reasons to the public. Ideally, it would include substantial public input, in part because public trust and cooperation are essential. In short, there are strong reasons for vigorous public engagement, with all potential stakeholders—both professionals and members of the public—in the process of developing and implementing surveillance policies. Such public engagement has become even more urgent in the context of concerns about health security and securitization.

PRACTICE VS. RESEARCH: IS THE DISTINCTION ETHICALLY SIGNIFICANT FOR SURVEILLANCE?

The Practice/Research Distinction in Public Health Surveillance

Lawrence Gostin, a public health lawyer and ethicist at the Georgetown University Law Center, observes that if the generation of information in public health—for instance, through surveillance—were to be viewed as research on human subjects, it would be difficult to respond rapidly and effectively to public health threats. Yet it is sometimes difficult to determine *when* routine public health activities, such as surveillance, epidemiological investigations, and evaluation and monitoring, fall into the category of research rather than practice. Gostin notes,

> [W]hen these routine practices become a form of population-based research ... is a vexing and important problem, because if routine public health practices were classified as "research," health departments would have to submit this activity for review by institutional review boards (IRBs) and obtain informed consent from participants. Classification of practice as research, therefore, could impede rapid and effective responses to community health threats.[19 (p. 309)]

In short, when public health surveillance is classified as public health research, it could entail both formal IRB review and informed consent by participants, which could cause risky delays in generating valuable information. But what exactly is the ethical significance, if any, of the distinction between surveillance as public health *practice* and surveillance as public health *research*?

As a public health practice, surveillance is intended to produce knowledge that can protect and promote public health. At first glance, this generation of knowledge through surveillance appears to be quite similar to what occurs in research. After all, research is frequently defined as "a systematic investigation ... designed to develop or contribute to generalizable knowledge."[20] And, in some cases, that generalizable knowledge may be used to protect and promote public health.

We will start this analysis of research and practice by glancing at medicine before returning to public health. In medical practice, there are various diagnostic and therapeutic interventions, some established and some experimental. These interventions are often subjected to clinical trials to determine their safety and efficacy. Such trials are forms of research that can enable clinicians, patients, and insurers to make well-grounded decisions about the use of these interventions. In the U.S., such research involving human subjects generally requires formal ethical review by institutional review boards (IRBs) in light of some broad ethical principles—for instance, beneficence, justice, and respect for persons, articulated in the Belmont Report—and more specific regulations.[21]

Central to these ethical principles and regulations is the voluntary and informed consent of the person engaged as a research subject or participant—terms that need further clarification. The federal regulations governing research use the term "subject," and, historically, the term "subject" was used to distinguish the human individuals being studied from "objects." As "subjects," rather than "objects," they were to be treated, in language drawn from the philosopher Immanuel Kant, as ends in themselves rather than merely as means to generate scientific knowledge; hence, their consent was required, and so forth. Over time, concerns arose that the term "subject" suggests subordination, being *subject to* and under the control of, others. As a result, the term "participant" has become increasingly common as a way to indicate the voluntary participation of individuals in research. This term, too, has its difficulties because not every individual (e.g., a child or a mentally ill person) is voluntarily enrolled in research—they may be enrolled by others (e.g., parents or guardians). Moreover, "participant" seems too broad because researchers are also participants. In view of this debate, we will use both terms interchangeably, while noting that the federal regulations governing research mainly use the term "subject."

Independent review and informed consent are often considered to be the two main pillars of the system for protecting the rights and welfare of human subjects in research. This system is designed to prevent harms, abuses, and exploitation in public health research as well as in clinical research. Indeed, its evolution was accelerated by the notorious U.S. Public Health Service syphilis study among nearly 400 African-American males in and around Tuskegee, Alabama. These men were diagnosed with syphilis but left untreated in order to determine the natural history of untreated syphilis among African-American males. Although the study started in the 1930s, it continued even after penicillin—an effective treatment for syphilis—was developed in the 1940s; the Tuskegee study only ended in the early 1970s, after public revelations and widespread outrage. Untold suffering and a number of deaths occurred in this untreated population. Furthermore, these men did not give their voluntary, informed consent to participation in research because they were deceived about the study—many thought they were being treated for "bad blood."[22]

If a particular activity of collecting information and generating data in public health is deemed to be *research* involving human subjects or participants, then it falls under the ethical principles and regulations for the protection of human subjects or participants. So the distinction between research and practice (i.e., nonresearch) is practically important, even though, as we will see, it faces serious conceptual and ethical challenges. Its practical role is evident in the CDC policy, "Distinguishing Public Health Research and Nonresearch."[3] This policy stresses that this distinction is important in determining legal and ethical obligations in public health activities:

> CDC has an ethical and legal obligation to ensure that individuals are protected in all public health research activities it conducts. All CDC activities must be reviewed to determine whether they are research involving human participants. When an activity is classified as research involving human participants, CDC and its collaborators will comply with Title 45, Code of Federal Regulations, Part 46 in assuring human research protections.[3]

Classifying as research a particular activity that produces data, information, or knowledge about human individuals does not necessarily bring it under the full formal review of an IRB, because some research does not involve *living* subjects (e.g., the individuals are deceased) and some research that does involve living participants may be exempt from formal review or subject to expedited review. The CDC takes its definition of human subjects/participants research from the Code of Federal Regulations (45 CFR 46. 102(f)): It involves "a living individual about whom an investigator ...conducting research obtains (1) data through intervention or interaction with the individual, or (2) identifiable private information."[3]

The CDC policy recognizes that, in public health, some emergency responses and some program evaluations as well as some surveillance projects may constitute research involving human subjects/participants, but we are here focusing only on surveillance projects. In the absence of definitive and exhaustive criteria for classifying surveillance projects as either research or nonresearch, the CDC indicates that the determination must be made on a case-by-case basis in light of the specific project's *purpose*.[3]

> If the purpose is to develop or contribute to generalizable knowledge, the project is research. If the purpose is to prevent or control disease or injury or to improve a public health program, and no research is intended at the present time, the project is nonresearch. If the purpose changes to developing or contributing to generalizable knowledge, then the project becomes research.[3 (p. 2)]

The CDC policy further indicates that surveillance systems

> are likely to be nonresearch when they involve the regular, ongoing collection and analysis of health-related data conducted to monitor the frequency of occurrence and distribution of disease or a health condition in the population. Data generated by these systems are used to manage public health programs. They have in place the ability to invoke public health mechanisms to prevent or control disease or injury in response to an event. Thus, the purpose of these surveillance systems is to prevent or control disease or injury in a defined population by producing information about the population from whom the data were collected.[3 (p. 2)]

The CDC policy notes several challenges to this approach, particularly in applying the federal regulations governing research, which do not address all public health activities. While some public health activities can be clearly classified as either research or nonresearch (i.e., practice), it is not easy to classify others. Moreover, research regulations do not recognize "the statutory authority of state and local health departments to conduct public health activities using methods similar to those used by researchers."[3] So some borderline activities are difficult to classify.

While recognizing all these difficulties, the CDC policy statement still attempts to distinguish what we can call *surveillance as practice* from *surveillance as research*, in part as a way to specify appropriate legal and ethical obligations to people from whom information is derived. One example of surveillance as public health practice, as distinguished from public health research, is the national diabetes surveillance system, which uses data from a number of national surveys to portray the burdens and complications of diabetes on both state and national levels. This surveillance system is designed for a public health purpose—to provide information to be used to develop and/or improve public health programs and services in order to prevent and control diabetes. The intended beneficiaries of the surveillance are persons with diabetes or at risk of developing diabetes.[3]

A more extensive surveillance system, also an example of practice rather than research, is the National Notifiable Diseases Surveillance System (NNDSS), which the CDC, at the request of the states and territories, developed to offer a central point of collection of data on the hundred or so diseases that are nationally notifiable, such as botulism, measles, syphilis, and tuberculosis, and to publish the data in the *Morbidity and Mortality Weekly Report* and in the annual *Summary of Notifiable Diseases in the U.S.* A notifiable disease is "one for which regular, frequent, and timely information regarding individual cases is considered necessary for the prevention and control of the disease."[23] The purpose of the NNDSS, according to the CDC policy statement, is "to provide CDC and state and local health officials with information to prevent, detect, and control outbreaks of disease."[3]

An Enhanced Approach to Distinguishing Public Health Practice and Research

In view of the difficulties of distinguishing the public health practice of surveillance from public health research, James Hodge, a public health lawyer at Arizona State University, seeks to develop an "enhanced approach" to drawing this distinction. In ways largely consistent with other approaches, he defines human subjects *research*, in the context of public health, as "the collection and analysis of identifiable health data by a public health authority for the purpose of generating knowledge that will benefit those beyond the participating community who bear the risks of participation."[24] He then defines—again, largely consistently with other approaches—public health *practice*, involving identifiable health information, as "the collection and analysis of identifiable health data by a public health authority for the purpose of protecting the health of a particular community, where the benefits and risks are primarily designed to accrue to the participating community."[24] We can summarize the basic distinctions Hodge draws between public health practice and public health research involving human subjects in **Tables 5.3** and **5.4.**

TABLE 5.3 Public Health Practice

• There is a specific legal authorization for the activity as public health practice
• The activity falls under a governmental duty to protect the public's health
• A governmental public health authority (or authorized partner), which is accountable to the public, undertakes or oversees the activity
• Informed consent is not a necessary requirement for the activity
• The activity is supported "by principles of public health ethics that focus on populations while respecting the dignity and rights of individuals"

Data from: James G. Hodge Jr., "An Enhanced Approach to Distinguishing Public Health Practice and Human Subjects Research," The Journal of Law, Medicine, and Ethics Spring 2005.

TABLE 5.4 Human Subjects Research

• The activity involves living individuals
• It includes identifiable private health information
• Those involved consented to participate (or their guardian consented) or there was a waiver of informed consent
• The activity is "supported by principles of research ethics that focus on the interests of individuals while balancing the communal value of research."

Data from: James G. Hodge Jr., "An Enhanced Approach to Distinguishing Public Health Practice and Human Subjects Research," The Journal of Law, Medicine, and Ethics Spring 2005.

Several differences merit further attention. Local, state, and federal laws authorize and often require public health practices, including surveillance and other activities. Public health practice, in short, involves governmental public health authorities and their partners in a context of public accountability. Furthermore, much public health surveillance involves information that does not identify particular individuals, as we have seen, while the regulations for the protection of human subjects/participants consider *only* the use of identifiable information from living individuals to be human subjects research.

There is also an important difference in emphasis between the two ethical frameworks: In the ethical framework for human subjects research, as reflected in federal and other regulations, the applicable principles "focus on the interests of individuals while balancing the communal value of research." By contrast, in the ethical framework of public health practice, the applicable principles "focus on populations while respecting the dignity and rights of individuals." Both ethical frameworks attend to both (1) individual rights and interests and (2) communal, population benefits. But the individual rights and interests are featured and implemented in somewhat different ways in these frameworks, and the balancing process differs somewhat in each one. These differences are important and are particularly evident in the centrality of voluntary and informed consent in human subjects research (unless there is a waiver of consent under certain specified conditions), in contrast to its general absence in the practice of public health surveillance.

Privacy and confidentiality are important in both of these contexts. Yet, as we have seen, these are *prima facie* or presumptively binding, rather than absolute. And their weights and limits may be specified differently in these two contexts. It is reasonable to view the protections of privacy and confidentiality (involving personally identifiable information) as more extensive and binding in public health research than in public health practice. For instance, it may be important to disclose personally identifiable information to prevent the spread of an infectious disease, such as tuberculosis. Furthermore, human subjects research generally involves a promise (though obviously not an absolute guarantee) of the protection of privacy and confidentiality as part of participant's informed consent to research. It is thus generally harder—though not impossible—to justify breaches of privacy and confidentiality in the context of research than in the context of public health. For instance, the Privacy Rule implementing the Health Insurance Portability and Accountability Act of 1996 (HIPAA) allows the disclosure of personally identifiable health information for public health purposes without the individual's specific authorization.[25]

According to Hodge, the criteria listed in **Table 5.3** and **Table 5.4** will enable us to distinguish simple cases of public health practice and public health research involving human subjects. However, they will not enable us to draw a clear line among more complex cases. They provide some suggestions for line drawing, but they are not always conclusive. Fully engaging Hodge's "enhanced criteria" for the difficult cases would take us too far afield. Nevertheless, the basic discussion is important in the process of determining whether and when the principles and regulations to protect human research subjects kick in. As we have seen, the judgment that a particular surveillance project in public health is actually human subjects research brings that project under the formal system of review for human subjects research, which generally includes scrutiny by an IRB (except for exempt research) and often ethical requirements related to voluntary, informed consent (except for waivers).

Concluding Problems

However important the distinction between practice and research has been—and still is, from a practical standpoint—it is sufficiently problematic to require caution in using it. There are inconsistencies in interpretation and application of the distinction—for instance, states tend to interpret most of their surveillance as practice, rather than research, while the CDC may view some of this surveillance as research. Furthermore, on each of these levels, there are discrepancies in the way the distinction between research and practice is drawn.[26]

The biggest problem is that the distinction between research and practice fails to reveal which activities are justified and when. As Rubel puts it, "whether an activity is research or practice tells us nothing whatever about what actions are justified as part of that activity"—the distinction thus lacks independent moral significance.[27] Hence, each activity of practice or of research still requires close ethical scrutiny to determine its consistency with relevant ethical principles.

Ethical Review of the Public Health Practice of Surveillance

In view of the conceptual/normative difficulties, inconsistencies in application, and unclear implications of the distinction between surveillance as practice and surveillance as research, are there helpful alternative approaches? One approach calls for more systematic ethical review and oversight of public health surveillance that involves name-based reporting, even if it is practice rather than research. According to Amy Fairchild and Ronald Bayer, who teach public health ethics at Mailman School of Public Health at Columbia University,

> It is time to resolve the matter by acknowledging the necessity of ethical review of public health surveillance activities at both state and federal levels, whether such activities fall neatly under the classification of research or practice or exist in a gray borderland.[26 (p. 632)]

They call for "explicit" and "systematic" review of surveillance, whether it is practice or research, but stress that this review need not mirror what is involved in the IRB's examination of research. Lest they be misunderstood, Fairchild and Bayer rightly stress that the ethical principles involved in this review cannot simply replicate those employed in either clinical practice or human subjects research, because those principles are oriented primarily to the individual whereas public health ethics must give "first priority to the communal welfare."[26 (p. 632)] Yet they do not neglect individual rights and interests—indeed, attending to these rights and interests as expressed in liberty, privacy, and confidentiality, in relation to communal welfare that surveillance may protect and promote, would be one major task of the proposed ethical review or oversight. Moreover, Fairchild and Bayer contend, the balancing required cannot be captured in simple rules for making the unavoidable and necessary ethical trade-offs.[26]

Even though some changes may be important in the legal or regulatory context for public health surveillance—in part because ethics and law may sometimes conflict—Fairchild and Bayer are mainly concerned to ensure a transparent ethical review, rather than merely relying on the public health's legal authority. They recognize the commitment of public health officials to ethical principles, such as the ones embodied in the Code of Ethics of the American Public Health Association. But they also claim, without providing substantial evidence, that the public health community is not enthusiastic about "proposals to establish mechanisms to assure ethical review."[26 (p. 632)]

Some critics charge that Fairchild and Bayer fail "to substantiate the need for major reform," particularly in light of the existing ethical review/oversight by public health agencies and professionals, which is "robust and open," though different from the system for research involving human subjects.[28] In response, Fairchild and Bayer stress that, while the ethical review they have in mind need not occur "outside of public health," it should be more "explicit, systematic."[29] And it should avoid focusing so much on whether the surveillance is practice or research in considering what is required and permitted.

It may be reasonable to go even further than Fairchild and Bayer suggest and include some public involvement in the ethical review process. Throughout our discussion, we have suggested the potential value of public engagement in, for instance, setting the criteria for allocating scarce resources in a public health emergency. Public engagement can operate at several levels. The most general level involves explaining to the public the nature and value of surveillance practices. A more specific level engages the public on particular surveillance practices, including what will be done to protect privacy and confidentiality. Both forms of public engagement can contribute to public trust and to effective and ethical surveillance in public health. Finally, we should note that public health officials have to justify their actions to elected officials, representing the public, and often directly to the public itself.

CHEERS: A Case of Ethically Unjustified Research?

Of course, ethical review or oversight does not guarantee that either practice or research will be ethically justifiable. It is designed to increase the odds of ethical acceptability. Following is a case of *surveillance as research*, rather than surveillance as practice, which was reviewed and approved by a number of oversight bodies, including several IRBs, and involved parental consent. Nevertheless, this study was cancelled because of its perceived ethical deficiencies.

Known as the Children's Environmental Exposure Research Study (CHEERS),[a] it was intended to help the U.S. Environmental Protection Agency (EPA) determine unsafe and safe levels of infant and toddler (age 3 and younger) exposure to pesticides used indoors.[30,31] This study was designed to follow 60 children in their homes in and around Jacksonville, Florida for two years to determine how pesticides get into their bodies. In this surveillance, parents would track and report their use of pesticides in the home and their children's activities—partly through the use of a camcorder provided to the family—as well as their food consumption. Additionally, in 30 home visits, field teams were to collect samples from the floors and other surfaces and obtain children's urine to test for evidence of pesticide ingestion (through the analysis of metabolites). Children would also wear an ankle electronic monitor of their activities during certain periods.

CHEERS received the approval of several bodies, including a special committee at the EPA, the IRBs of the Battelle Memorial Institute, the University of Florida, and the Florida Department of Health. The CDC and the Duval County Department of Health were co-sponsors of the study. Nevertheless, and despite its (unfortunate) acronym,

[a] The summary of this case is pieced together from information presented in References 30 and 31.

CHEERS received such severe ethical criticisms that it was cancelled.

The criticisms focused on several features of the study. The fact that the study would have had high rates of participation of low-income people of color—in part because of the composition of the populations served by the health department clinics and hospitals helping with recruitment—brought charges of unfair selection of participants. The study also appeared to many critics to entail *intentional exposure* rather than mere *observation*; after all, to be eligible to participate in this study, the parents had to indicate that they were using pesticides in the home. They were told that they were not required to continue using pesticides throughout the study, but they may have reasonably thought that continued pesticide use in the home was a condition of their ongoing participation (and by inference, their chance of receiving compensation for participation). Because the study offered each family participating in CHEERS a sum of $970 and allowed them to keep the camcorder used for surveillance, some critics worried that the financial incentives to families for their participation might encourage continued use of household pesticides.

Worries also surfaced about the quality of the informed consent for study participation. Parents were not specifically warned about pesticides' special risks to young children, which stem from their susceptibilities to neurotoxic substances at their stage of development combined with normal activities such as crawling on the floor and putting their hands in their mouths. The investigators' rationale was that the use of pesticides as labeled is considered safe, and participants were not being asked to change their pattern of use. Yet the safe level of exposure of children to pesticides is not known, and, indeed, the study was designed to contribute information that could help determine safe levels. Another ethical controversy erupted as the scope of the study expanded as a result of a commercial grant: CHEERS was originally designed to study only pesticide exposure, but the American Chemistry Council provided a grant of $2 million to include other chemicals, to be selected by EPA.

In light of these and other ethical concerns, commentators on this case have drawn several lessons for future observational or surveillance studies of children's exposure to hazards, such as pesticides, in the home (**Table 5.5**). One is the necessity to clarify the distinction between research that involves the intentional dosing of hazardous agents, such as pesticides, and research that merely observes the use of those agents. In both cases, there is an effort to determine the effects of exposures. In line with our emphasis on public participation, Resnik and Wing stress the importance of community input and involvement in developing the design and implementation of such studies.[31] They also emphasize the importance of standard ethical requirements in research, including observation or surveillance as research. These include fairly selecting research participants to avoid "unfair representation of the poor or people of color" and ensuring adequate disclosure and understanding of the risks involved in the activities under observation, such as pesticide use. Another lesson is the avoidance of conflicts of interests and appearances of such conflicts.

TABLE 5.5 Lessons from CHEERS

Seek community consultation and participation
Seek to set compensation levels that are not unduly influential, on the one hand, or exploitative, on the other hand
Seek to ensure that studies do not have "unfair representation of the poor or people of color"
Inform participants about all the risks associated with the research (including uncertainties about the risks of hazardous agents being studied)
Clarify that the studies will not intentionally expose participants to hazardous environmental agents
Avoid conflicts of interest and appearances of such conflicts

Data from Resnik D and Wing S. Lessons Learned from the Children's Environmental Exposure Research Study. American Journal of Public Health 2007 (March);97(3):414–418. The second row is our addition.

Questions also arise about appropriate levels of compensation for participation in research. On the one hand, investigators need to avoid exploiting populations that are financially less well-off. Exploitation may involve taking advantage of the immediate needs of potential participants by offering small amounts of money that almost certainly would not attract economically better-off participants. On the other hand, investigators need to avoid excessively large amounts that might constitute undue influence.[32 (Chap. 5)] Resnik and Wing do not draw a specific lesson about setting fair levels of compensation, but they rightly emphasize that community consultation and input can be helpful in the process of setting the appropriate level.[31] (For various reasons discussed elsewhere—and in contrast to the language used by Resnik and Wing—we do not view even high financial incentives as coercive. We share the concern that financial incentives may sometimes be unduly influential in decisions, but influencing decisions is not the same as coercing decisions.)

As we have seen, the judgment that a particular surveillance project in public health is actually human subjects research brings that project under the formal system of review for human subjects research, which generally includes scrutiny by an IRB (except for exempt research) and ethical requirements related to voluntary, informed consent (except for waivers of consent). This formal review includes a wide range of ethical considerations assessing human subjects research. We featured some of these in our analysis of the CHEERS protocol, but, in conclusion, it is useful to indicate the range of considerations. These include the value of the generalizable knowledge that is sought; the likelihood that the research will generate that knowledge—here scientific design merges with ethics; the balance of probable benefits of the research and the risks to research participants; the minimization of risk to participants; the fair selection of participants; voluntary, informed consent; and protection of privacy and confidentiality.[33,34]

CASE STUDY: NONCONSENSUAL NAME-BASED SURVEILLANCE OF DIABETES CONTROL

New York City's Surveillance Program for Inadequately Controlled Diabetes

We now turn to surveillance in public health practice by looking at a controversial case: the nonconsensual name-based surveillance program New York City (NYC) developed in 2005 to help address uncontrolled or poorly controlled blood sugar levels among residents with diabetes. This "radical new form"[35] of surveillance is controversial in part because it targets and tracks a chronic, noncommunicable disease. The question we will consider in this case study is whether the different components of this surveillance program are ethically justifiable.

Chronic disease now accounts for a huge proportion of the disease burden in the U.S.—as much as two-thirds of the disease burden according to some estimates. The public health community strongly believes that the tools of public health are not being adequately and effectively used to prevent and control these diseases. Among the underused tools are surveillance, monitoring of patients' conditions and clinical care, and education of patients, the public, and professionals, all of which play roles in the NYC surveillance program.

In 2005, Thomas Frieden, then NYC Health Commissioner, stressed that diabetes is "the only major health problem in this country that's getting worse and getting worse quickly."[35] In NYC over the previous decade, the percentage of the adult population with diabetes had doubled to more than 9%—approximately half a million people—resulting in more than 20,000 hospitalizations each year and close to 3,000 lower extremity amputations each year, and, altogether, accounting for close to $500 million dollars in medical costs.[36] Nationwide, diabetes has now become the seventh leading cause of death and the source of untold morbidity and suffering.[37]

A major obstacle to reducing mortality and morbidity from diabetes is that so many people with diabetes do not have adequate blood glucose control. Evidence of a lack of adequate control appears in their high blood sugar level, as indicated by a hemoglobin A1C level greater than 9% (an A1C level of 6% is considered ideal for patients with diabetes). In NYC, it appears that perhaps 30–40% of people with diabetes have an A1C level greater than 9%, and yet only 10% of those who have diabetes even know their A1C levels.[35]

The NYC surveillance program requires that laboratories with electronic reporting capability submit the hemoglobin A1C test results of all city residents; these results are entered into a registry. The mandate falls on the laboratory, not on the physician or healthcare facility. Patients who are being tested as part of their treatment are not asked to consent to this tracking. When they are tested, their personally identifiable data, including their test results, are entered into the registry without their consent or even against their objections.[36]

The surveillance program was citywide from the outset but the follow-up interventions—contacting patients who have A1C test results greater than 9% or who have not had a recent test and also notifying their healthcare providers and facilities—were first piloted in the South Bronx. An opt-out provision accompanies the intervention program, but not the tracking program. This complex case raises several ethical issues related to patient consent, privacy and confidentiality of patient data, and incursion into the physician-patient relationship, as well as concerns about vulnerability and empowerment and the legitimate scope of public health. We will examine the ethical arguments offered by supporters and opponents on several of these key issues.

Ethical Issues Raised by the NYC Diabetes Surveillance Program

Public Health Goals

In part because the NYC diabetes surveillance program targets a noncommunicable disease and breaches privacy and confidentiality without consent, public officials and other defenders from the outset mounted a vigorous campaign of public justification. Their justifications often rested on claims of an "epidemic." Even though the term "epidemic" is used most commonly for outbreaks of infectious diseases, it is not technically inappropriate for NYC's diabetes problems. Rhetorically, the term evokes an image that can support expansive public health authority and interventions, which are allegedly needed and intended to address a disease that is spreading very rapidly and extensively, thus putting the public at risk.

In a letter to *The American Journal of Public Health*, Thomas Frieden stressed that "Diabetes and HIV/AIDS are major epidemics of our era, disabling and killing millions in this country, particularly people who are poor, Black, or Hispanic. Public health agencies have an obligation to intervene to try to reverse these epidemics and to reduce their impact."[38] Without questioning this obligation to intervene, based on principles of beneficence and justice, we must at least note that it is not an unlimited obligation. There are ethical limits, even if only *prima facie* or presumptive ones, and they too need to be considered. Not even an "epidemic" justifies *all* possibly effective means of action; for instance, it would not warrant extreme acts such as killing infected individuals.

Even if rhetoric of an "epidemic" is warranted in cases of noncommunicable diseases, public health officials should recognize, as Goldman argues, a duty "to provide resources for prevention and treatment of disease and to implement meaningful safeguards that protect patients from undue exposure to risk and harm" before they try to justify "heightened surveillance and intervention."[39 (p. 17)] She charges that NYC public health officials failed to provide the needed resources and safeguards.

Whether we believe that the term "epidemic" obscures more than it illuminates in this case, the health problems associated with diabetes are indeed real, extensive, burdensome, and costly. Diabetes that is not adequately controlled can cause major health problems for individuals, including kidney disease, heart disease, and stroke. These create huge burdens for the individuals affected and for their families and caregivers. In addition, these health problems have tremendous social and economic impacts, including heavy financial costs the city must bear.

There has been a "mission creep" in public health, Mariner contends, parallel to what has happened in intelligence surveillance since the 9/11 attacks.[40] (See our discussion of health security and securitization earlier in this chapter.) In public health, there has been a movement from communicable diseases—the first laws in the 19th century required doctors to report smallpox and other contagious diseases—to chronic diseases, such as diabetes. We do not deny the legitimacy of incorporating all these under the rubric of "public health" as inclusive of "population health." However, "public health" (or "population health") is by itself too broad to serve as an adequate justification of overriding liberty, privacy, and confidentiality. It is not sufficient to appeal to "public health" as the rationale for nonconsensual infringements of liberty, privacy, and confidentiality. Whether these infringements are ethically justified depends in part on the nature and magnitude of the specific public health problem being addressed. Instead of invoking a vague (and malleable and expansive) notion of public health to be balanced against privacy, confidentiality, and consent, we need to identify more specific goals of public health and then ask whether they warrant using means that dispense with consent and that override privacy and confidentiality. Clearly, a number of specific goals in public health do warrant such means—we do not at all question that in many efforts to control infectious and communicable diseases. But the case is less clear in diabetes control.

Focusing on principles of constitutional law in a way that also applies to ethical analysis, Mariner stresses the problems in a simple balancing test: "When an undefined public good is balanced against one person's immediate, concrete harm, there is little opportunity to seriously evaluate the merits of any possible invasion of privacy. The deck is stacked before the game begins."[40 (p. 347)] Instead, Mariner proposes that we balance "the present value of the particular information to achieve specific public health functions against the dignitary cost of invading privacy," contending that this "may better align basic constitutional principles with the real world of public health today."[40] This analysis also applies to ethical balancing.

Let's recall that the generation of data through surveillance may be a necessary condition but it is not a sufficient condition for protecting or promoting public health—actions must follow. Upon closer examination, there appear to be two distinguishable, though not unrelated, justifications for how this NYC surveillance program could promote public health. On the one hand, it could generate data for determining the scope of the problem of uncontrolled diabetes and for developing effective public health responses. For instance, Thomas Frieden justified the surveillance in a way that presumably could avoid the use of personally identifiable information (even though he did not suggest that): "The advantage is that for the first time, we'll know the scope of the problem. We're in the middle of an epidemic. Cases have nearly tripled in the past 10 years. I can't tell you what portion of how many people are in poor control. Ninety percent don't know themselves."[41] Beyond knowing the scope of the problem, as a basis for further public health planning, Frieden and others had a second goal: Changing individuals' conduct now to ensure better diabetes control. Pursuing this goal requires personally identifiable information so that contact can be made. This goal, as Frieden put it in a public hearing, is "to help strengthen ... physicians' efforts to better manage their patients, and to empower patients with more information."[42 (p. 6)] Even though these two goals are distinguishable, Frieden and other public health officials stressed that "personal identifiers are essential to enable both accurate surveillance and actions to improve the care of individual patients."[36 (p. 555)]

The strongest argument for collecting information about and reporting diseases, through named reporting, is to protect others who might be at risk from individuals' uncontrolled diseases. Examples include infectious tuberculosis and syphilis. These arguments represent versions of John Stuart Mill's "harm-to-others principle," which is discussed elsewhere. However, narrowly understood, the "harm-to-others principle" offers no warrant for the diabetes surveillance and intervention program, since diabetes is not communicable.[b]

Nevertheless, there may be other harms to others in a much more interdependent society than existed in Mill's day, a century before the welfare state. In our context, the financial burdens associated with diseases are borne in part by taxpayers, and NYC officials may have been concerned about the increases in government Medicaid and other costs of caring for patients with diabetes.

Still another possible goal of the NYC surveillance program is at least in part paternalistic. From a paternalistic standpoint, liberty, privacy, and confidentiality are justifiably breached in order to protect the individuals themselves. Of course, these individuals are part of the "public," but the goal in this weak paternalistic intervention is to empower them as individuals to control their diabetes, through using such soft tools as providing information and nagging through notification.

We will explore this conception in the next section. For now, we should note that these goals may be combined in a mixed justificatory argument. However, bringing several more specific goals together may not strengthen the arguments for overriding privacy and confidentiality without regard for consent.

Vulnerability and Empowerment

Vulnerability and empowerment are concepts that appear on both sides of the debate about the justifiability of the NYC diabetes surveillance program. Particularly important is the vulnerability of the populations most significantly affected by diabetes and by the surveillance program: poor, largely African-American and Hispanic populations in the South Bronx, where the intervention program was piloted.

Defenders of NYC's diabetes surveillance program often stress individuals' and groups' vulnerability because of their limited medical relationships and contacts (even though the program is obviously building on some relationships and contacts that lead to A1C tests). Fairchild praises this measure as "groundbreaking in that public health is responding to what it has taken to be a moral duty to meet the needs of and, indeed, empower populations that have been inadequately served by the existing healthcare system."[43] Here the focus is on the empowerment of vulnerable persons through providing information, even without their consent.[35] If this is paternalism, Fairchild suggests, it is what might be called a weak or soft paternalism, and it is warranted—after all, it enables people to make choices and nudges them to make good choices. In Frieden's words, it aims "to empower patients with more information."[42 (p. 6)]

By contrast, critics of the NYC surveillance program stress the need for safeguards of privacy and confidentiality because of risks of stigmatization and other harms to vulnerable people and the need for resources to empower them to address their inadequately controlled diabetes.[39] In particular, these critics call for attention to the "underlying social, environmental, and economic factors that contribute to disease."[39] Unfortunately, these critics observe, the surveillance program generates personally identifiable information to be used for follow-up with patients, but it does not provide resources for their treatment or to bring others with uncontrolled diabetes into the healthcare system for diagnosis and treatment. As an article in *The Lancet* notes, "in the absence of an infrastructure to provide comprehensive care for diabetes in the USA, this registry-based initiative can offer only a small step forwards for treatment of patients with diabetes."[44]

These positions need not be locked in implacable opposition. Surely, most could agree that, in the context of different vulnerabilities, both information and other resources can be empowering. First, information can often be empowering—if individuals know that their diabetes is not being adequately controlled, they may be better able to take appropriate actions. Second, other resources, such as financial resources, can also enable individuals to take actions, for example, to improve their diets, which might otherwise be difficult. It is possible to debate which vulnerability most urgently needs attention and which empowerment is most urgently needed for vulnerable people in these circumstances.

Consent/Nonconsent to Surveillance

The NYC diabetes surveillance program does not require patients' consent for the reporting of the A1C laboratory data and the entry of the data into the registry, and patients

[b] For a version of the Millian principle, see Rubel A. Justifying public health surveillance: basic interests, unreasonable exercise, and privacy. *Kennedy Institute of Ethics Journal*, 2012;22:1–33.

cannot opt out of participation in this phase of the program. Whatever their preferences, individuals' personally identifiable test results will be reported and entered into the registry.

Defenders of the program insist that there is no need for consent for A1C tracking, whether through opt-in or opt-out. They also argue that a consent process would be problematic for several reasons. First, it would result in incomplete reporting, and that would compromise the analysis of data for public health purposes. Second, consent processes vary greatly among providers and facilities, and it is simply unreasonable to suppose that everyone would be asked for consent. As a result, some people who would want to be included in the A1C reporting and registry would be excluded, simply because they had not been asked to consent. Finally, requiring consent for reporting A1C test results "could set a hazardous precedent for other notifiable disease reporting, severely hindering the control of communicable disease outbreaks and the detection of environmental exposures."[36 (pp. 559–560)]

Critics stress that these arguments are not compelling. First, even if complete reporting is deemed essential—a claim that needs to be established rather than merely asserted—there is at least an argument that some persons with diabetes will avoid treatment (and hence testing) because of concerns about the disclosure of their personally identifiable information. The second argument above suggests a reason for improving the consent process, rather than abandoning it altogether, especially when privacy and confidentiality are being compromised. Finally, the third argument above is implausible in part because much of the opposition to the NYC diabetes surveillance program hinges on the fact that diabetes is noncommunicable. This suggests that people can reasonably distinguish between (a) name-based reporting of a *communicable* disease to prevent the spread of that disease to others, and (b) name-based reporting of a *noncommunicable* disease. Hence, it is implausible to argue that requiring consent for A1C reporting would create a "dangerous precedent." Instead, critics charge, the NYC surveillance program creates a really "dangerous precedent" because of its compromise of privacy and confidentiality without consent and without adequate public health justification in the context of this particular chronic, noncommunicable condition.[c]

By contrast, the intervention phase of the program does allow patients with diabetes to opt out. Essentially, as Frieden explains, this is similar to a "do-not-call" registry.[42] However, objectors at the public hearing noted that opting out was possible only after their information had been "seized" and their privacy "invaded."[42] Printed materials about the letter service and about patients' right to opt out are provided to facilities for display in patient care areas,[36] but it is not known how many do so. Many patients may not even be aware of their right to opt out of the intervention program until they receive their first notification from the Department of Health and Mental Hygiene informing them that they have fallen behind in getting their blood sugar levels tested or that, according to the tests, their blood sugar levels are too high. Not surprisingly, there were calls at the public hearing for an opt-in approach rather than an opt-out approach or, at a minimum, an opt-out option up front rather than later.

Privacy and Confidentiality

Critics of the proposed diabetes surveillance program frequently appeal to individuals' privacy and rights to privacy. At a public hearing in 2005, one opponent stated:

> To me diabetes is a very private matter that would become a public matter. What gives New York City the right to take my private information from me without my consent and usurp it as their own? Do I pose a bioterrorist threat? No. Is there some type of infectious disease threat? No. Is there an imminent threat that I will harm someone else? No. Am I a criminal? No. And am I an idiot who needs to have the great City of New York babysit for me? No.[42]

The problem, this individual protested, is that diabetes "is being treated like a communicable disease, and patients' names and lab results are being entered into a public health database or registry." "What is next?" he asked.[42] One witness at the hearing ended his remarks: "In closing, I want to say that as a diabetic, I am not a threat to the City's public health, nor do I wish to be treated as one."[42]

At the hearing, Frieden emphasized that there are stronger protections for privacy and confidentiality in the NYC diabetes surveillance program than for communicable diseases. Specifically, this program "would not allow the information with anyone other than the treating physician or the patient, essentially under any circumstances."[42] However, the ethical issue concerns not only the security after the data and information have been obtained but the initial capture of personally identifiable information without consent—which constitutes a breach of privacy.

In line with Frieden's comment, the NYC health department also stresses the confidentiality of the information. It emphasizes that the information about hemoglobin A1C

[c] Of course, there are precedents for reporting of chronic, noncommunicable conditions; such precedents include registries of cancer and workplace injuries, as Mariner[40] notes.

levels is provided only to patients and medical providers, including both facilities and professionals, involved in the treatment of the patients being tested. In responding to concerns, the NYC health department indicates that information will not be provided to other agencies, such as the agency that issues driver licenses. Nor will it be provided to other individuals or institutions even with the patient's consent. The patient, of course, has the right to disclose that information himself or herself.

Impact on the Doctor–Patient Relationship

In discussing the NYC diabetes surveillance program, Fairchild predicts that "if New York City comes to serve as a model, public health surveillance in the United States will take on a radical new form, entailing a reconfiguration of the relation between public health and medicine."[35] We have already observed that physicians and others in health care are also agents in public health surveillance, in part because they are often legally and ethically obligated to provide information about patients' conditions. However, in the NYC program they do not face a mandate to provide information about patients; indeed, they are not even directly involved in the provision of information, because the public health department obtains the data from the laboratories doing the testing. All they do is order a hemoglobin A1C test; the rest is out of their hands.

Instead, the reconfiguration of the relationship between public health and medicine comes from the public health monitoring of the care provided and of patient compliance through tracking the A1C results and then providing information back to patients, physicians, and facilities. There are significant concerns about these intrusions into the doctor-patient relationship and the threat they pose to trust in health care. Following is one possible unintended negative result: Some patients with diabetes who receive a letter telling them that they are behind in their testing or are not adequately controlling their A1C levels will not seek medical care when they should in order to avoid implicit blame and other perceived, even if mistaken, threats from the governmental intervention.[39] A letter from the Association of American Physicians and Surgeons strenuously objected to the tracking of A1C lab test results "without patient consent" and "the proposed unauthorized contact with each patient's physician to discuss treatment plan and education," contending that this "blatant invasion of patient privacy ... will cause many patients to avoid testing and treatment" and result in harm to them as well as increased costs.[45] This letter further stressed the potentially "catastrophic" "chilling effects on patient's [sic] voluntary and preventive visits to physicians."

Many patients live in fear of their medical information falling into the hands of the government, employers, insurance companies, political rivals, or even ex-spouses. The mere chance that strangers will be able to access their lab results will cause many to decline having tests performed. Even those who do not fear embarrassment or a loss of benefits will still want to keep private their most personal medical information.[45]

Another possible unintended negative outcome is that physicians will seek to avoid difficult, noncompliant patients because of the implicit criticism in the notification.[39] At the time of the initiative, these were speculative concerns, and we are not aware of any studies that indicate whether these negative results have occurred and, if so, at what rate.

Ethical Analysis and Assessment of the NYC Diabetes Surveillance Program

Now we will use the justificatory conditions we developed elsewhere (**Table 5.6**) to pull together the elements of ethical analysis and assessment of the NYC diabetes surveillance program presented above. The NYC diabetes surveillance program—as well as its proposed HIV surveillance program—encounters a strong, though not absolute, ethical constraint: the rights to privacy and confidentiality. Even in the absence of individual consent, the right to keep personally identifiable medical information private is not absolute and must be balanced against other ethical principles and rules. The question is how this balance is undertaken.

TABLE 5.6 Justificatory Conditions

Effectiveness: Is the action likely to accomplish the public health goal?
Necessity: Is the action necessary to override the conflicting ethical claims to achieve the public health goal?
Least infringement: Is the action the least restrictive and least intrusive?
Proportionality: Will the probable benefits of the action outweigh the infringed moral norms and any negative effects?
Impartiality: Are all potentially affected stakeholders treated impartially?
Public justification: Can public health officials offer public justification that citizens, and in particular those most affected, could find acceptable in principle?
Data from: Childress JF, Faden RR, Gaare RD, et al. Public Health Ethics: Mapping the Terrain. *Journal of Law, Medicine, & Ethics* 2002;30(2):169–177, at 172.

Evaluating the surveillance program as a *means*, rather than an end in itself, presupposes the legitimacy of a specific public health goal, not simply public health or population health in general terms or the rhetorically powerful language of "epidemic." NYC's broad, overall goal is legitimate and important—addressing uncontrolled or poorly controlled diabetes. This is a major health problem for NYC and beyond. Hence, there is a specific, defined, legitimate public health goal in terms of which we can assess the surveillance program to determine whether it can pass rigorous ethical review. But the justification will also depend on the actions that will follow from the data and information derived through the surveillance—the data and information will not be sufficient by themselves.

Critics contend that the surveillance program is not likely to be effective overall because it involves report and notification *without* additional resources for prevention and treatment services. It also seeks to address uncontrolled or inadequately controlled diabetes of persons who are already, to some extent, in the healthcare system, but does not identify persons with undiagnosed diabetes or prediabetes, another large population. The goal, as we earlier quoted Frieden, is "to help strengthen ... physicians' efforts to better manage their patients, and to empower patients with more information."[42 (p. 6)] (This goal, in contrast to getting a picture of the scope of the problem, entails the use of information with identifiers.) The main burden of the program falls on the patients, with uncontrolled or poorly controlled diabetes, who receive the warning information. In effect, critics charge, a nagging system has been put in place, without sufficient attention to other sources of empowerment for diabetes control. We are not aware of any systematic follow-up evaluation.

The question of necessity focuses not merely on the surveillance program itself but on its infringement of rights of privacy and confidentiality in the absence of consent. Is the infringement of the rights of privacy and confidentiality necessary in this case? However valuable and even necessary surveillance might be in accomplishing NYC's specific public health goal, the infringement of rights of privacy and confidentiality is arguably not necessary in this case. With patients' consent there would be no breach of rights of privacy and confidentiality—patients could voluntarily grant others access to their personal information, under the terms indicated by the requesters of consent. Of course, the process would be costly, some would not consent, and so forth.

The points about necessity also apply to the condition of least infringement. There would have been no infringement of patients' rights of privacy and confidentiality if their consent had been obtained. If we suppose for purposes of argument that infringements can be justified in this case, a further ethical question concerns the adequacy of security measures to protect personal information once obtained and entered into the registry, as well as the measures undertaken to safeguard this personal information when disclosed to healthcare providers. Strong security measures could obviate some of the potential negative effects of overriding the rights to privacy and confidentiality in the first instance. However, avoiding or eliminating the negative effects of the infringements of rights of privacy and confidentiality would not justify the infringements themselves.

A judgment about proportionality requires attention to all of the features of the surveillance program, including the probable positive and negative effects previously noted. This requires determining whether the surveillance program's probable benefits outweigh the infringed moral norms along with any negative effects of their breach to medical relationships (e.g., damage to patients' trust), many of which are somewhat speculative. A judgment of proportionality also requires attention to cost-effectiveness and cost-benefit analysis. The surveillance program cost at least $1 million to establish and there are continuing implementation costs. Early on, public health officials concluded that the "program's potential benefit and reach outweigh the potential harm to individuals" and that the early experience "suggests that the benefits will outweigh the potential harms." [36 (pp. 548, 559)] We are not aware of up-to-date cost-effectiveness and cost-benefit analyses.

Another question is whether the surveillance program is impartial with regard to potentially affected stakeholders. Even though there is no reason to challenge the surveillance program's impartiality, important questions can be raised about the program's actual (as contrasted to its intended) effects on poor people and minority groups, as we discussed earlier.

The last question concerns whether public health and other officials can offer public justifications of the surveillance program that citizens, and in particular those most affected, could in principle find acceptable. Some commentators note that broad engagement with a variety of stakeholder groups and the public was limited, at least in the early stages of the development of the surveillance proposal.[35] Later in the process, public comments were received and a public hearing was held.

Even though we have raised several critical questions about the program, reasonable people of good will may come to quite different ethical judgments about it. Our ethical framework—and other such frameworks—can help us better see and analyze the issues at stake but resolving those issues requires practical judgment and each resolution can be only tentative and provisional. This case study is particularly important because it illustrates the complexity of ethical analysis and reasoning in real-world cases with complex features, involving a wide range of ethical considerations.

In sum, in determining whether a public health policy or practice that infringes privacy and confidentiality, without consent, is ethically justifiable, all things considered, there are several relevant factors. The first factor is the importance of the specific goal itself (public health or population health, along with the avoidance or reduction of social and economic burdens); whether the surveillance program would probably realize the goal; whether the infringement of rights of privacy and confidentiality is necessary, is proportionate, and is the least intrusive means consistent with realizing the goal; whether adequate security measures are in place to protect personal information (which would minimize the negative effects of overriding the rights of privacy and confidentiality); whether the program is impartial; and so forth.

PUBLIC DISCLOSURE OF SURVEILLANCE DATA

Questions sometimes arise about the disclosure of surveillance data: How much should be disclosed to whom, including the public, and when? An example of the controversies that may arise comes from the outbreak of the deadly bacterium *Klebsiella pneumoniae* at the National Institutes of Health's (NIH) 234-bed research facility in Bethesda, Maryland, in 2011–2012.[46] The outbreak started with the arrival of a New York patient who needed a lung transplant; by the time it apparently ended in September, 2012, the superbug had infected a total of 18 patients, many already very ill, and caused or contributed to 12 deaths, seven of which were considered to be directly caused by the bacterium.[46] The public was not notified about this outbreak, and Montgomery County officials, including public health officials, did not learn about it until NIH researchers published a scientific article in August 2012. Factors in the nondisclosure included the following: The NIH determined that there was minimal risk to the public; this infection does not appear on the list of infections notifiable to the CDC; and, as a federal facility, NIH is not licensed by the state of Maryland. Nevertheless, as information about the outbreak emerged over a year after its first appearance, some NIH employees, as well as residents and workers near the NIH campus, protested the lack of notification. As a result of this controversy, the NIH engaged in discussion with Montgomery County and the state of Maryland and reached an agreement to consult with the Maryland Department of Health and Mental Hygiene about any infection cluster or outbreak at the clinical center and to inform the state and county health departments about any cases the state deems to represent public health risks.[46] The NIH also agreed to alert the county when patients in its clinical center have communicable diseases, such as measles, that could create a risk for county residents or workers. This cooperative agreement is an effort to address the major concerns of public health and other officials in the state and county and the public itself. As reported, this agreement does not appear to address another important question: Whether there is also an obligation to disclose to patients and their families, as well as prospective patients, the spread of an infectious agent in the facility. Arguably there is such an obligation.

Disclosures of surveillance data are legally required in some circumstances. In addition, some disclosures can be based on and justified by a risk assessment that considers the probability of harm's occurrence and the magnitude of that harm if it does occur. In the absence of legal obligations to disclose this particular outbreak—for reasons noted above—the NIH determined that the risk was not significant enough to warrant disclosure to public health and other officials or to the public in the vicinity. If the risk had been significant, disclosure of the relevant data presumably would not have required the use of personally identifying information and thus would not have infringed any ethical principles, even in the absence of individual consent.

CONCLUSIONS

This chapter has examined surveillance as the first tool in public health—the "foundation" or "eyes"—because it generates the information necessary for a variety of interventions. By itself surveillance is not sufficient for public health—its value depends on the uses of the information that is generated. And those intended and probable uses in part justify the surveillance. Using human data without personal identifiers can obviate some of the ethical problems associated with privacy and confidentiality; however, personal identifiers are sometimes essential for public health purposes. It is not a violation of ethical rights of privacy and confidentiality to collect, analyze, store, use, and share personal health-related information if the individual source has given his or her consent. In public health, however, consent is not always possible, may lead to less complete information, and is time consuming and costly.

We focused attention on two major and controversial cases. One used surveillance in a research context: the CHEERS study. The other involved surveillance in public health practice: NYC's program to control diabetes, a noncommunicable disease, through obtaining identifiable information about individuals' diabetes control without their consent. The latter case in particular reveals the wide array of arguments about privacy, confidentiality, and consent in the context of public health surveillance and provides an opportunity to consider possible ways to reduce the salient ethical problems in surveillance in public health practice.

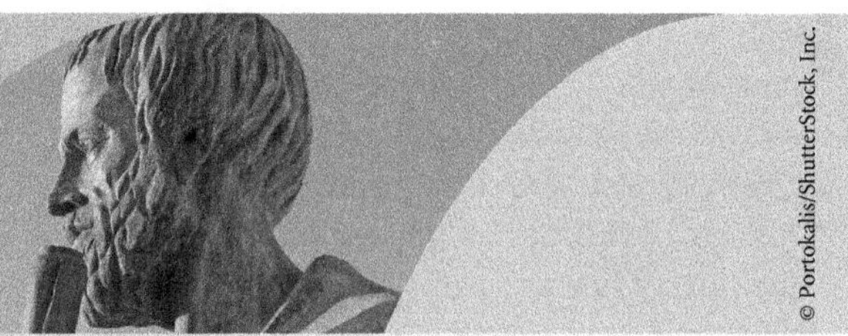

Discussion Questions

1. What are the distinctions and relations between privacy and confidentiality?
2. How important are these principles and values in the context of public health surveillance?
3. What are the respective advantages and disadvantages in public health surveillance of using anonymous or anonymized data versus data with personal identifiers?
4. Do you believe the ethical problems identified in the CHEERS study were serious enough to cancel the study? Why or why not?
5. In view of the conflicting arguments about the NYC diabetes surveillance program, do you believe that it is ethically justified? If not, what changes would make it ethically acceptable? In particular, should there have been consent (either opt-in or opt-out) for sending test results to the public health department and registry?

REFERENCES

1. Dillow C. How the largest health surveillance system ever created is preventing an Olympic-size pandemic: How do you tell if a flu is dangerous enough to bring down the Olympics? Map diseases in real-time, throughout the entire country. *Popular Science*, 08/03/12. Available at: http://www.popsci.com/science/article/2012-07/how-it-works-worlds-largest-health-surveillance-system (accessed August 12, 2012).

2. Lee LM, Heilig CM, White A. Ethical justification for conducting public health surveillance without patient consent. *American Journal of Public Health*, 2012;102:38–44.

3. Centers for Disease Control and Prevention. *Policy 557. Distinguishing Public Health Research and Public Health Nonresearch.* CDC-SA-2010-02. Date of Issue: 07/29/2010 (This supersedes the *Guidelines for Defining Public Health Research and Public Health Non-research,* revised October 1999.) Available at http://www.cdc.gov/od/science/integrity/docs/cdc-policy-distinguishing-public-health-research-nonresearch.pdf (accessed August 7, 2013).

4. Buehler JW. Introduction. In: Centers for Disease Control and Prevention, CDC's Vision for Public Health Surveillance in the 21st Century. *Morbidity and Mortality Weekly Report*, 2012;61(Suppl):1–2.

5. Garcia-Abreu A, Halperin W, Danel I. *Public Health Surveillance Toolkit: A Guide for Busy Task Managers.* Washington, DC: The World Bank, 2002.

6. Teutsch SM. Considerations in planning a surveillance system. In: Lee LM, Teutsch SM, Thacker SB, St. Louis, ME (eds.) *Principles and Practice of Public Health Surveillance*, 4th ed. New York: Oxford University Press, 2010:18–23.

7. Presidential Commission for the Study of Bioethical Issues. *Safeguarding Children: Pediatric Medical Countermeasure Research.* Washington, DC: Presidential Commission for the Study of Bioethical Issues, 2013.

8. United States Government Accountability Office. *Emerging Infectious Diseases: Review of State and Federal Disease Surveillance Efforts.* Washington, DC: Government Accountability Office, 2004.

9. Hall HI, Correa A, Yoon PW, Braden CR. Lexicon, definitions, and conceptual framework for public health surveillance. In: Centers for Disease Control and Prevention, CDC's Vision for Public Health Surveillance in the 21st Century. *Morbidity and Mortality Weekly Report*, 2012;61(Suppl):10–14.

10. Thacker SB. Historical development. In: Lee LM, Teutsch SM, Thacker SB, St. Louis, ME (eds.). *Principles and Practice of Public Health Surveillance*, 4th ed. New York: Oxford University Press, 2010:1–17.

11. Thacker SB, Qualters JR, Lee LM. Public health surveillance in the United States: Evolution and challenges. In: Centers for Disease Control and Prevention, CDC's Vision for Public Health Surveillance in the 21st Century. *Morbidity and Mortality Weekly Report*, 2012;61(Suppl):3–9.

12. Fairchild AL, Bayer R, Colgrove J. Privacy, democracy and the politics of disease surveillance. *Public Health Ethics*, 2008;1:30–38.

13. Fairchild AL, Bayer R, Colgrove J. *Searching Eyes: Privacy, the State, and Disease Surveillance in America.* Berkeley, CA: University of California Press, and New York: The Milbank Fund, 2007.

14. Glynn MK and Backer LC. Collecting public health surveillance data: creating a surveillance system. In: Thacker SB. Historical Development. In: Lee LM, Teutsch SM, Thacker SB, St. Louis, ME (eds.) *Principles and Practice of Public Health Surveillance*, 4th ed. New York: Oxford University Press, 2010:44–64.

15. Rein DB. Economic and policy justification for public health surveillance. In: Lee LM, Teutsch SM, Thacker SB, St. Louis, ME (eds.) *Principles and Practice of Public Health Surveillance,* 4th ed. New York: Oxford University Press, 2010:32–43.

16. Kelle, A. Securitization of international public health: implications for global health governance and the biological weapons prohibition regime. *Global Governance*, 2007;13:207.

17. Annas, GJ, Mariner WK, Parmet WE. *Pandemic Preparedness: The Need for a Public Health—Not a Law Enforcement/National Security—Approach.* New York: American Civil Liberties Union, 2008.

18. Verity C, Nicoll A. Consent, confidentiality, and the threat to public health surveillance. *British Medical Journal*, 2002;324:1210–1203.

19. Gostin L. *Public Health Law: Power, Duty, Restraint*, 2nd ed. Berkeley, CA: University of California Press, 2008.

20. Department of Health and Human Services. Code of Federal Regulations. Title 45: Public Welfare, Part 46, Protection of Human Subjects (45 *C.F.R* 46.102(d). Available at http://www.hhs.gov/ohrp/humansubjects/guidance/45cfr46.html (accessed August 7, 2013).

21. National Commission for the Protection of Human Subjects of Biomedical and Behavioral Research. *The Belmont Report: Ethical Principles and Guidelines for the Protection of Human Subjects of Research.* DHEW Publication No. (OS) 78-0012. September 30, 1978. Available at http://www.hhs.gov/ohrp/archive/nationalcommission.html (accessed August 7, 2013).

22. Jones JH. *Bad Blood.* New York: Free Press, 1993.

23. Summary of Notifiable Diseases—United States, 2010. *Morbidity and Mortality Weekly Report*, 2012;59(3):1–111.

24. Hodge JG Jr. An enhanced approach to distinguishing public health practice and human subjects research. *The Journal of Law, Medicine, and Ethics*, 2005;33(1):125–141.

25. Department of Health and Human Services. Code of Federal Regulations. Title 45: Public Welfare, Subchapter C, Administrative Data Standards and Related Requirements, Parts 160 and 164 (45 *C.F.R.* 160 and 164). Available in simplified form at http://www.hhs.gov/ocr/privacy/hipaa/administrative/combined/hipaa-simplification-201303.pdf (accessed August 7, 2013).

26. Fairchild AL, Bayer R. Ethics and the conduct of public health surveillance. *Science*, 2004;304:631–632.

27. Rubel A. Justifying public health surveillance: basic interests, unreasonable exercise, and privacy. *Kennedy Institute of Ethics Journal*, 2012;22:1–33.

28. Middaugh JP, Hodge JG, and Cartter ML. The ethics of public health surveillance (Letter to the Editor). *Science*, 2004;304:681–682.

29. Fairchild AL, Bayer R. Response (to Letter to Editor). *Science*, 2004;304:683.

30. Stokstad E. EPA criticized for study of child pesticide exposure. *Science*, 2004;306:961.

31. Resnik DB, Wing S. Lessons learned from the Children's Environmental Exposure Research Study. *American Journal of Public Health*, 2007 (March);97(3):414–418.

32. National Research Council, Committee on the Use of Third Party Toxicity Research with Human Research Participants. *Intentional Human Dosing Studies for EPA Regulatory Purposes: Scientific and Ethical Issues.* Washington, DC: The National Academies Press, 2004.

33. Beauchamp TL and Childress JF. *Principles of Biomedical Ethics*, 7th edition. New York: Oxford University Press, 2013.

34. Emanuel EJ, Wendler D, Grady C. What makes clinical research ethical? *JAMA*, 2000;283:2701–2711

35. Fairchild AL. Diabetes and disease surveillance. *Science*, 2006;313:175–176.

36. Chamany S, et al. Tracking diabetes: New York City's A1C registry. *Milbank Quarterly*, 2009;87(3):547–570.

37. Centers for Disease Control and Prevention. *2011 National Diabetes Fact Sheet.* http://www.cdc.gov/diabetes/pubs/factsheet11.htm (accessed December 31, 2012).

38. Frieden TR. New York City's diabetes reporting system helps patients and physicians [Letter to the Editor]. *American Journal of Public Health*, 2008;98:1543–1544.

39. Goldman J, Kinnear S, Chung J, Rothman DJ. New York City's initiative on diabetes and HIV/AIDS: Implications for patient care, public health, and medical professionalism. *American Journal of Public Health*, 2008;98:16–19.

40. Mariner WK. Mission creep: Public health surveillance and medical privacy. *Boston University Law Journal*, 2007;87:347–395.

41. Goldman H. New York City to register, monitor 500,000 diabetics (Update 3). *Bloomberg News*, December 14, 2005. http://www.bloomberg.com/apps/news?pid=newsarchive&sid=aJn10Kwi_MVg (accessed April 13, 2013).

42. *Public Hearing on Intention to Amend Articles Article 13 of the New York City Health Code.* August 16, 2005. Available at the following website: http://www.stopnyca1ctracking.org/downloads/nyc-a1c-hearing-08162005.PDF.

43. Fairchild AL. Commentary: Beyond historical precedent. *The Milbank Quarterly*, 2009;87.

44. [Editorial] Monitoring diabetes treatment in New York City. *The Lancet*, 2006;367(9506):183.

45. Association of American Physicians and Surgeons, Inc. *Letter to the New York City Department of Health and Mental Hygiene.* April 17, 2005. http://www.aapsonline.org/confiden/schlafly-8-16-05.php (accessed December 31, 2012).

46. Sun L. Montgomery, Md. to be told of outbreaks. *The Washington Post*, November 22, 2012, pp. B2 and B5.

© Portokalis/ShutterStock, Inc.

CHAPTER 6

Case Finding: Screening, Testing, and Contact Tracing

by Alan L. Melnick

LEARNING OBJECTIVES

By the end of this chapter, the reader will be able to

- Understand the nature and purposes of public health screening and of case contact tracing and notification.
- Distinguish the goals of primary and secondary prevention
- Effectively use a framework of ethical decision making for cases of newborn screening and case contact tracing
- Describe and employ the justificatory conditions for public health interventions that restrict individual liberties, such as mandated screening and contact notification
- Analyze and assess the key ethical issues raised by screening and treating pregnant women, for instance, for HIV infection.
- Analyze and assess the key ethical issues raised by contact investigation and partner contact for individuals infected with HIV and syphilis

INTRODUCTION

As healthcare has evolved from a wholly curative to a preventive approach, screening, case contact tracing, and case contact notification have become routine parts of medical and public health practice. Screening, tracing, and contact notification involve the detection of a disease, the detection of risk factors for a disease, the detection of exposure to a disease or the notification of a person exposed to a disease early enough so that clinical intervention can prevent or mitigate adverse health outcomes. Commonly, the person receiving screening or notification has no symptoms, is unaware of risk factors or is unaware of exposure. Screening methods can include specific questions, specific items on physical examination, and diagnostic tests.[1]

Primary prevention includes screening programs accompanied by clinical or community-based interventions, such as case contact notification, that can prevent a condition or disease from ever occurring. For example, screening for sexual risk behaviors combined with counseling to reduce the identified risk behaviors can prevent the acquisition of sexually transmitted disease. Alternatively, with secondary prevention, screening can identify a disease early in its course, before it becomes symptomatic, and allow clinical interventions that modify the disease process to prevent symptoms and complications. For example, questioning patients about potential substance abuse, measuring blood pressure, performing microbiologic tests for sexually transmitted disease, and diagnostic examinations to detect cancer, such as mammography or colonoscopy, can lead to clinical interventions that prevent complications and even death from these conditions. One goal of primary and secondary prevention is to reduce the need for and cost of tertiary prevention, which involves clinical interventions that modify the disease process that has already progressed and mitigate the consequences of late stage disease outcomes, such as functional loss due to stroke.

To be effective, primary and secondary prevention screening programs and the diseases screened for must meet several criteria. First, the disease the screening addresses should be common and severe. If the disease is rare, screening large populations might be costly yet ineffective in improving overall population health. For example, although men can get breast cancer, the disease is so rare in men that offering mammography to men would incur a great expense yet would do little toward improving male health outcomes or life expectancy. Likewise, if the disease is common but mild, screening for the disease or its attendant risk factors might not do much to improve individual or community health. Secondly, any method used for screening should be accurate. Screening methods that too frequently fail to identify risk factors or early disease (false negatives) or conversely that too frequently positively identify risk factors or early disease when they're not present (false positives) can either provide a false sense of security or lead to unnecessary anxiety and unnecessary, yet potentially harmful, follow-up evaluations. Preventive or treatment measures available at the time of screening or case contact notification, before persons screened or exposed have symptoms, must also be more effective than measures available later, when symptoms or complications develop. In addition, the screening tests and preventive measures available must be safe, and the cost of screening, tracing, or contact notification must be low enough to justify any potential benefits.[1]

Many public health officials and healthcare reform advocates believe that screening, tracing, and case contact notification programs directed at primary and secondary prevention can reduce healthcare costs by preventing diseases and their costly complications. Consequently, state governments, businesses, and health insurers are beginning to implement primary and secondary prevention strategies that include screening activities. For example, using health information technology, Kaiser Permanente was able to increase colorectal cancer screening among its members.[2] However, the claims of cost savings are not without controversy. Some studies have shown that while preventing illness can sometimes save money, in other cases it can increase healthcare costs.[3] One reason is that screening programs directed at even relatively common diseases must target many more people than those with either early disease or risk factors for the disease. For example, screening large populations for cancer and treating those with early disease can be more costly than doing nothing.[2, 3]

In this chapter, we will first describe two examples of preventive services, newborn screening and case contact tracing and notification. Next, we will present two case studies illustrating the use of ethical analysis in helping public health officials make better decisions regarding case finding, screening, contact tracing, and contact notification. The first case involves screening and coerced treatment for a pregnant woman infected with HIV. The second case involves contact investigation and contact (partner) notification for an individual infected with HIV and syphilis. In each case study, we will illustrate a three-step decision-making framework, which includes an analysis of the ethical issues, an evaluation of the ethical dimensions of public health options, and the justification for choosing one particular public health action. Using the framework, this chapter will focus on debates about whether, which, and when public health interventions that restrict civil liberties, such as mandated screening, treatment, or contact notification, are necessary to protect the public, what public health officials should consider when contemplating restrictive measures, and what processes they should use to justify their decisions and promote trust. The chapter will also address how officials, using ethical analysis, can recognize whether alternative less restrictive measures are available, whether proposed measures disproportionately affect specific and vulnerable populations, and how they can include relevant stakeholders in their decision-making process. This ethical analysis can also help public health officials determine when and which laws and regulations are ethically justifiable for mandating screening, treatment, and contact tracing and notification.

NEWBORN SCREENING

Newborn Screening (NBS) programs are examples of secondary prevention activities promoted to improve health, prevent disease, and save healthcare costs. NBS programs developed over 50 years ago, following development of a test for phenylketonuria (PKU), a genetic metabolic condition that causes severe developmental delay. If identified early, eliminating phenylalanine from the infant's diet can prevent symptoms and complications. PKU is a very rare disorder, occurring in about 1/15,000 individuals.[4] The screening test is easy to perform, requiring only a small sample of blood taken from the newborn's heel. Newborns with positive screening tests receive confirmatory testing to determine whether the tests are true positives, and if so, they receive referral for treatment. Treatment involves feeding the infant phenylalanine-free medical formula as soon as possible after birth and having the individual maintain a low-protein diet for life. Although newborn screening for PKU has nearly eliminated adverse neurologic outcomes from PKU, there is some evidence that treated individuals have a higher incidence of neuropsychological problems.[4] Newborn screening for PKU began as a voluntary program in one state. Based on the effectiveness of the NBS program for PKU, technological advances, and due to strong advocacy and lobbying efforts from organizations such as the National Association for Retarded Children (NARC), now known as the ARC (Association for Retarded Citizens), over time NBS programs expanded to other states and began to cover many other inherited and congenital disorders. In addition, most states began to mandate the testing without requiring parental consent.[5]

Today, all states have NBS programs that provide initial testing and some follow-up. All 50 states and the District of

Columbia test for PKU, sickle cell disease, congenital hypothyroidism, and galactosemia, but vary somewhat in other conditions they screen for and the specific follow-up they provide, such as diagnostic services, case management, and education. In addition, states vary by how much families of the screened newborns pay for the cost of the NBS program. Almost all states mandate the screening and do not obtain consent from the parents. Most states allow parents to opt out of screening, but in reality, few parents do so, and many do not know they have that option.[5, 6] Today, 48 states have mandatory NBS programs, although in most states, some or all parents may opt out.[6 (p. 302)]

As NBS programs have expanded in scope, critics have raised concerns over mandated screening, particularly concerns about opportunity costs, effectiveness evidence, and parental rights. Opportunity costs are concerning because states choosing to screen entire populations for rare diseases sometimes draw funding away from other preventive programs that might be more cost effective. For example, following NBS advocacy efforts, Mississippi expanded NBS from five disorders to 40, and created teams in nine state districts to manage cases with abnormal results. Because funding came from a fee for each newborn screened, Mississippi doubled the fee to cover the expanded testing. Given that Medicaid covered more than half of the births in the state, most of the funding for the NBS expansion came from Medicaid funds. At the same time Mississippi expanded NBS, it cut Medicaid funding by increasing eligibility requirements and eliminating some programs. Also at the same time, while the NBS program identified a small number of infants with inherited and congenital disorders, it suffered a significant increase in infant mortality. While there is no evidence pointing to a connection between Medicaid cuts and the increase in infant mortality, it is clear that decisions to fund screening programs should consider their opportunity costs and the potential stakeholders involved. For example, decision makers should consider that limited funds could be used to fund other needed preventive services, such as asthma control and prevention, car seat programs, or smoking cessation and prevention for pregnant women.

Before the rapid expansion of NBS programs, states often justified the use of public health powers to mandate screening based on the Wilson–Jungner criteria, which require that the condition screened for should be an important health problem, the natural history of the disease should be well understood, there should be a suitable test, the test should be acceptable to the population, and there should be an accepted treatment and agreed-upon policy regarding who should receive treatment.[6, 7] As new technologies have expanded the number of inherited and congenital problems addressed by NBS, critics have pointed out that these conditions are less likely to be met. Not meeting these criteria can present the potential for harm for the infants and their families. For example, increasing the number of conditions screened for, especially for rare conditions, increases the likelihood of false positives. False-positive results can cause unnecessary psychological and emotional trauma for the families involved, require additional costly diagnostic testing, and result in unnecessary and expensive treatment. Without understanding of the natural history of some rare diseases, and without evidence on treatment effectiveness, infants can be subjected to ineffective and unnecessary treatment. For example, Wisconsin identified over 20 Hmong children with a rare genetic enzyme deficiency and treated them with restrictive diets, only to discover later that the "disorder" was actually a normal variant requiring no treatment at all.[6]

The uncertainties surrounding opportunity costs, test accuracy, and its attendant risk for false-positive results, and the lack of evidence of treatment effectiveness for newly added conditions, highlight the concerns about requiring parental consent for NBS. There are alternatives to mandated screening. For example, pilot programs could offer voluntary screening for newly identified conditions, which could help generate evidence for effectiveness and inform decisions regarding whether it should be mandated later. Alternatively, for newly identified conditions, rather than screen in the hospital after birth, physicians can offer the screening in the office after clinical consultation and after obtaining consent. States could make screening available to all newborns, but on a voluntary basis with informed consent.

Opponents to voluntary consent for NBS have raised concerns about costs and time involved, whether the parents would act in their infants' best interests, and whether the consent would be perfunctory. However, a 1978 study in all 39 Maryland hospitals with obstetrical units revealed that these concerns were not justified. Two-thirds of the nurses surveyed noted that obtaining consent or refusal took between 1 and 5 minutes,[8] and over a 1-year period, only 27 of 50,000 mothers refused testing. Researchers were able to find seven who refused, and discovered that they did not understand the purpose of screening. Two of the seven did not speak English, and one later consented to the screening during a pediatric visit.[6] In addition, the researchers found that the mothers who gave informed consent had a higher knowledge score than those given a standard form.[9]

One author has suggested a two-tiered approach, using opt-out or opt-in consent. With opt-in consent, often used with vaccination programs, the screening or treatment will occur unless the parents actively refuse. With opt-in consent, the screening is offered but will not occur without the parents' consent. The two-tiered approach for NBS would use opt-out consent for known conditions that meet the Wilson–Jungner criteria, and an opt-in consent for newly identified conditions for which evidence was lacking and the benefits and risks of testing were less clear.[6]

CASE CONTACT TRACING AND CONTACT (PARTNER) NOTIFICATION

Case contact tracing, combined with case contact notification, involves screening of a population to detect diseases, risk factors for diseases or disease exposures early enough so that clinical intervention can prevent or mitigate adverse health outcomes. In this case, the diseases are sexually transmitted infections, including but not limited to HIV, syphilis, gonorrhea, chlamydia, and hepatitis B, and the contacts are partners of the sexually transmitted disease cases. These conditions are notifiable in most if not all states, which means that healthcare providers, laboratories, and hospitals identifying these conditions must notify public health officials. When health officials learn of an individual with a sexually transmitted infection (STI), they can use contact tracing to discover the identities of that individual's sexual contacts (and, in cases of HIV or hepatitis B, needle-sharing contacts as well).

Partner notification involves sharing exposure information with the individual's identified contacts so they understand their risk of either already being infected or acquiring the disease. Partner notification has been an accepted part of public health law and practice throughout the 20th century and has recently expanded to include a range of services such as counseling and medical treatment. Consequently, preferred terminologies have evolved such as *partner notification support services* (PNSS)[10] and, for HIV, *partner counseling and referral services* (PCRS).[11]

The goal of contact investigation and partner notification, supported by the ethical justification that sexual partners would seek treatment and change their behaviors if they knew they were at risk for infection, is to reduce the incidence of STI in the community. Contact tracing evolved in Europe in the mid-nineteenth century, when authorities began tracking prostitutes and their contacts, and the practice spread to the United States in the 1930s. For both, the goal was to curb the spread of syphilis.[10]

Like for most public health interventions, there is some uncertainty about whether contact tracing and partner notification are effective in preventing the spread of STIs, including HIV.[10] For example, one 1990 study showed that partner notification efforts were helpful in controlling the incidence of gonorrhea in at-risk patients in Oregon, but not the incidence of syphilis. Authors of the study attributed their findings to the fact that patients infected with syphilis tended to have a larger number of sexual encounters, and a larger number of *anonymous* sexual encounters, than those with gonorrhea, so that it simply was not possible to track sexual partners of people with syphilis, and other strategies were needed to control syphilis outbreaks.[12] If patients infected with HIV have a large number of anonymous sexual or needle-sharing partners, attempts at partner notification may prove similarly ineffective.

Once public health officials have interviewed an individual with a sexually transmitted disease or HIV and have identified their contacts, they have several alternatives for partner notification, each with ethical challenges. The most preferable approach for ethicists, public health officials, and healthcare providers is to ask the infected individual, also known as the "index case," to contact his or her sexual or needle-sharing partners, inform them of their exposure risk, and encourage them to see a healthcare provider for testing and treatment. A new variant on this approach is known as *expedited partner therapy*, in which public health officials provide antibiotic medications to individuals with gonorrhea and/or chlamydia infections to give to their partners. While the index case loses some degree of privacy, it is done so by choice, and the index case's healthcare provider is able to maintain confidentiality. In addition, infected individuals might be willing to identify and contact more partners if they provide the notification themselves.

Of course, some individuals will not be willing or able to notify all, or even some, of their partners to advise them of risks. Instead, either the healthcare provider or, in most cases, public health officials could notify the identified partners. In these cases, healthcare providers and public health officials must decide how to balance an individual's right to and desire for privacy against the right of his or her partners to know their risks, as well as the public-health goal of decreasing the spread of STIs and HIV. With medications now available that allow patients to live with HIV as a chronic disease and even to lower their viral loads so as to decrease significantly the risk of transmission to others, it has become even more important to contact people at risk as soon as possible. Though concerns still exist, the privacy considerations are less compelling, since partners who are contacted have treatment options and will not immediately assume that the index patient is infected with, and has passed on, a disease that is a death sentence.[13]

Some states have laws giving healthcare providers permission or privilege (but not requiring them) to warn partners of infected patients about their risks without risking liability for breaching confidentiality. In these cases, the laws require the providers to notify the infected individual about their intent to notify their contact(s). Regardless of the legal issues, healthcare providers must consider the moral issue of whether the duty to warn should override the duty to maintain confidentiality for a patient who may be at risk of stigma or abuse, loss of community support, or even certain types of discrimination.

Healthcare providers have responsibilities to respect the autonomous decisions of their patients. They may even have a responsibility of nonmaleficence in not harming patients by revealing their infection status to their families or communities, which may reject or discriminate against them. However, healthcare providers might also have a responsibility to protect the health of partners of infected persons, even though the partners might not be their patients and even if their patients have not consented to such notification.

At a 1990 board meeting, the American Academy of Family Physicians suggested that "if a physician failed to convince a patient to inform a partner at risk about his or her HIV infection, the imperative that these persons be informed 'supersedes the patient's right to confidentiality.'"[13] In this case, a physician would be "ethically obligated to warn partners at risk."[13] One concern about this practice, however, is that the patients might be less likely to give permission for testing or will not follow up with their physicians if they fear that their partners will be notified without their consent.[13] In addition, healthcare providers in a busy practice might be less likely to interview their infected patients about their contacts if they are required to track down and counsel patients' partners.[13, 14]

One way to address these concerns is for public health officials to provide contact tracing and partner notification, thereby relieving healthcare providers of these responsibilities. Most if not all states already require healthcare providers to notify public health officials when they diagnose patients with syphilis, gonorrhea, chlamydia, HIV, and hepatitis B. Designating public health officials as responsible for contact tracing and partner notification may, at least in part, sidestep the issue of provider-patient confidentiality, and public health officials who are trained in counseling and partner notification may be better able to work with patients to notify their partners who are at risk. In addition, unlike private healthcare providers, the chief obligation for public health officials is protection of the entire community. Of course, public health officials implementing contact tracing and partner notification must still maintain confidentiality, and by doing so, will encourage more at-risk individuals to seek testing and cooperate with any investigation.[14]

SUMMARY: NEWBORN SCREENING AND CONTACT TRACING/NOTIFICATION

It is common in public health practice for conflicts to arise among important moral considerations. In case finding, screening, and contact tracing programs, the conflicts are often between producing population benefits and respecting individual liberty. To help determine whether promoting public health with a particular program warrants overriding conflicting values such as individual liberty, Childress et al propose five "justificatory conditions" or criteria. These are: (1) *effectiveness*—the public health program will likely realize its goal; (2) *proportionality*—the probable benefits of the program outweigh the infringed general moral considerations; (3) *necessity*—the program is essential to achieve the public health goal; (4) *least infringement*—the program is the least restrictive alternative; and (5) *public justification*—adequate public justification can be given.[15] An ethical analysis of newborn screening and contact tracing and partner notification programs using these criteria would be aided by empirical data, as well as public consultation. For example, information about parents' willingness to give consent if the screening programs were voluntary would provide evidence about whether the mandatory programs satisfy the least infringement condition.

SCREENING AND COERCED TREATMENT OF A PREGNANT WOMAN FOR HIV INFECTION

Overview of Prenatal HIV Screening and Treatment

HIV transmission from mothers to their children during pregnancy, known as perinatal or vertical transmission, was responsible for nearly all pediatric cases of AIDS (93%) reported in the United States from 1985–2005.[16, 17] In 1995, after a multicenter trial found that administering zidovudine, an antiretroviral (ARV) drug, to HIV-infected pregnant women and their newborns could reduce perinatal HIV transmission by two-thirds, the CDC recommended that all pregnant women receive counseling, testing, and if indicated, treatment for HIV.[18, 19] At that time, the CDC recommended that healthcare providers obtain voluntary consent before testing, that providers should not deny services to women testing positive, and that providers should not report women refusing testing to child protective service agencies.[19]

Implementation of these recommendations led to a dramatic decline in perinatal HIV transmission (**Figure 6.1**). By 1999, perinatal AIDS cases had declined by 83% compared

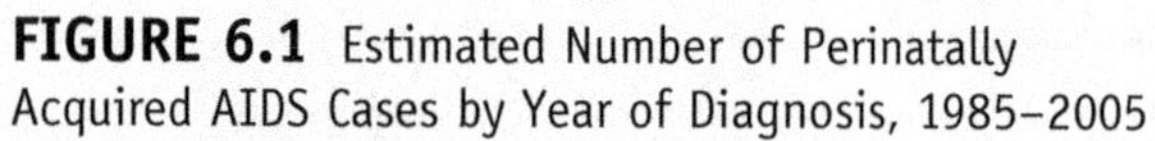

FIGURE 6.1 Estimated Number of Perinatally Acquired AIDS Cases by Year of Diagnosis, 1985–2005

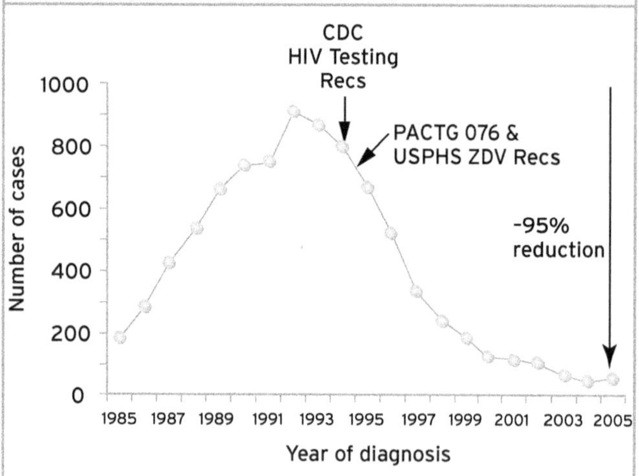

Reproduced from: Estimated Number of Perinatally Acquired AIDS Cases by Year of Diagnosis, 1985–2005 CDC Retrieved from http://www.cdc.gov/hiv/topics/perinatal/pdf/perinatal_graph2005.pdf

to 1992.[20, 21] Clearly, many healthcare providers were following the recommendations and their HIV-infected pregnant patients were accepting treatment. The screening program had met all the criteria related to effectiveness. The infection was common enough during pregnancy yet undetectable without screening, the test was accurate and inexpensive, treatment was safe yet effective in preventing transmission to the newborn, and the disease outcomes that treatment prevented were severe. However, for several reasons, perinatal HIV infection remained a significant problem affecting approximately 280–370 children each year in the United States. One reason the problem persisted was that many women—especially women at risk for HIV, such as intravenous drug users—lacked prenatal care, so they did not have an opportunity for screening and treatment.[22] In other cases, women refused testing when their healthcare providers, perhaps unaware of the universal recommendations, did not recommend screening strongly enough. In addition, some providers did not offer screening because they perceived the women to be low risk, they misunderstood the counseling requirements, or they felt that the logistics of counseling and testing were too onerous.

Consequently, the Congress commissioned the Institute of Medicine (IOM) to study the problem and make additional recommendations. The IOM concluded that many pregnant women were unaware of their HIV status for a couple of reasons. Some healthcare providers, believing that they could predict which women were at risk, failed to follow the universal screening recommendations. Other healthcare providers believed that extensive pretest counseling requirements were too onerous to employ with all of their patients. Based on these findings, the IOM recommended that HIV screening become a part of routine prenatal testing whether or not patients had risk factors and regardless of the prevalence of HIV in the community. In reinforcing previous policy, the IOM recommended healthcare providers inform women when they perform HIV screening and that women have the right to refuse (opt-out) testing.

In 1999, the CDC gathered HIV specialists and obtained public comment, including input from women living with HIV, to revise the guidelines set 4 years earlier. The resulting 2001 guidelines differed from the 1995 guidelines in several ways. The new guidelines emphasized routine, universal HIV screening in pregnancy, simplified screening by making the counseling requirement less onerous, and increased the flexibility of the consent process to allow for different types of informed consent, including oral consent. In addition, the new guidelines recommended that healthcare providers work with patients to address reasons for refusing screening and emphasized testing and treatment at labor and delivery for women who did not receive screening earlier in their pregnancies.

The new recommendations reiterated that HIV screenings should be voluntary, un-coerced, and include informed consent in language understandable to the patient. In addition, the new recommendations stated that healthcare providers should allow women to refuse screening; that such refusal should not affect the receipt or quality of care; and that women should not receive screening without their knowledge.

By 2006, national surveillance data revealed that perinatal HIV transmission had doggedly persisted, primarily due to lack of prenatal care or failure of providers to offer screening during pregnancy.[23] The CDC concluded that many of the estimated 144–236 perinatal HIV infections in the United States each year were due to lack of screening and treatment during pregnancy.[23] Earlier, recognized problems remained. These problems included language barriers, late entry to prenatal care, healthcare provider misunderstanding about universal screening and perceptions that specific patients were at low risk of HIV infection, lack of time available for counseling and testing, and onerous state regulations requiring counseling and separate informed consent.[24] At the same time, other studies revealed possible solutions. For example, studies showed that women were more likely to receive screening if their healthcare providers strongly recommended it.[28]

In addition, opt-out screening rather than opt-in screening held additional promise for preventing perinatal HIV transmission. With opt-out screening, providers would obtain HIV tests after notifying patients that they will perform the test and that patients may decline or defer testing. When doing so, providers could infer that unless patients declined, they had agreed to have the test even without explicit consent from the patients. By comparison, opt-in programs require pre-test counseling and explicit written or oral consent for HIV testing. Prenatal and STD settings using opt-out HIV screening achieved higher rates of screening compared to opt-in programs.[25, 26, 27, 29–34] Despite losing an opportunity to provide written consent, pregnant women expressed less anxiety with opt-out HIV screening and did not find it difficult to decline a test.[29, 36] A 2006 survey revealed that nearly two-thirds of U.S. adults agreed that healthcare providers should consider HIV screening no differently than any other disease screening and should not require specific procedures such as written consent.[35]

By 2006, evidence revealed that the combined approach (**Figure 6.2**) of universal screening during pregnancy, administration of ARV medication to pregnant women found infected with HIV, scheduled cesarean section delivery when indicated, and avoidance of breastfeeding could reduce perinatal HIV transmission from 25% to less than 2%.[36–40] Consequently, the CDC issued new recommendations for HIV screening during pregnancy (**Table 6.1**).

These new recommendations differed from earlier recommendations in several key ways. First, the new recommendations included universal opt-out screening. This meant that healthcare providers should (1) include HIV screening in the routine panel of prenatal screening tests; (2) inform their patients that all pregnant women should receive HIV testing; and (3) perform the tests unless the patients declined. The recommendations added that healthcare providers should perform rapid HIV testing on all pregnant women who did not have documentation of previous screening. If the rapid tests were positive, the recommendations directed providers to begin immediate ARV prophylaxis without waiting for confirmatory testing. In addition, the new recommendations directed providers to repeat HIV testing in the third trimester for all women in communities with elevated HIV/AIDS incidence or

FIGURE 6.2 HIV Diagnostic Outcomes Among Infants, by Time of Antiretroviral (ARV) Treatment, Birth Years 2007–2010 46 States

	Infected		Exposed but Not Infected	Total
Time of ARV Treatment	No.	% of Row Total	No.	No.
During Pregnancy (DP) only	2	2.7	71	73
During Labor and Delivery (L&D) only	6	3.9	147	153
Infant received ARV after birth (infant ARV) only	64	6.6	902	966
DP and L&D	3	1.6	186	189
DP and Infant ARV	13	2.9	438	451
L&D and Infant ARV	64	2.8	2,235	2,299
DP and L&D and Infant ARV	85	1.7	5,048	5,133
No known treatment	122	11.0	992	1,114
Total	359	3.5	10,019	10,378

Courtesy of the CDC.

TABLE 6.1 2006 CDC Recommendations: HIV Screening for Pregnant Women and Their Infants (CDC, MMWR, 2006/55(RR14)

Universal Opt-Out Screening
• All pregnant women in the United States should be screened for HIV infection.
• Screening should occur after a woman is notified that HIV screening is recommended for all pregnant patients and that she will receive an HIV test as part of the routine panel of prenatal tests unless she declines (opt-out screening).
• HIV testing must be voluntary and free from coercion. No woman should be tested without her knowledge.
• Pregnant women should receive oral or written information that includes an explanation of HIV infection, a description of interventions that can reduce HIV transmission from mother to infant, and the meanings of positive and negative test results, and should be offered an opportunity to ask questions and to decline testing.
• No additional process or written documentation of informed consent beyond what is required for other routine prenatal tests should be required for HIV testing.
• If a patient declines an HIV test, this decision should be documented in the medical record.
Addressing Reasons for Declining Testing
• Providers should discuss and address reasons for declining an HIV test (e.g., lack of perceived risk; fear of the disease; and concerns regarding partner violence or potential stigma or discrimination).
• Women who decline an HIV test because they have had a previous negative test result should be informed of the importance of retesting during each pregnancy.
• Logistical reasons for not testing (e.g., scheduling) should be resolved.
• Certain women who initially decline an HIV test might accept at a later date, especially if their concerns are discussed. Certain women will continue to decline testing, and their decisions should be respected and documented in the medical record.
Timing of HIV Testing
• To promote informed and timely therapeutic decisions, healthcare providers should test women for HIV as early as possible during each pregnancy. Women who decline the test early in prenatal care should be encouraged to be tested at a subsequent visit.
• A second HIV test during the third trimester, preferably < 36 weeks of gestation, is cost-effective even in areas of low HIV prevalence and may be considered for all pregnant women. A second HIV test during the third trimester is recommended for women who meet one or more of the following criteria: • Women who receive health care in jurisdictions with elevated incidence of HIV or AIDS among women aged 15–45 years. In 2004, these jurisdictions included Alabama, Connecticut, Delaware, the District of Columbia, Florida, Georgia, Illinois, Louisiana, Maryland, Massachusetts, Mississippi, Nevada, New Jersey, New York, North Carolina, Pennsylvania, Puerto Rico, Rhode Island, South Carolina, Tennessee, Texas, and Virginia.[†] • Women who receive health care in facilities in which prenatal screening identifies at least one HIV-infected pregnant woman per 1,000 women screened. • Women who are known to be at high risk for acquiring HIV (e.g., injection-drug users and their sex partners, women who exchange sex for money or drugs, women who are sex partners of HIV-infected persons, and women who have had a new or more than one sex partner during this pregnancy). • Women who have signs or symptoms consistent with acute HIV infection. When acute retroviral syndrome is a possibility, a plasma RNA test should be used in conjunction with an HIV antibody test to diagnose acute HIV infection.
Rapid Testing During Labor
• Any woman with undocumented HIV status at the time of labor should be screened with a rapid HIV test unless she declines (opt-out screening).
• Reasons for declining a rapid test should be explored (see Addressing Reasons for Declining Testing).
• Immediate initiation of appropriate antiretroviral prophylaxis should be recommended to women on the basis of a reactive rapid test result without waiting for the result of a confirmatory test.

TABLE 6.1 2006 CDC Recommendations: HIV Screening for Pregnant Women and Their Infants (CDC, MMWR, 2006 / 55(RR14) (*Continued*)

Postpartum/Newborn Testing
• When a woman's HIV status is still unknown at the time of delivery, she should be screened immediately postpartum with a rapid HIV test unless she declines (opt-out screening).
• When the mother's HIV status is unknown postpartum, rapid testing of the newborn as soon as possible after birth is recommended so antiretroviral prophylaxis can be offered to HIV-exposed infants. Women should be informed that identifying HIV antibodies in the newborn indicates that the mother is infected.
• For infants whose HIV exposure status is unknown and who are in foster care, the person legally authorized to provide consent should be informed that rapid HIV testing is recommended for infants whose biologic mothers have not been tested.
• The benefits of neonatal antiretroviral prophylaxis are best realized when it is initiated ≤ 12 hours after birth.
Confirmatory Testing
• Whenever possible, uncertainties regarding laboratory test results indicating HIV infection status should be resolved before final decisions are made regarding reproductive options, antiretroviral therapy, cesarean delivery, or other interventions.
• If the confirmatory test result is not available before delivery, immediate initiation of appropriate antiretroviral prophylaxis should be recommended to any pregnant patient whose HIV screening test result is reactive to reduce the risk for perinatal transmission.
Similarities and Differences Between Current and Previous Recommendations for Pregnant Women and Their Infants
Aspects of these recommendations that remain unchanged from previous recommendations are as follows:
• Universal HIV testing with notification should be performed for all pregnant women as early as possible during pregnancy.
• HIV screening should be repeated in the third trimester of pregnancy for women known to be at high risk for HIV.
• Providers should explore and address reasons for declining HIV testing.
• Pregnant women should receive appropriate health education, including information regarding HIV and its transmission, as a routine part of prenatal care.
• Access to clinical care, prevention counseling, and support services is essential for women with positive HIV test results.
Aspects of these recommendations that differ from previous recommendations are as follows:
• HIV screening should be included in the routine panel of prenatal screening tests for all pregnant women. Patients should be informed that HIV screening is recommended for all pregnant women and that it will be performed unless they decline (opt-out screening).
• Repeat HIV testing in the third trimester is recommended for all women in jurisdictions with elevated HIV or AIDS incidence and for women receiving health care in facilities with at least one diagnosed HIV case per 1,000 pregnant women per year.
• Rapid HIV testing should be performed for all women in labor who do not have documentation of results from an HIV test during pregnancy. Patients should be informed that HIV testing is recommended for all pregnant women and will be performed unless they decline (opt-out screening). Immediate initiation of appropriate antiretroviral prophylaxis should be recommended on the basis of a reactive rapid HIV test result, without awaiting the result of confirmatory testing.
Data from 2006 CDC Recommendations: HIV Screening for Pregnant Women and Their Infants (CDC, MMWR, 2006 / 55(RR14) http://www.cdc.gov/mmwr/preview/mmwrhtml/rr5514a1.htm

for women receiving care in facilities with an incidence of at least one HIV case per 1,000 pregnant women each year.[23] As previously stated, the new recommendations explicitly stated that the screening should be voluntary, uncoerced, and that providers should not test women without their knowledge. In addition, the recommendations stated that healthcare providers should give pregnant women oral or written information about HIV, about treatments that can reduce perinatal transmission and about the meaning of positive or negative tests, and that providers should offer women opportunities to ask questions and refuse testing.[23] (Although not the focus of this section, it should be noted that the recommendations for routine HIV testing also have been extended to all persons aged 13–64, with similar challenges in implementation in practice.)

Case Description

In one jurisdiction, a local obstetrical provider reported a positive HIV result in a 25-year-old Indonesian woman screened through the opt-out policy. This was her first pregnancy. She was 30 weeks pregnant and had been without previous prenatal care. The test results surprised her because she did not believe she was at risk for HIV, and she was unaware she had been tested. The provider consulted with specialists who recommended that she begin highly active ARV therapy (HAART) immediately and that she not nurse the baby. With the aid of an interpreter, the provider had explained the benefits and risks from HAART to the woman, who expressed understanding about what she had heard. However, the woman refused medical treatment and told the provider she intended to nurse her newborn baby. The woman was skeptical about the results, and at any rate, believed that natural remedies would suffice even if she were infected, and that natural remedies and breastfeeding would be safer for her baby than HAART. The healthcare provider asked local health officials to require the woman to undergo HAART treatment while pregnant and to require her to refrain from breastfeeding.

Ethics Framework

Step 1: Analysis of the Ethical Issues

The analysis includes the following considerations:

- What are the public health goals?
- What are the public health risks and harms of concern?
- What are the ethical conflicts and competing moral claims of stakeholders in the situation?
- Is the source or scope of authority in question? Are laws and regulations otherwise relevant?
- Are precedent cases or the historical context relevant?
- Do professional codes of ethics provide guidance?

As a first step, local health officials first need to clarify the risks or harms of concern in the situation, as well as the goal(s) of public health action. While answers to these questions often seem obvious, careful analyses may reveal separable concerns or unclear goals that limit good decision-making and cloud justification. In this example, is the public health goal primarily to prevent perinatal HIV transmission in this patient, to prevent perinatal transmission in the community, to provide appropriate care for the mother, or to provide appropriate care for the child? As in the other cases in this book, the purpose of this question is not to challenge any one goal, but rather to clarify each goal to reason about and provide justification for any public health decision.

In most settings involving a communicable disease such as HIV, the public health goals are to prevent transmission and to ensure that people with the disease receive the appropriate care. In addition, public health goals and medical goals overlap in the case of pregnant women in that both public health professionals and physicians treating pregnant women have an overlapping commitment to ensuring that appropriate prenatal care is available for pregnant women in the community, including access to many kinds of early education and counseling, as well as medical assessments and treatment, even without a risk of disease transmission.

Regarding the risks of HIV transmission during pregnancy, without the combination of drug treatment, cesarean section, and avoidance of breastfeeding, the risk of the newborn acquiring the infection could be as high as 25%. Without further treatment, the newborn infant has a 20% chance of developing rapidly progressive AIDS or death within the first year.[46] Compared to uninfected children, children born with HIV who survive past the first year have a significantly increased mortality rate and suffer a variety of ailments, including recurrent infections associated with AIDS.[46] To prevent these complications, infected children require ARV treatment, which has particular challenges for children compared to adults. For example, pediatric formulations of some drugs might not be available, the dosages must change with growth, the poor taste of some formulations as well as a lack of understanding of the infection might compromise adherence, and there are fewer drug choices for children. In addition, data on drug toxicity in childhood are limited, and children starting ARV treatment face a much longer duration of treatment with potential side effects compared to adults.[46] Given the clear benefit from ARV treatment during pregnancy, national experts continue to recommend that HIV infected pregnant women receive ARV treatment.[36]

On the other hand, allowing the woman to forgo HIV treatment during pregnancy and beyond, also has potential risks and harms for herself, the child, and the community. The woman herself is at risk for disease progression, which could ultimately compromise her ability to care for her child. In addition, if she decides later at delivery that she agrees with measures to avoid transmitting the infection to her newborn, she is at risk from complications from recommended cesarean delivery. Without effective treatment during pregnancy, high blood levels of the virus at the time of delivery increase the risk of HIV transmission to the newborn from vaginal delivery.[23, 36] By reducing the amount of circulating virus, treatment during pregnancy can avoid the need for cesarean delivery to prevent HIV transmission to the newborn. Compared to vaginal delivery, cesarean delivery—especially urgent cesarean delivery—has higher rates of complication, including postoperative infections.[36, 47]

Requiring this pregnant woman to take HAART could create potential risks and harms for the mother, the child, and the community, however. The risk and harms for the mother from requiring treatment include the side effects of HAART as well as the risks and harms related to the coercion itself. HAART side effects can include, among other things, gastrointestinal symptoms such as nausea, vomiting, and diarrhea; peripheral neuropathy, a painful condition affecting the hands and feet; liver and kidney damage; high blood sugar and blood lipids; bone marrow suppression; and an increased risk for heart disease. However, clinicians can minimize toxicity through careful monitoring and selection of alternative medications as appropriate. In addition, the required treatment would only continue for the remainder of pregnancy (postpartum treatment would be voluntary), thereby making some of these long-term complications less likely. On the other hand, development of antiviral drug resistance, if the pregnant woman started and then stopped treatment, could present another potential complication for the mother, compromising her treatment choices later.

Although data regarding adverse effects of combination ARV therapy are limited, observational studies of pregnant women receiving combination retreatment have found no differences in birth defects or low birth weight for children born to women receiving it.[36, 41, 43] However, receipt of HAART during pregnancy may increase the risk of preterm birth. In addition, available data do not provide sufficient information to address any potential long-term risk of cancer or other organ toxicities in children exposed to ARV treatment in utero.[36]

The risks and harms from coercing this woman into accepting treatment could also be significant. For example, restricting the woman or even confining her in jail or a medically suitable location in order to force her to take the medication or refrain from breastfeeding could harm both the mother and the child by separating them from each other.[36, 44] If authorities confine the woman or remove the infant from her care, the child might face risks related to foster care, such as the failure of foster parents to meet the child's medical, psychological, and emotional needs.[45] Coercive measures could also threaten the physician-patient relationship. As a result, the pregnant woman might be less likely to follow other medical and behavioral recommendations to maximize her health, the health of her fetus, and (subsequently) the health of her newborn. In addition, requiring the woman to take the medication creates a potential community risk related to driving potential cases "underground," leading to delayed prenatal care, delayed HIV identification, and delayed treatment for potentially many other women and children.[44] For example, if other women believe that they could face similar sanctions, they may choose to avoid prenatal care or refuse screening, thereby increasing the risk of poor birth outcomes and increasing the risk of HIV transmission in the community.

Prohibiting breastfeeding without separating the woman from her infant would be intrusive at the least and likely impossible. Infants feed many times daily in private settings, making it difficult to monitor whether or not the child is breastfeeding.[45] Interference or disregard of the parents' cultural values and beliefs by prohibiting women from breastfeeding their infants could present additional harm. For example, the Koran requires Islamic women to breastfeed their babies for 2 years,[45] although women can wean their children earlier if their husbands agree. Forcing an Islamic woman to wean earlier could interfere with her relationship with her baby as well as with her husband. Consequently, the woman could risk loss of housing or other support.[45]

In this case, there are several stakeholders: the pregnant woman who has an interest both in her own care and in the wellbeing of her fetus, her sexual partner, the family, the particular community, other pregnant women who might have HIV infection, and the public. The pregnant woman has expectations of freedom of movement and respect for her rights to make her own choices about medical treatment. However, these claims are not absolute, and competing moral claims could supersede them. By refusing treatment, the pregnant woman is potentially harming herself and, if she develops complications from HIV/AIDS, her ability to care for herself and her family. In addition, by not treating her HIV infection, the increased viral load could increase her chance of transmitting the infection, potentially putting any sexual partners at risk.[48, 49] In this case, the public might have a moral claim based on two expectations: (1) that the health department will protect the community from HIV infection, and (2) that people contagious for HIV and other infectious diseases will protect others by behaving in an appropriate manner, including cooperating with treatment recommendations. Furthermore, by refusing to take HAART, this pregnant woman is potentially harming her fetus, although the presumption is that she wants to take pregnancy to term and has an interest in the wellbeing of the fetus. Given that health officials disagree with her regarding the danger to her fetus and the need for medical treatment, should they require or even coerce her to take therapy while pregnant for the sake of her fetus?

This question has become more salient in the last 20 years as medical treatments, such as HAART, have become available and studies have shown their effectiveness in preventing vertical transmission of HIV. To address the question, ethicists and legal scholars have looked for older cases and arguments that deal with analogous concerns. For example, this case has similarities with other personal control measure cases (described elsewhere) in which a person is expected to take measures to avoid infecting others with an infectious disease, such as tuberculosis. In both cases, refusal of treatment or refusal to comply with some other health measure, such as quarantine, may harm another. Although a competent patient has a right to make autonomous decisions, the state clearly has the authority in some circumstances to intervene coercively to prevent transmission and offer treatment for noncompliant TB patients. While public health officials cannot force medication practically speaking, they can restrict liberty in a number of ways in order to protect others from harm.

That being said, then, can health officials override the choices of a pregnant woman for the sake of the fetus she is carrying? For some, this question may raise controversial, unresolved philosophical tensions in society about the status of and state's interest in the fetus. Court decisions, for example, have addressed the state's interest in the abortion context, and while the state's interest in the fetus is said to be compelling post-viability, the only significance of that characterization is that the state can override a woman's right to *terminate* the pregnancy. But that is not the issue here. The woman in this case intends to bring her child to term. In such cases, both the state's interest and the woman's interest in a healthy newborn are aligned all the way through the pregnancy. When considering the ethical perspectives of a case when a pregnant woman refuses medical treatment that could benefit the fetus, however, arguments presented in abortion court cases and in political forums demonstrate the tremendous and heightened sensitivity in the public to protecting the health and welfare of the unborn fetus in the last trimester.

What is at stake for the woman is (1) her autonomy to make medical decisions regarding her own treatment; (2) her parental autonomy to make decisions about the treatment of her fetus; and (3) her bodily autonomy, which limits what the state can do to override her parental decision-making autonomy because it is intertwined with her personal autonomy. A starting place for analysis is medical neglect—and the authority of the state to displace parental autonomy, even if grounded in religious belief, if the parent refuses life-saving treatment. That precedent is difficult to extend to a pregnant woman to make her accept treatment herself for the sake of the fetus, however. The woman has a nearly absolute right to refuse treatment for her own condition, even if it were life threatening. (It should be recognized, though, that there are some circumstances in which treatment can be forcibly imposed in psychiatric care, and the state's interests are accentuated if the woman is pregnant. Again, however, that is not the case here.)

While there is no case directly on point, one case on a related question held that a pregnant woman could not be compelled to undergo a cesarean section to save the fetus. In the District of Columbia Court of Appeals decision upholding a pregnant cancer patient's right to refuse a cesarean delivery surgery to save her fetus, the court determined that "in virtually all circumstances, the pregnant woman should make medical decisions on behalf of herself and her fetus."[50] An analysis concluded that physicians and health officials should respect a pregnant woman's refusal to accept HIV treatment, and that after delivery, health officials could seek a court order, if necessary, to determine the treatment the newborn should receive.[50]

Most state statutes and administrative codes give health officials the authority to conduct investigations and institute disease control and contamination control measures, including medical examination, testing, counseling, treatment, vaccination, decontamination of persons or animals, isolation, quarantine, vector control, condemnation of food supplies, and inspection and closure of facilities, or other measures he or she deems necessary based on his or her professional judgment, current standards of practice, and the best available medical and scientific information. Based on this code, and previous court rulings,[51] it is possible that health officials could compel an HIV-infected woman to accept treatment to protect her fetus.

However, regardless of whether administrative code and case law address a health officer's authority to compel HIV infected women to accept treatment, specifically stating what the health officer can do, the Public Health Code of Ethics (**Table 6.2**) provides some guidance for deliberation about what the Health Officer should do. Several of the 12 principles in the Code (Principles 1, 2, 4, 5, 6, 7, 8, 10, and 12) are particularly relevant for Step 2 and Step 3 of the framework.

Step 2: Evaluate the Ethical Dimensions of the Public Health Options

The case evaluation, directed at determining whether one or more public health decisions/actions are more justifiable ethically than other decisions, includes the following considerations with the corresponding principle(s) from the Code of Ethics (see **Table 6.3**).

State statutes and administrative codes might permit, but do not require, the health officer to order the woman to take HAART while pregnant and to refrain from breastfeeding after birth. Given the risk to the fetus from vertical transmission of HIV infection, given the risk to the newborn

TABLE 6.2 Principles of the Ethical Practice of Public Health (Public Health Leadership Society)

1	Public health should address principally the fundamental causes of disease and requirements for health, aiming to prevent adverse health outcomes.
2	Public health should achieve community health in a way that respects the rights of individuals in the community.
3	Public health policies, programs, and priorities should be developed/evaluated with community members' input.
4	Public health should advocate and work for the empowerment of disenfranchised community members, aiming to ensure that the basic resources and conditions necessary for health are accessible to all.
5	Public health should seek the information needed to implement effective policies and programs that protect and promote health
6	Public health institutions should provide communities with the information they have that is needed for decisions on policies or programs and should obtain the community's consent for their implementation.
7	Public health institutions should act in a timely manner on the information they have within the resources and the mandate given to them by the public.
8	Public health programs and policies should incorporate a variety of approaches that anticipate and respect diverse values, beliefs, and cultures in the community.
9	Public health programs/policies should be implemented in manner that most enhances the physical and social environment.
10	Public health institutions should protect the confidentiality of information that can bring harm to an individual or community if made public. Exceptions must be justified based on the high likelihood of significant harm to the individual or others.
11	Public health institutions should ensure their employees' professional competence.
12	Public health institutions and their employees should engage in collaborations and affiliations in ways that build the public's trust and the institution's effectiveness.

Reproduced from: Public Health Leadership Society (2002). Principles of the ethical practice of public health version 2.2. New Orelans, LA. PHLS.

from breastfeeding, and given the woman's refusal to receive treatment and to insist on breastfeeding, is there any justification for *not* compelling her to take HAART or to refrain from breastfeeding? On the other hand, the woman's perspective is that requiring her to comply with HAART is a violation of her autonomy and privacy and an insult to her ability to decide what is best for herself, her future child, and her infant. Given that the woman believes and states strongly

TABLE 6.3 Ethical Considerations and Accompanying Ethical Principles for Pregnancy/HIV Case

Considerations	Principle(s) Relevant for Pregnancy/HIV Case
Utility: Does a particular public health option produce a balance of benefits over harms?	1, 2, 4, 7, 8
Justice: Are the benefits and burdens distributed fairly (distributive justice), and do legitimate representatives of affected groups have the opportunity to participate in making decisions (procedural justice)?	1, 2, 4, 8
Respect for liberty: Does the public health action respect individual choices and interests (autonomy, liberty, privacy)?	2, 4, 8
Respect for legitimate public institutions: Does the public health action respect professional and civic roles and values, such as transparency, honesty, trustworthiness, promise-keeping, protecting confidentiality, and protecting vulnerable individuals and communities from undue stigmatization?	2, 4, 8, 12

Reproduced from: Public Health Leadership Society (2002). Principles of the ethical practice of public health version 2.2. New Orelans, LA. PHLS.

that her primary goals are that her baby is born and remains healthy, is there any justification for requiring her to take HAART and to formula-feed her newborn?

When deciding whether to require compliance with HAART and formula feeding, the health officer might focus his or her deliberation on the following questions the framework raises, specifically:

1. "Does the option of requiring the woman to accept HAART and formula-feed her newborn produce a balance of benefits over harms?"
2. "Are the benefits and burdens distributed fairly?"[24]

The answers to these questions would depend in part on the values and relationships in the particular context, including the degree of trust and cooperation between the pregnant woman, her family, her physicians, and public health officials, including public health nurses that might be visiting the mother at home. Given the priority or presumption for liberty over coercion in the United States, health officials would have the burden of showing that the public health value of utility overrode the liberty interest of the pregnant woman and her family and the burdens imposed on them.

When considering restrictive actions, health officials could mitigate potential harm and promote justice in several ways. They could assign a culturally competent nurse case manager to work with the patient and her family to identify and address cultural and other barriers affecting their decisions. Nurses can serve as patient advocates, provide teaching and support, and ensure that the pregnant woman and her subsequent child receive appropriate care and referrals.[52] There is no evidence in this case that the pregnant woman intends to harm her fetus or her newborn child. A skilled, culturally competent nurse could work with the woman to continue prenatal care and to try to persuade her to accept HAART treatment by listening, understanding her concerns, and emphasizing how accepting HAART treatment while pregnant and abstaining from breastfeeding could promote her child's health.[52] In addition, health officials can mitigate harm by ensuring that the woman had access to culturally proficient counseling and medical care.

Health officials can promote justice and avoid stigmatizing groups or populations by ensuring that the screening program, including the response to screening results, applies universally to all pregnant women. In the past, policies that coerced or punished pregnant women, particularly those related to screening pregnant women for illicit drug use, have raised questions about justice and fairness, because physicians and law enforcement officials have implemented them differently based on race and income.[53] For example, in the 1980s, a hospital in Charleston, South Carolina developed a policy for screening women for cocaine use during pregnancy that disproportionately affected low-income and minority women. The hospital, which was the only hospital in the state implementing the policy, was a public hospital located in a low-income community. The policy included criteria for selecting women for screening, such as women who had received late, inadequate, or no prenatal care, or women who had a history of drug or alcohol abuse. Many women not using illicit drugs underwent screening without their consent. Positive screening results prompted a report to the police, and authorities threatened prosecution for women testing positive for cocaine use unless they accepted treatment. Physicians made social service referrals rather than police reports for women testing positive for methamphetamine and heroin, drugs more likely associated with middle or upper class and white populations. Subsequently, of the 41 women arrested, 40 were African American.

This case is particularly salient because it involves an immigrant facing language barriers who was unaware she had been tested. Although the CDC recommendations for opt-out testing emphasize that the testing be voluntary, eliminating pretest counseling and a separate consent for the test might undermine the voluntary nature of the test, and might cause disproportionate application of testing.[54, 55] For example, an Arkansas study found that 16% of women tested through the opt-out policy were unaware they had been tested.[25] Healthcare providers and public health officials could consider opt-out policies that include pre-test counseling and explicit consent procedures.

It might be possible to demonstrate that either voluntary or forced compliance with HAART during pregnancy and avoidance of breastfeeding are ethically defensible options. The question then becomes, "how does one choose and justify one option over another?" Step 3 of the framework poses questions to help public health decision makers justify a particular option.

Step 3: Provide Justification for One Particular Public Health Action

Justifying the final decision when several options are available includes the following questions, with the corresponding principles from the Code of Ethics (**Table 6.4**). Choosing one option usually means that one value, such as public health benefit, overrides another value, such as individual liberty.

In public health, as in medicine, there is often uncertainty about the effectiveness of specific interventions. Compelling a pregnant woman to take HAART and avoid breastfeeding after the child is born is no exception. There is evidence that

TABLE 6.4 Justification Questions and Accompanying Ethical Principles for Pregnancy/HIV Case

Questions	Principle(s) Relevant for Pregnancy/HIV Case
Effectiveness: Is the action likely to accomplish the public health goal?	1, 2, 4, 7, 8, 10, 12
Proportionality: Will the probable benefits of the action outweigh the infringed moral considerations?	1, 2, 4, 10
Necessity: Is it necessary to override the conflicting ethical claims to achieve the public health goal?	1, 2, 4, 7, 8
Impartiality: Are the burdens and benefits of the action distributed fairly?	2, 4, 8
Least infringement: Is the action the least restrictive and least intrusive?	2, 4, 8, 10, 12
Public justification: Can public health officials offer public justification that citizens, and in particular those most affected, could find acceptable in principle?	1, 2, 6, 12

Reproduced from: Public Health Leadership Society (2002). Principles of the ethical practice of public health version 2.2. New Orleans, LA. PHLS.

HAART treatment while pregnant, cesarean section when appropriate (high viral load) and avoidance of breastfeeding can reduce transmission of HIV infection from mother to baby from about 25% to about 2%. However, it is not clear how officials could compel the woman to receive treatment, and it is not clear how they could keep her from breastfeeding. For example, we do not know how effective the threat of confinement would be to induce the pregnant woman to comply with medical measures. In addition, if health officials confined her, it is not clear how they could force her to take medication. Attempts at coercion could interfere with the physician-patient relationship, making treatment even more difficult and discouraging the woman from further prenatal care and discouraging her from obtaining care for her infant.[44, 51] The reduced trust the patient has for her provider might also discourage her from sharing health concerns with her provider, further threatening the quality of care for her and her child. In addition, other patients in similar positions might avoid prenatal care, resulting in potential adverse outcomes for other mothers and children.

If the threat of coercion during pregnancy were ineffective, some officials might consider punishing the woman for vertical transmission of HIV after the child is born, hoping that such punishment would deter other HIV-infected women from refusing HAART or breastfeeding their children. This is similar to the South Carolina policy discussed earlier, that prosecuted pregnant women testing positive for cocaine. However, there is no evidence that such a policy would be effective. If authorities imprison the woman after birth, the separation of the mother from the child could lead to poorer health and social outcomes for the child. In addition, as in the South Carolina example, some authorities might implement the policy differentially by targeting low-income and minority women, and the policy might drive the patient away from prenatal care while potentially discouraging other women from seeing prenatal care[56] or pediatric care of their children.

Health officials contemplating a coercive approach might consider the Intervention Ladder proposed by the Nuffield Council on Bioethics.[a] The ladder highlights the relationship between the degree that a proposed intervention infringes on individual freedoms and the requirement for justification of that intervention. In general, health officials can justify their actions to the extent that they will be effective while having the least impact on personal liberties. In this case, public health officials should ensure that they and the patient's healthcare providers have given the patient adequate, culturally relevant information and that they have provided access to quality prenatal and pediatric care. Incentives, such as transportation to office visits, home visits by nurse case managers, and adequate, safe housing might help. Our communities do not need jail time or other criminal punishments for women, but communities would benefit from better education, counseling, access to quality healthcare, and compassionate treatment for women with HIV who are pregnant or might become so.[56]

Explicitly addressing these questions is essential in justifying public health policy decisions, especially decisions that

[a] Nuffield Council on Bioethics report, *Public Health: Ethical Issues* (London: Nuffield Council, November 2007) Available at: www.nuffieldbioethics.org (accessed January 17, 2013).

could affect personal liberties for specific populations. Public health officials should justify policy decisions with rhetorical strategies that build not only community support and trust, but also build support and trust from the individuals and families directly affected. Certainly, even incarcerating pregnant women to get them to comply with HAART requires patient cooperation, since public health officials do not have the right to force people to take medication. In justifying their decisions, health officials might appeal to principles, rights, and duties, and by acknowledging that while a particular action overrides important values, the action is likely to be effective and the least restrictive infringement, given the situation.[57]

HIV/SYPHILIS CONTACT INVESTIGATION AND PARTNER NOTIFICATION

Overview of Contact Investigation and Partner Notification

Ever since people recognized that sexual activity could transmit disease, many of those suffering from sexually transmissible disease have tried to keep their maladies secret from their friends, partners and communities.[10] Unfortunately, these attempts at secrecy have contributed to the spread of the disease by keeping sexual partners uninformed of their exposure and by preventing public health authorities from tracking the infection and intervening to prevent further transmission.[10] As early as 200 years ago, realizing that state involvement might be necessary in controlling sexually transmitted disease, authorities began developing strategies to identify sexual contacts and notify them about their potential exposures. The moral theory supporting public health authorities in violating case individuals' privacy rights was that disclosure of the exposures would allow sexual partners to seek treatment and change their behaviors to avoid spreading the infection further. Beginning in the 18th century, public health authorities in Denmark began working with priests to notify the sex partners of people with syphilis, and by the 1940s, contact tracing, also known as partner notification, had become a responsibility of public health authorities in the United States.[58]

In most states, sexually transmitted diseases such as chlamydia, gonorrhea, syphilis and HIV are notifiable conditions. State law requires healthcare providers diagnosing these conditions to report each case to local or state public health authorities. Once public health authorities receive the reports, they contact cases and ask them to provide the names and contact information for each of their sexual contacts, and in the case of HIV, to report any drug using contacts as well.[59] To protect case privacy and to promote case cooperation, health authorities do not reveal the names of cases to their contacts. Instead, they tell the contacts about their exposures, they provide counseling and testing, and they ensure that contacts receive prophylaxis and if necessary, treatment. If health authorities determine that contacts are infected, they repeat the process by asking the contacts to provide the names and contact information for each of their sexual contacts. Health authorities repeat the process until they believe they have notified all contacts, until they have offered counseling, prophylaxis and treatment to all contacts as appropriate, and until they are unable to identify any additional contacts. While doing so, their guidelines recommend that they act professionally, without bias or judgment, at all times while acting to prevent the spread of sexually transmitted disease.[59] Because many of these infections can be asymptomatic, especially early in the course of the infection, partner notification might be the only way that contacts discover their exposure to a sexually transmissible disease.[60]

There are three types of partner notification: provider referral, patient referral, or contact referral. Having public health authorized to notify partners is a type of provider referral, in which healthcare providers rely on a third party—in this case, the local or state health department—to notify exposed contacts. Another approach to partner notification is patient referral, in which health officials or healthcare providers encourage the index cases to notify their partners. A third approach is contact referral, a hybrid of the first two approaches. With contact referral, healthcare providers or health officials encourage index cases not notify their partners, with an understanding that healthcare providers or health officials will inform exposed partners who have not come in for evaluation or treatment by a given date.

Unfortunately, evidence that any type of partner notification is effective in preventing the spread of HIV or other sexually transmitted diseases is limited.[10] As noted earlier, one 1990 study showed that partner notification efforts were helpful in controlling gonorrhea but not syphilis, possibly because patients infected with syphilis tended to have a larger number of sexual encounters, and a larger number of *anonymous* sexual encounters, than those with gonorrhea.[12] Therefore, it was not possible to reach all the sexual partners of people with syphilis, and health authorities needed other strategies to control syphilis outbreaks.[54] Likewise, if patients infected with HIV have a large number of anonymous sexual or needle-sharing partners, attempts at partner notification may prove similarly ineffective. According to the CDC, "Data are limited regarding whether partner notification effectively decreases exposure to STDs and whether it reduces the incidence and prevalence of these infections in a community."[61]

A recent systematic review found "moderately strong" evidence that contacts notified through provider referral were more likely to present themselves for evaluation than contacts notified through patient referral.[62]

Case Description

A healthcare provider notifies local public health officials about a case of primary syphilis and HIV infection in a 45-year-old married Latino male. The provider has treated the syphilis infection and has counseled the patient about HIV. During the case investigation, local health officials discover that the man, who lives with his wife and two children in a suburban county, has been having anonymous sexual encounters with men in a bathhouse located in a nearby city. The man has contemplated beginning HIV treatment, but does not want his wife to know about his HIV and syphilis infections. The man insists that he and his wife had not had any sexual relations for several years. He refuses to provide contact information for his wife or to allow health officials to contact his wife, and he has intercepted health department attempts to contact her through phone calls and mailings. The healthcare provider asks health officials to compel the man to allow health officials to notify the wife.

Ethics Framework

Step 1: Analysis of the Ethical Issues

The analysis includes the following considerations:

- What are the public health goals?
- What are the public health risks and harms of concern?
- What are the ethical conflicts and competing moral claims of stakeholders in the situation?
- Is the source or scope of authority in question?
- Are laws and regulations otherwise relevant?
- Are precedent cases or the historical context relevant?
- Do professional codes of ethics provide guidance?

As with the other cases in this book, health officials must clarify the risks and harms of concern as well as the goals of any intervention. Again, a careful analysis might identify separate concerns and unclear goals that could make it more difficult to make justifiable decisions. In this case, is the primary public health goal to prevent, and if necessary, treat HIV infection in the wife, or is the primary goal to prevent HIV and syphilis transmission in the community? The object of this analysis is not to challenge any specific goal but to clarify each goal to deliberate about and provide justification for any intervention health officials decide to take.

As in most settings involving communicable diseases such as HIV and syphilis, the public health goals are to prevent transmission and to ensure that people with the disease receive the appropriate care. Having public health staff contact the man's wife, interview her, and notify her about potential exposure to HIV and syphilis creates potential risks and harms for the man, his wife, their family, and the community. Although health officials would not report the name of the index case to the wife, if she had no other sexual contacts, she would likely correctly conclude that her husband was the index case. The resulting risks and harms to the man could therefore include loss of privacy for the man and possibly stigmatization by his wife, his family, his friends and the community. Potential risks and harms to the wife and the family include a possible increased risk of domestic violence, family dissolution with attendant loss of income and housing, and stigmatization. The community could be at risk because the man might decide to cooperate even less with health officials, denying them information about other potentially exposed contacts and refusing treatment for syphilis and HIV. If he refused treatment, his viral load could remain high, increasing the risk of HIV transmission to his wife and other sexual contacts.[63] In addition, if other men learn in similar situations heard about the case, they might less likely to come forward for screening, testing and treatment, thereby increasing the risk of transmission within the community. This is especially concerning given that many HIV-infected people are not aware they are infected.[63] The CDC has reported that up to 25% of people infected with HIV are unaware of their infection,[63, 64] with the problem even greater for men who have sex with men (MSM), with 77% of MSM in five cities unaware of their infection.[63, 65]

On the other hand, *not* notifying the man's wife could also present risks to the man, his wife, his family, and the community. It is possible that the wife is unaware of her risk for sexually transmitted disease. One reason for using partner notification strategies is that not all patients with sexually transmitted disease, including HIV, are the same, nor are all in identical social circumstances. For example, as HIV incidence has shifted from MSM to other populations, many of these new populations, especially women, might be less aware of their risks.[13, 59] Without outside intervention from partner notification programs, persons from some demographic groups, such as low-income Latina women, might not know about their risk of exposure. Compared to men, women are more likely to be monogamous, and their only risk factors might be their male partners' behaviors.[59] Consequently, women are less likely to seek testing for HIV. Additional reasons that women might not seek testing are their risks for domestic violence and loss of social support if their partners find out, and their fears about losing their children or facing stigma due to their infection.[59]

In this case, even though treated, the man is at risk of reacquiring syphilis post-treatment if his wife has the infection yet is asymptomatic and unaware. If the wife already has syphilis, she is at risk for complications from the infection if it goes undetected and untreated. In addition, if she has syphilis and is (or becomes) pregnant, her fetus is at risk for congenital syphilis. The wife, if currently uninfected with syphilis or HIV, is at risk for future exposure to both syphilis and HIV. If she already has an HIV infection, she is at risk for complications from the infection, and if she is pregnant or breastfeeding, she is at risk for transmitting the infection to the fetus or her breastfeeding child. In addition, if the wife has other sexual contacts besides her husband, these sexual contacts and their other sexual contacts in the community are at risk for acquiring either infection.

There are several stakeholders involved: the index case, his wife, their family, and the public. Regarding moral claims, the index case has expectations about privacy, respect for his freedom, and responsibility to notify his wife about her exposure, if he has exposed her, without outside interference. The wife has moral claims that could compete with her husband's claims. She has expectations that her husband notify her about his infection, particularly if he has exposed her. In addition, she has expectations that any notification, whether it comes from her husband, his healthcare provider, or health authorities, contains accurate information about any exposure risks that could affect her health, the health of her family, and the health of any possible sexual partners she might have. The wife also has expectations about privacy and respect for freedom to decide what actions to take to protect her family and any other sexual partners she might have. The public has a moral claim based on two expectations: first, that the health department will protect the community from sexually transmitted disease, and second, that people with sexually transmitted diseases such as syphilis and HIV will protect others by behaving in an appropriate manner, including practicing safe sex and by notifying their sexual partners if they have an infection.

In deliberating about what to do, health officials should consider previous cases, their scope of authority and the ethical norms and tensions within their community. Individuals infected with sexually transmitted disease have a moral duty, and increasingly a legal duty, to inform their sexual partners. The infamous case of Nushawn Williams, who exposed at least 71 women to HIV through unprotected sex, set off calls for laws prosecuting HIV-infected people for knowingly exposing others to the infection. In 1998, without HIV-specific state laws, New York authorities jailed Williams for statutory rape and reckless endangerment. Subsequently, by tying certification to receipt of funds for AIDS treatment and care, the federal government prompted every state to certify that it has criminal laws to prosecute any HIV-infected person who knowingly exposes another person to the disease. By 2000, all states had certified that they had such laws on their books.[10] By 2010, authorities continued to imprison Williams under the State's Civil Confinement Law as a "danger to society."[66] Individuals now have a legal as well as a moral duty to warn others with whom they have engaged in sexual or needle-sharing activities about the risk of transmission.

Of course, patients are not always willing to notify all, or even some, of their partners to advise them of risks. In these cases, when investigation reveals that a person with sexually transmitted disease has partners who might be unaware of their risk, public health officials must decide how to balance a patient's right to and desire for privacy against the right of his partners to know their risks, and the public-health goal of decreasing the spread of HIV. Partner notification for HIV has become more salient now that exposed persons have access to medications that can reduce their risk of acquiring the infection, and once infected, improve their health and reduce the likelihood that they will transmit the infection to others.[13]

Healthcare providers and public health officials might have a moral and even a legal duty to warn those whom they know to be at risk of acquiring sexually transmitted infections. In *Tarasoff v. Regents of the University of California*, the Supreme Court of California held that a psychologist treating a patient who had expressed his intention of murdering a particular woman had a legal duty to warn the intended victim. This case established a precedent for a legal duty on the part of any healthcare provider, in at least some cases, to warn a third party who is at risk of harm from a person that provider treated.[9] On the other hand, can a case involving violent intentions compare with a case involving consensual sexual or needle-sharing behavior? Do healthcare providers or public health officials have a duty to warn those who know that their behavior is risky or, even if they are unaware of the risks, who engage in their behavior freely?

In most states, healthcare providers have a legal permission or privilege to warn the partners of infected patients of their risks.[11] This means that providers do not have a legal obligation to warn, but they are not liable for breaching confidentiality when doing so. For example, California and New York allow but do not obligate a physician to notify a patient's sexual contacts if the physician reasonably believes a significant risk of transmission exists and if the physician believes that the patient will not warn the contacts. However, the physician must have notified the patient of the physician's intent to warn the third party. Washington State statute (RCW 70.24.105) is a bit more restrictive in that it allows healthcare providers to notify exposed persons, but only if the local health officer or authorized representative believes that the exposed persons were unaware that a risk of disease exposure existed and that the disclosure of the identity of the infected person was necessary. According to Washington State guidelines, local health officials have the responsibility to identify exposed contacts, counsel them regarding risk, and facilitate screening. In addition to partner notification, Washington State administrative code gives state and local health officials additional authority in addressing people with sexually transmitted disease who refuse to cooperate with recommendations to avoid infecting others. A local or state health officer can "issue orders for medical examination, testing, and/or counseling, as well as orders to cease and desist specific activities, when he or she knows or has reason to believe that a person has a sexually transmitted disease and is engaging in conduct endangering the public health." Local and state health authorities may issue these orders only after they meet three criteria. First, "all other efforts to protect public health have failed, including reasonable efforts to obtain the voluntary cooperation of the person to be affected by the order," second, "health officers have sufficient evidence to reasonably believe that the person has HIV," and third, "[health officers] have investigated and confirmed the existence of conduct endangering the public health." For HIV, "conduct endangering the public health means unprotected anal, oral, vaginal intercourse; sharing of injection equipment; and/or donating blood, blood products, body tissues, or semen."

These statutes and administrative codes appear to give health officials the authority to warn contacts and to require infected individuals to cooperate with recommendations. "In contrast, duty to warn statutes create an affirmative, legal obligation to warn, either directly or indirectly, when a physician knows of a third party's risk."[11] Statutes and guidelines vary by state, so whether health officials have the authority or the affirmative obligation to warn might differ by jurisdiction. While most state statutes address the health official's authority but not duty, specifically stating what the health officer can do, the Public Health Code of Ethics (**Table 6.1**) provides some guidance for deliberation about what the Health Officer should do. Several of the 12 principles in the Code (Principles 1, 2, 4, 5, 8, 10) are particularly relevant to the decision to require the man to notify his wife or to have public health staff do so, and are relevant for Step 2 and Step 3 of the framework.

Step 2: Evaluate the Ethical Dimensions of the Public Health Options

The case evaluation, directed at determining whether one or more public health decisions/actions are more justifiable ethically than other decisions, requires considering several ethical dimensions (**Table 6.5**) along with the corresponding principle(s) from the Code of Ethics (**Table 6.1**):

TABLE 6.5 Ethical Considerations and Accompanying Ethical Principles for HIV/Syphilis Contact Investigation and Partner Notification Case

Considerations	Principle(s) Relevant for HIV/Syphilis Notification Case
Utility: Does a particular public health option produce a balance of benefits over harms?	1, 2, 4, 5, 7, 8, 10, 12
Justice: Are the benefits and burdens distributed fairly (distributive justice), and do legitimate representatives of affected groups have the opportunity to participate in making decision (procedural justice)?	1, 2, 4, 8
Respect for liberty: Does the public health action respect individual choices and interests (autonomy, liberty, privacy)?	1, 2, 7, 8, 10
Respect for legitimate public institutions: Does the public health action respect professional and civic roles and values, such as transparency, honesty, trustworthiness, promise-keeping, protecting confidentiality, and protecting vulnerable individuals and communities from undue stigmatization?	1, 2, 8, 10, 12

Reproduced from: Public Health Leadership Society (2002). Principles of the ethical practice of public health version 2.2. New Orleans, LA. PHLS.

As noted earlier, most state statutes permit, but do not require, the health officer to compel the man to notify his wife or compel him to allow public health workers to notify his wife. However, given the potential risk to the wife and the community from HIV infection and syphilis, and given the index case's refusal to cooperate with partner notification, is there any justification for not compelling him to cooperate? On the other hand, the index case does not believe his wife is at risk since he and his wife are not sexually active, and therefore forcing him to comply with notification would be a violation of his rights to autonomy and privacy. Assuming this is true, is there any justification for compelling him to cooperate by ensuring either he or health workers notify his wife?

When deciding whether to require compliance with partner notification, the health officer might focus his or her deliberation on the following questions the framework raises, specifically,

1. "Does the option of compelling partner notification produce a balance of benefits over harms?"
2. "Are the benefits and burdens distributed fairly?"[57]

The answers to these questions would depend in part on the values and relationships in the particular context, including the degree of trust and cooperation between the case and public health workers, including the public health staff conducting partner notification. Leaving legal issues aside, health officials have the burden of showing that the public health value from compelling cooperation would overcome the liberty interests of a patient who might be at risk for stigma, loss of community support, and discrimination. In addition, health officials would need to consider the additional risk that other men facing similar situations who became aware of this case might choose to avoid screening, further increasing risk to the community.

When considering restrictive actions, health officials could tip the balance away from potential harm and towards justice in several ways. First, they can ensure that the public health workers involved in investigating the case and notifying partners are professionally and culturally competent, especially in working with Latino men who have sex with men. The health workers should be capable of listening effectively, understanding the case's concerns and identifying cultural and other barriers impeding the index case's willingness to cooperate. In addition, the health workers can advocate for the index case in ensuring that he receives the appropriate care and referrals. At this point, based on earlier interviews, health officials have no evidence that the index case has knowingly exposed his wife to HIV infection without her knowledge, as he has insisted that he and his wife are not sexually active. A skilled, culturally competent health worker working with the case could identify timelines and risk behaviors that might have put his wife at risk of exposure. In doing so, the health worker could help him understand the necessity for notifying his wife about her risk of exposure. Additionally, health officials can increase the likelihood of cooperation by ensuring the index case that his wife would have access to appropriate counseling, testing, and health care.

It might be possible to demonstrate that either voluntary or forced compliance with partner notification are ethically defensible options. The question then becomes, "How does one choose and justify one option over another?" Step 3 of the framework poses questions to help public health decision makers justify a particular option.

Step 3: Provide Justification for One Particular Public Health Action

Justifying the final decision when several options are available includes the questions in **Table 6.6,** with the corresponding principles from the Code of Ethics (**Table 6.1**).

Choosing one option usually means that one value, such as public health benefit, overrides another value, such as individual privacy. When overriding an important value, it is important that an action address the conditions underlying these questions.

As described earlier, there is uncertainty whether any type of partner notification is effective in preventing the spread of HIV or other sexually transmitted diseases.[11] However, based on the results a systemic review,[63] the index case's wife might be more likely to seek screening or testing following notification by health officials rather than by her husband. As public health officials weigh their alternatives, they should again consider the Intervention Ladder, which highlights the relationship between the degree that a proposed intervention infringes on individual freedoms and the requirement for justification of that intervention. Accordingly, health officials should contemplate a menu of options. Such options might start with those that infringe least on the index case's choices. For example, health officials might first provide additional information and assurance regarding confidentiality while allowing the index case to notify his wife and other sexual partners voluntarily alone or with the help of public health workers. If this proves unsuccessful at persuading the index case to cooperate, health officials could consider using incentives, such as assistance with the costs associated with obtaining screening and treatment. Health officials could also consider notifying the index case's wife without the case's knowledge or consent, but if they choose to do so, they must be prepared to identify, prevent,

TABLE 6.6 Justification Questions and Accompanying Ethical Principles for HIV/Syphilis Contact Investigation and Partner Notification Case

Questions	Principle(s) Relevant for HIV/Syphilis Notification Case
Effectiveness: Is the action likely to accomplish the public health goal?	1, 2, 4, 7, 8, 10, 12
Proportionality: Will the probable benefits of the action outweigh the infringed moral considerations?	1, 2, 4, 7, 8, 10, 12
Necessity: Is it necessary to override the conflicting ethical claims to achieve the public health goal?	1, 4, 7, 8
Impartiality: Are the burdens and benefits of the action distributed fairly?	2, 4, 7, 10
Least infringement: Is the action the least restrictive and least intrusive?	2, 4, 8, 12
Public justification: Can public health officials offer public justification that citizens, and in particular those most affected, could find acceptable in principle?	1, 2, 4, 7, 8, 10

Reproduced from: Public Health Leadership Society (2002). Principles of the ethical practice of public health version 2.2. New Orleans, LA. PHLS.

and address possible adverse outcomes for the wife, such as domestic violence, loss of income, or loss of housing. If the index case continues to refuse to cooperate, and health officials remain concerned that the case might be exposing his wife without her knowledge, officials could consider threatening the index case with restrictions, such as isolation and incarceration. However, in doing so, health officials risk their ability to gain his trust and cooperation, and become less likely to obtain information necessary to identify and protect other possible sexual partners.

Partner notification can be most effective if the index case is willing to provide health officials the names and contact information of all of his partners. This requires health officials to avoid coercive measures and to work closely with the index case. Frequently, health officials can gain cooperation and trust by promising never to reveal the name of the index patient to any partner, although in this situation, the wife is likely to conclude that her husband is the index case. However, by allowing the husband to notify his wife and other partners, rather than forcing him to do so or by doing the notification without him, and by not revealing he is infected, health officials allow him to maintain some control over the process, thereby demonstrating that they respect his autonomy and liberty. The historic effectiveness of contact investigation and partner notification has relied on voluntary cooperation and a commitment to not revealing an index case's identity.[13]

Explicitly addressing the questions in Step 3 is essential in justifying interventions that could affect personal liberties such as privacy and freedom of movement. Public health officials should justify their decisions with deliberations that build not only community support and trust, but also build support and trust from the individuals and families directly affected. In this case, using the most restrictive approach not only harms the case, but also has potential adverse outcomes for his family. In justifying their decisions, health officials might appeal to principles, rights, and duties, and by acknowledging that while a particular action overrides important values, the action is likely to be effective and the least restrictive infringement, given the situation.[57]

CONCLUSIONS

Public health interventions directed at screening and notifying otherwise healthy individuals for early disease or exposure present some of the same ethical challenges to health officials as the other interventions discussed in this book. These challenges result from the conflicting goals frequently associated with screening, contact tracing and notification, particularly screening and notification for diseases spread through intimate contact, such as sexually transmitted disease. In addition, given limited resources, a decision to fund a screening or contact notification program means less funding is available for other public health interventions. Certainly one screening goal—detection of disease or exposure early enough to prevent complications—might benefit the individual screened, but only if the individual has access to effective treatment. Contact notification goals, directed at protecting others from sexually transmitted disease, can threaten the privacy rights of those screened. Sexually transmitted disease screening and partner notification efforts clearly require balancing individual rights with community benefit. Health officials considering alternative interventions, especially interventions that restrict individual rights, must address questions about effectiveness, proportionality, necessity, and fairness when justifying their decisions to affected individuals and to the public, especially since individual cooperation is essential in preventing the spread of infection and protecting at-risk contacts. To build community trust, health officials must build support and trust from individuals and families directly affected, some of whom come from vulnerable populations, such as low-income populations or minorities, or groups already distrustful of government. Health officials can begin with an assumption that most people with sexually transmitted disease, including HIV, understand they have a duty to protect their intimate contacts, and that women, regardless of whether they suffer from HIV infection, are devoted to the well-being of their children. Attempts to force pregnant women to receive HIV screening or, if infected with HIV, to take HAART, are likely to be ineffective and difficult to enforce. In addition, such efforts could possibly encourage at-risk women to avoid prenatal care, thereby increasing the risk for poor birth outcomes and HIV transmission in the community. Likewise, efforts to force women to refrain from breastfeeding would be difficult to enforce and could interfere with family relationships, causing other adverse outcomes for women and their children. The effectiveness of partner notification programs depends on the willingness of patients with sexually transmitted disease to share information about their intimate contacts with health officials. This willingness depends on trust. By using the least restrictive interventions, by listening, and by respecting privacy and cultural differences, health officials can build support and trust that can be effective in protecting at-risk contacts and ultimately protecting the community.

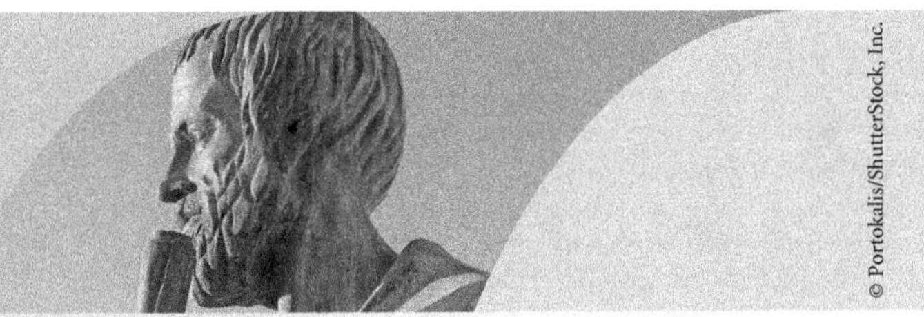

Discussion Questions

1. What should public health officials consider before adding new conditions to newborn screening programs for inherited or congenital disease?
2. When is it ethically justifiable to mandate newborn screening? What conditions need to be met?
3. When mandating newborn screening, what can health officials do to reduce any imposed burdens?
4. What are the advantages and disadvantages for mandatory and voluntary newborn screening programs?
5. When, if ever, is voluntary consent for newborn screening programs acceptable, and when should public health officials consider using an opt-in or opt-out methodology?
6. What should health officials do to increase the likelihood that women get tested for HIV during pregnancy?
7. Should testing be voluntary, opt-in or opt-out, or mandatory, and why? What should public health officials consider before mandating that pregnant women infected with HIV receive treatment?
8. What are the benefits and harms from mandated HIV treatment during pregnancy, and how are they distributed?
9. What are the benefits and harms of contact tracing and partner notification for individuals with sexually transmitted infections including HIV, and how are these benefits and harms distributed?
10. What should health officials consider when deciding to rely on individuals to identify and notify their contacts or doing so themselves?
11. How should public health officials intervene and what should they consider when they learn that individuals with sexually transmitted disease, including HIV, are engaged in risky behaviors with contacts who are unaware of their risks?
12. What process should health officials use to justify their chosen interventions? What can health officials do to mitigate the negative consequences of any restrictive interventions?
13. How can public health officials use professional codes of ethics, such as the Public Health Code of Ethics, in guiding their decision making related to screening, case finding, contact tracing, and partner notification?

REFERENCES

1. Dans LF, Asuncion M, Silvestre A, Dans AL. Trade-off between benefit and harm is crucial in health screening recommendations. Part I: General principles. *Journal of Clinical Epidemiology*, 2011;64:231–239.

2. Alliance for Health Reform. *The Case for Prevention: Tales from the Field.* Available at http://allhealth.org/publications/Public_health/The_Case_for_Prevention_90.pdf, 2009 (accessed April 26, 2013).

3. Cohen JT, Neumann PJ, Weinstein MC. Does preventive care save money? Health economics and the presidential candidates. *New England Journal of Medicine*, 2008;358(7):661–663.

4. Mitchell JJ, Trakadis YJ, Scriver CR. Phenylalanine hydroxylase deficiency. *Genetics in Medicine*, 2011;13(8):697–707.

5. Baily MA, Murray TH. Ethics, Evidence and Cost in Newborn Screening. *Hastings Center Report*, 2008;38(3): 23–31.

6. Ross LF. Mandatory versus voluntary consent for newborn screening? *Kennedy Institute of Ethics Journal*, 2011;20(4):299–328.

7. Wilson JM, Jungner G. Principles and practice of screening for disease. *Public Health Papers*, Vol. 34. Geneva: World Health Organization, 1968.

8. Faden R, Chwalow AJ, Holtzman NA, Horn SD. 1982a. A survey to evaluate parental consent as public policy for neonatal screening. *American Journal of Public Health* 72: 1347–52.

9. Holtzman NA, Faden R, Chwalow AJ, Horn SD. Effect of informed parental consent on mothers' knowledge of newborn screening. *Pediatrics*, 1983;72:807–812.

10. Gostin LO, Hodge JG Jr. Piercing the veil of secrecy in HIV/AIDS and other sexually transmitted diseases: Theories of privacy and disclosure in partner notification. *Duke Journal of Gender Law and Policy*, 1998;5(9):9–88. Available at http://scholarship.law.duke.edu/cgi/viewcontent.cgi?article=1014&context=djglp (accessed August 13, 2013).

11. Bernheim RG, Nieburg P, Bonnie RJ. Ethics and the Practice of Public Health. In: Goodman RA, ed. *Law in Public Health Practice*, 2d edition. Oxford, UK: Oxford University Press, 2007.

12. Andrus JK, Fleming DW, Harger DR, et al. Partner notification: can it control epidemic syphilis? *Annals of Internal Medicine*, 1990;112(7):539–543.

13. Bayer R, Toomey KE. HIV prevention and the two faces of partner notification. *American Journal of Public Health*, 1992;82(8):1158–1164.

14. Pottker-Fishel CG. Improper bedside manner: why state partner notification laws are ineffective in controlling the proliferation of HIV. *Health Matrix: Journal of Law Medicine*, 2007;17:147–179.

15. Childress JF, Faden RR, Gaare RD, et al. Public health ethics: mapping the terrain. *Journal of Law, Medicine, & Ethics*, 2002;30(2):170–178.

16. Centers for Disease Control and Prevention. Pregnancy and Childbirth: Perinatal HIV Transmission. Available at http://www.cdc.gov/hiv/topics/perinatal/overview_partner.htm (accessed August 13, 2013).

17. Centers for Disease Control and Prevention. *HIV/AIDS Surveillance Report, 2005.* Atlanta: U.S. Department of Health and Human Services 2006, revised 2007.

18. Connor EM, Sealing RS, Gelber R, et al. Reduction of maternal-infant transmission of human immunodeficiency virus type 1 with zidovudine treatment. *New England Journal of Medicine*, 1994;221:1173–1180.

19. Centers for Disease Control and Prevention. U.S. public health service recommendations for human immunodeficiency virus counseling and voluntary testing for pregnant women. *Morbidity & Mortality Weekly Report* 1995;44:RR-7. Available at http://www.cdc.gov/mmwr/PDF/rr/rr4407.pdf (accessed August 13, 2013).

20. Centers for Disease Control and Prevention. Revised recommendations for HIV screening of pregnant women. *Morbidity & Mortality Weekly Report*, November 9, 2001;50(RR19):59–86. Available at http://www.cdc.gov/mmwr/preview/mmwrhtml/rr5019a2.htm (accessed August 13, 2013).

21. Lindegren ML, Byers RH, Thomas P, et al. Trends in perinatal transmission of HIV/AIDS in the United States. *JAMA*, 1999;282:531–538.

22. Cooper ER, Nugent RP, Diaz C, et al. After AIDS clinical trial 076: the changing pattern of zidovudine use during pregnancy, and the subsequent reduction in the vertical transmission of human immunodeficiency virus in a cohort of infected women and their infants. *Journal of Infectious Disease*, 1996;174:1207–1211.

23. Centers for Disease Control and Prevention. Revised recommendations for HIV testing of adults, adolescents, and pregnant women in health-care settings. *Morbidity & Mortality Weekly Report*, September 22, 2006;55(RR14):1–17. Available at http://www.cdc.gov/mmwr/preview/mmwrhtml/rr5514a1.htm (accessed August 13, 2013).

24. U.S. Department of Health and Human Services. Reducing obstetrician barriers to offering HIV testing. Washington, DC: U.S. Department of Health and Human Services; 2002. Report OEI-05-01-00260. Available at http://oig.hhs.gov/oei/reports/oei-05-01-00260.pdf (accessed August 13, 2013).

25. Centers for Disease Control and Prevention. HIV testing among pregnant women—United States and Canada, 1998–2001. *Morbidity & Mortality Weekly Report*, 2002;51:1013–1016.

26. Stringer EM, Stringer JS, Cliver SP, Goldenberg RL, Goepfert AR. Evaluation of a new testing policy for human immunodeficiency virus to improve screening rates. *Obstetrics & Gynecology*, 2001;98:1104–1108.

27. Lindsay MK, Johnson N, Peterson HB, Willis S, Williams H, Klein L. Human immunodeficiency virus infection among inner-city adolescent parturients undergoing routine voluntary screening, July 1987 to March 1991. *American Journal of Obstetrics and Gynecology*, 1992;167:1096–1099.

28. Royce RA, Walter EB, Fernandez MI, Wilson TE, Ickovics JR, Simonds RJ. Barriers to universal prenatal HIV testing in 4 US locations in 1997. *American Journal of Public Health*, 2001;91:727–733.

29. Simpson WM, Johnstone FD, Goldberg DJ, Gormley SM, Hart GJ. Antenatal HIV testing: assessment of a routine voluntary approach. *British Medical Journal*, 1999;318:1660–1661.

30. Breese P, Burman W, Shlay J, Guinn D. The effectiveness of a verbal opt-out system for human immunodeficiency virus screening during pregnancy. *Obstetrics & Gynecology*, 2004;104:134–137.

31. Jayaraman GC, Preiksaitis JK, Larke B. Mandatory reporting of HIV infection and opt-out prenatal screening for HIV infection: effect on testing rates. *Canadian Medical Association Journal*, 2003;168:679–682.

32. Branson BM, Lee JH, Mitchell B, Nolt B, Robbins A, Thomas MC. Targeted opt-in vs. routine opt-out HIV testing in STD clinics [Abstract]. Presented at the 13th meeting of the International Society for Sexually Transmitted Diseases Research; July 11–14, 1999; Denver, Colorado.

33. Stanley B, Fraser J, Cox NH. Uptake of HIV screening in genitourinary medicine after change to "opt-out" consent. *British Medical Journal*, 2003;326:1174.

34. Perez F, Zvandaziva C, Engelsmann B, Dabis F. Acceptability of routine HIV testing ("opt-out") in antenatal services in two rural districts of Zimbabwe. *Journal of Acquired Immune Deficiency Syndrome*, 2006;41:514–520.

35. Kaiser Family Foundation. Survey of Americans on HIV/AIDS. Washington, DC: Kaiser Family Foundation; 2006. Available at http://www.kff.org/kaiserpolls/7521.cfm (accessed August 13, 2013).

36. Panel on Treatment of HIV-Infected Pregnant Women and Prevention of Perinatal Transmission. Recommendations for Use of Antiretroviral Drugs in Pregnant HIV-1-Infected Women for Maternal Health and Interventions to Reduce Perinatal HIV Transmission in the United States. Available at http://aidsinfo.nih.gov/contentfiles/lvguidelines/PerinatalGL.pdf (accessed August 13, 2013).

37. Cooper ER, Charurat M, Mofenson L, et al. Combination antiretroviral strategies for the treatment of pregnant HIV-1–infected women and prevention of perinatal HIV-1 transmission. *Journal of Acquired Immune Deficiency Syndrome*, 2002;29:484–494.

38. International Perinatal HIV Group. The mode of delivery and the risk of vertical transmission of human immunodeficiency virus type 1: a meta-analysis of 15 prospective cohort studies. *New England Journal of Medicine*, 1999;340:977–987.

39. American College of Obstetricians and Gynecologists. Scheduled cesarean delivery and the prevention of vertical transmission of HIV infection. *International Journal of Gynaecology & Obstetrics*, 2000;73:279–281.

40. World Health Organization. *HIV and Infant Feeding: Guidelines for Decision-Makers*. Geneva, Switzerland: World Health Organization, 2003.

41. Chou R, Smits AK, Huffman LH, Fu R, Korthuis PT. Prenatal screening for HIV: A review of the evidence for the U.S. Preventive Services Task Force. *Annals of Internal Medicine*, 2005;143:38–54.

42. European Collaborative Study. HIV-infected pregnant women and vertical transmission in Europe since 1986. *AIDS*, 2001;15:761–770.

43. Tuomala RE, Shapiro DE, Mofenson LM, Bryson Y, Culnane M, Hughes MD, et al. Antiretroviral therapy during pregnancy and the risk for an adverse outcome. *New England Journal of Medicine*, 2002;346:1863–1870.

44. Grizzi MA. Compelled antiviral treatment of HIV positive pregnant women. *UCLA Women's Law Journal*, 1995;5(2):483–500.

45. Wolf LE, Lo B, Beckerman KP, Dorenbaum A, Kilpatrick SJ, Weintrub PS. When parents reject interventions to reduce postnatal human immunodeficiency virus transmission. *Archives of Pediatric and Adolescent Medicine*, 2001;155:927–933.

46. Prendergast A, Tudor-Williams G, Jeena P, Burchett S, Goulder P. International perspectives, progress, and future challenges of paediatric HIV infection. *Lancet*, 2007;370:68–80.

47. Read JS, Newell MK. Efficacy and safety of cesarean delivery for prevention of mother-to-child transmission of HIV-1. *Cochrane Database of Systematic Reviews*, 2005(4):CD005479. Available at http://www.ncbi.nlm.nih.gov/pubmed/16235405 (accessed August 13, 2013).

48. Montaner JS, Hogg R, Wood E, et al. The case for expanding access to highly active antiretroviral therapy to curb the growth of the HIV epidemic. *Lancet*, 2006;368(9534):531–536.

49. Cohen MS, Chen YQ, McCauley M, et al. Prevention of HIV-1 infection with early antiretroviral therapy. *New England Journal of Medicine*, 2011;365(6):493–505.

50. Garber M, Hunt S, Arnold R. Ask the ethicist: Can an HIV-positive woman be forced to take medicine to protect her fetus? *Lahey Clinic Medical Ethics*, 2004:11(3):3.

51. Kaplan M. "A special class of persons": Pregnant women's right to refuse medical treatment after *Gonzales v. Carhart*. *Journal of Constitutional Law*, 2010;13(1):145–206.

52. Foley EM. Drug screening and criminal prosecution of pregnant women. *Journal of Obstetric, Gynecologic & Neonatal Nursing*, 2002;31:133–137.

53. Gostin LO. The Rights of Pregnant Women: The Supreme Court and Drug Testing. *Hastings Center Report*, September 2001:8–9.

54. Fields L, Kaplan C. Opt-out HIV testing: An ethical analysis of women's reproductive rights. *Nursing Ethics*, 2011;18(5):734–742.

55. American Civil Liberties Union. Increasing access to voluntary HIV testing: the importance of informed consent and counseling in HIV testing. Available at http://www.aclu.org/files/images/asset_upload_file473_30248.pdf (accessed August 13, 2013), 2007.

56. Sprintz H. Criminalization of perinatal HIV transmission. *Health Matrix* (Cleveland, OH), 1993;3(2):495–537.

57. Bernheim R, Nieburg P, Bonnie RJ. Ethics and the Practice of Public Health. In Goodman R, ed. *Law in Public Health Practice*, 2d ed. Oxford, UK: Oxford University Press, 2007.

58. Golden MR. HIV partner counseling and referral services finally getting beyond the name. *American Journal of Preventive Medicine*, 2007;33(2S):S89–S100.

59. Kass NE, Gielen AC. The ethics of contact tracing programs and their implications for women. *Duke Journal of Gender Law and Policy*, 1998;5:89–102. Available at http://scholarship.law.duke.edu/cgi/viewcontent.cgi?article=1015&context=djglp (accessed August 13, 2013).

60. Hogben M, Kissinger P. A review of partner notification for sex partners of men infected with chlamydia. *Sexually Transmitted Diseases*, 2008;35(Suppl 11):S34–S39.

61. Centers for Disease Control and Prevention. Sexually Transmitted Disease Guidelines 2010. *Morbidity & Mortality Weekly Report*, December 17, 2010;59:RR-12. Available at http://www.cdc.gov/std/treatment/2010/STD-Treatment-2010-RR5912.pdf (accessed August 13, 2013).

62. Mathews C, Coetzee N, Zwarenstein M, Lombard C, Guttmacher S, Oxman AD, Schmid G. Strategies for partner notification for sexually transmitted diseases. *Cochrane Database of Systematic Reviews*, 2001:CD002843.

63. Dooley SW, Douglas JM, Janssen RS. Partner counseling and referral services for HIV infection. New endorsement of an old approach. *American Journal of Preventive Medicine*, 2007;33(2S):S81-S83

64. Centers for Disease Control and Prevention. Number of persons tested for HIV–United States, 2002. *Morbidity & Mortality Weekly Report*, 2004;53:1110–1113.

65. Centers for Disease Control and Prevention. HIV prevalence, unrecognized infection, and HIV testing among men who have sex with men—five U.S. cities, June 2004–April 2005. *Morbidity & Mortality Weekly Report*, 2005;54:597–601.

66. McNiff E. 'HIV Predator' Served Time for Crime but May be Confined for Life. July 21, 2010. Available at http://abcnews.go.com/TheLaw/hiv-predator-confined-jail-officials-confined-life/story?id=11210268 (accessed August 13, 2013).

© Portokalis/ShutterStock, Inc.

CHAPTER 7

Immunization: Protection Through Vaccination

by James F. Childress

Learning Objectives

By the end of this chapter, the reader will be able to

- Participate effectively in debates about which vaccinations should be voluntary and which should be mandated in mass immunization programs
- Determine whether to add new vaccinations, such as the HPV vaccination, to the mandatory list
- Evaluate whether, how, and to what extent the government should recognize religious, philosophical, or personal objections as grounds for exemption from mandatory immunizations
- Analyze the ethical issues on both sides of the debate about whether health care workers in a hospital or nursing home should be required to get an annual influenza vaccination
- Describe and evaluate various measures, such as incentives, for ensuring compliance with vaccination recommendations
- Understand the range and balance of ethical considerations in allocating scarce vaccines in a public health crisis

INTRODUCTION

In the early part of the 20th century, public health and medicine in the United States confronted a number of serious infectious diseases. Smallpox afflicted over 21,000 persons and resulted in almost 900 deaths in 1900; measles struck almost 470,000 persons, leading to over 7,500 deaths. Thousands of diphtheria cases and pertussis (whooping cough) cases were also reported, with the former causing over 13,000 deaths and the latter causing over 5,000 deaths in 1922.[1] In response, mass or collective immunization programs represent one of the greatest achievements of public health in the 20th century. Early in the century

> just a handful of vaccines had been developed, and only one, for smallpox, was commonly used in the United States. A loose patchwork of widely varying local and state laws governed the practice, some requiring it only during epidemics, and others for students in public schools. Enforcement was often haphazard, and large segments of the population, both adults and children, remained unimmunized.[2]

This picture had changed dramatically by 2006 when James Colgrove published his *State of Immunity: The Politics of Vaccination in Twentieth-Century America*:

> ... there are more than two dozen vaccines in use, fourteen of which are universally recommended for children. Levels of coverage among youth have topped 90 percent for most vaccines, and as a result, almost all of the conditions they protect against have declined to the vanishing point in the United States.[2]

Vaccination made the list of "Ten Great Public Health Achievements—United States, 1900–1999," released by the Centers for Disease Control and Prevention (CDC).[3] Immunization eradicated smallpox and eliminated poliomyelitis in the Americas, while also controlling measles, rubella, tetanus, diphtheria, *Haemophilis influenzae* type B (which causes a type of meningitis), along with other infectious diseases not only in the U.S., but also in many other parts of the world.[1, 3]

Throughout the 20th century, Colgrove further notes, public health officials and others used various strategies "to secure the trust, cooperation, and compliance of the public." Their strategies, which were widely though not uniformly successful, involved treading carefully "between respect for individual liberty in medical matters and the need to protect the community against disease." Legislative and public health decision making was generally guided by "pragmatism and political acuity, rather than doctrinaire adherence to epidemiological theory or ethical principles."[2]

Ongoing debates about vaccination policy and practice mark discourse in and about public health ethics, particularly in relation to the public philosophy of our liberal, pluralistic, democratic society. This public philosophy is liberal in that it puts a premium on individual and familial liberties; it is pluralistic because the society has a variety of views of the good life; and it is democratic in that public policies are generally formulated or authorized by democratically elected officials.

This chapter will focus on debates about whether, which, and when vaccinations are needed; which satisfy benefit-risk and benefit-cost assessments; which should be voluntary and which should be mandated in mass immunization programs; whether, how, and to what extent to recognize medical, religious, philosophical, and personal objections as grounds for exemption from mandatory immunizations; whether to add new vaccinations, such as the HPV vaccination to the mandatory list; and how to allocate vaccines in a crisis. This chapter will address these and other issues surrounding mass immunization programs in part through several case studies.

MASS IMMUNIZATION PROGRAMS: JUSTIFICATIONS

Jacobson v. Massachusetts

Early in the 20th century, the most famous public health legal case, *Jacobson v. Massachusetts*, addressed government-mandated vaccinations. In this case, the U.S. Supreme Court upheld a Massachusetts law that authorized local boards of public health to "require and enforce the vaccination and revaccination of all the inhabitants" of their city or town and provide them with free vaccination. Any person over 21 who failed or refused to comply would be fined five dollars (and could be confined until he or she paid the fine). In response to a smallpox outbreak in 1902, the Board of Health of the city of Cambridge, Massachusetts, required vaccination or revaccination of any inhabitants who had not been vaccinated successfully since March 1, 1897. Jacobson, a Lutheran minister, refused—not on religious grounds, but because of a variety of fears about the vaccination.[4]

This U.S. Supreme Court decision is obviously an important precedent in our public philosophy, which delineates citizens' rights and responsibilities in the context of public health. This public philosophy has been articulated in a variety of ways to justify mass immunization campaigns, backed by government-imposed sanctions when needed. We turn to some of those justifications.

Societal Self-Defense for the Common Good

In *Jacobson*, the U.S. Supreme Court wrote, "Upon the principle of self-defense, of paramount necessity, a community has the right to protect itself against an epidemic of disease which threatens the safety of its members."[4] This notion of self-defense, which includes both the community and its members, also appears in John Stuart Mill's seminal *On Liberty* in its justification of the government's and society's coercive intervention into individual liberties under the harm principle—or, more fully, the harm-to-others principle—which warrants such interference.[5] He argued that the "sole end for which mankind are warranted, individually or collectively, in interfering with the liberty of action of any of their number is *self-protection*"[5 (p. 10)] (italics added). Contrary to some interpretations, Mill did not limit justifiable interferences with individual liberties to their *actions* but also included their inactions or their *failures to act* (e.g., a failure to engage in the "positive act" of bearing a "fair share" of the "common defense").[5 (p. 12)]

This notion of societal self-defense or self-protection, encompassing both the society as a whole and its individual members, is a strong one in our public philosophy. As articulated in *Jacobson*, the "organized society" through the government has the right and responsibility to defend against dangers to "public health and public safety" using coercive means if necessary: "There are manifold restraints to which every person is necessarily subject for the common good. On any other basis organized society could not exist with safety to its members."[4] Four principles can be found in the *Jacobson* decision for determining the legitimacy of any compulsory vaccination law. These are presented in **Table 7.1**.

TABLE 7.1 Summary of *Jacobson* Principles

There must be a public health necessity.
There must be a reasonable relationship between the intervention and the objective.
The intervention may not be arbitrary or oppressive.
The intervention should not pose a health risk to its subject.

Data from Javitt G, Berkowitz D, and Gostin LO. Assessing Mandatory HPV Vaccination: Who Should Call the Shots? Journal of Law, Medicine & Ethics 2008;36(2):388–389.

While distinct from each other, these several principles are grounded in the public philosophy that the state has an ethical right and responsibility to provide societal self-defense on behalf of its citizens against life-threatening diseases, and that the "common good" may legitimately override personal liberties if the threat is severe enough. This approach is a *presumptivist approach* in that it identifies a presumption in favor of personal liberties but indicates that this presumption can be rebutted or outweighed under certain conditions—and it provides the justificatory conditions for doing so. This is not a mere weighing or balancing of several ethical principles. We will come back to this argument later, when we consider the case of a possible HPV (human papillomavirus) vaccine mandate, which Javitt and colleagues oppose on grounds of the *Jacobson* principles.[6] An ethical justification for mandatory immunization based on societal self-defense focuses attention on the meaning of "organized society" and on the state's proper rationale for its use of coercion, when deemed to be necessary, rather than on balancing shared ethical principles in particular cases.

An important analogy, though not complete or uncontroversial, exists between military conscription and mandatory immunization. While the U.S. currently has an all-volunteer military force, it has often had a conscripted force. In line with the model noted in *Jacobson*, military conscription provides personnel for waging a war against external enemies of the state, while public health wages war against infectious diseases as enemies. The war metaphor became quite prominent in our conceptions of medicine and of public health, especially with the emergence of the germ theory of disease in the latter part of the 19th century. In both military conscription and mandatory immunization, there are risks to the individuals involved, but those individuals also participate in societal benefits. The military draft and compulsory vaccination laws function to share the risks. As Salmon and Siegal note, "duties (to bear arms and to be vaccinated) are generally considered a potential obligation that goes hand in hand with enjoying the benefits of citizenry."[7 (p. 292)] This position is consistent with our public philosophy in the U.S.

To be sure, there are differences between state-mandated vaccinations and military conscription. The war against disease requires larger numbers to participate—preferably immunization of 90% or so of the population in order to ensure "herd immunity"—and vaccinations are much less risky than military combat. Moreover, beyond the shared indirect benefits of both military conscription and mandatory immunization, individuals may directly benefit through their participation in immunization programs because they receive strong (though not perfect or complete) protection from the vaccine-preventable disease.

Balancing Principles

The societal self-defense model requires that coercive measures be necessary to accomplish the public health goal of protecting the community and its members from serious infectious diseases. It sets a fairly high bar of justification, and probably would not admit all of the (coercive) mass immunization programs that would be justified under a model of balancing principles.

Some proponents of a model of balancing principles view the conflict over mandatory vaccinations as a conflict between respect for autonomy, on the one hand, and several other principles, including especially beneficence, but also utility, justice, and nonmaleficence, all of which have to be balanced against autonomy and liberty in setting vaccination policy. For Field and Caplan, "[t]he ethical analysis of vaccine mandates requires a delicate balance of cherished values."[8] They suggest that in the weighing or balancing of the two primary ethical principles of autonomy and beneficence, there is a "tipping point" at which the disease's contagiousness and its severity outweigh autonomy and liberty and thus support mandatory vaccination.

In the Field–Caplan ethical analysis, utility[a] provides "the most prominent and longstanding justification put forth by mandate proponents."[8] This is not surprising in view of the importance of maximizing benefit at minimal cost and achieving overall societal benefit. Consider, for instance, their analysis of "herd immunity"—the statistical point at which the eradication of a disease is possible because of population immunity (usually around 90%). This focus on eradication moves beyond the *Jacobson* focus on control. For Field and Caplan "the ultimate utilitarian benefit from vaccine mandates is to reach the threshold percentage of vaccinated individuals necessary to achieve herd immunity."[8] This is a "utility bonus." When this threshold is in jeopardy, then the case for "coercing widespread vaccination rises precipitously." The "utility bonus" of "herd immunity" is often sufficient to justify a coercive vaccination mandate even when the severity or burden of the disease is not severe.[8] Nevertheless, it is not exactly clear what conditions need to be met to bring about the "tipping point," when considering both the degree of

---

[a] Field and Caplan often write "utilitarianism," but we will use the language of the principle or value of "utility," since it is in competition with other principles and values. By contrast, utilitarianism is the overall philosophy, not just a principle or value.[8]

severity of the disease in terms of morbidity and mortality and the possibility of the "utility bonus" of "herd immunity."

Clearly, an important difference between the societal self-defense model and the balancing model is that the former sets stricter conditions for compulsory vaccinations, including necessity of control measures in the face of an imminent and serious public health problem of infectious disease spread. As Gostin and de Angelis put it, building on *Jacobson*, "In the absence of an immediate risk of serious harm, it is preferable to adopt voluntary measures, making state compulsion a last resort."[9] We will see below that these two different frameworks have different implications for HPV vaccine policy.

More Specific Guidance for Mass Immunization Programs

Seven principles to guide mass vaccination programs are presented in **Table 7.2**. These principles, formulated by Vermeij and Dawson,[10] are very similar to the general principles and justificatory conditions that we identified earlier. For the most part, their formulation can be viewed as specifying and concretizing our broad principles and justificatory conditions, and their list can be quite useful in deliberating about mass immunization programs in the name of public health.

TABLE 7.2 Seven Principles for Collective Vaccination Programs

1. Collective vaccination programs should target serious diseases that are a public health problem.
2. Each vaccine, and the program as a whole, must be effective and safe.
3. The burdens and inconveniences for participants should be as small as possible.
4. The program's burden-to-benefits ratio should be favorable in comparison with alternative vaccination schemes or preventative options.
5. Collective vaccination programs should involve a just distribution of benefits and burdens.
6. Participation should, generally, be voluntary unless compulsory vaccination is essential to prevent a concrete and serious harm.
7. Public trust in the vaccination program should be honored and protected.

Data from: Verweij M, Dawson A. Ethical Principles for Collective Immunization Programmes. Vaccine 2004; 22: 3122–3126. Spellings have been converted to American English.

VOLUNTARY AND MANDATORY IMMUNIZATION PROGRAMS

Now we turn to the specific issue raised by Vermeij and Dawson's sixth principle: "participation in mass immunization programs should, generally, be voluntary." In the selection of means of achieving mass immunization, voluntary participation has priority, "unless compulsory vaccination is essential to prevent a concrete and serious harm." This falls somewhat short of the strong societal self-defense model drawn from *Jacobson*, but nevertheless captures the (rebuttable) presumption in favor of liberty. This principle does not spell out the "concrete and serious harm," whether it can be individual or societal. It involves, as *Jacobson* noted, considerable deference to public health authorities in determining either necessity or concrete and serious harm.

Persuasion and/or Coercion?

According to James Colgrove's history of vaccination policy in the U.S., persuasion, rather than coercion, dominated vaccination policy until the late 1960s, when efforts to eradicate—not merely control—infectious disease, in the context of a campaign against measles, led to legal requirements of immunization for school attendance. Yet persuasion was not totally ignored.

> The belief that parents were basically willing, but needed special stimulus to help them act responsibly, provided a justification for the recourse to coercion .... The use of persuasion remained a cornerstone of vaccination programs, with school laws serving in the eyes of health officials as a kind of societal safety net to catch the children of the 'hard to reach.'[2 (p. 12)]

Over time, immunization patterns displayed a socioeconomic gradient—children in poor families were less likely to be vaccinated on schedule. The problem of delayed or incomplete immunization was increasingly viewed as a problem of social injustice and inequality, conceptions that have supported the retention of school immunization laws as well as changes in the system for delivering health care, including vaccinations.[2 (p. 13)] In addition to their efforts at persuasion and motivation through educational and advertising campaigns, governments have taken other steps, including eliminating or reducing the financial burdens to individuals or families by providing the vaccines or by covering their cost. For instance, since the 1990s, a federal program has provided free vaccinations to children who come from low-income families.[11]

Incentive Rewards or Monetary Sanctions?

The requirement of certain vaccinations as a condition for children's school attendance has been widely accepted—and upheld by the U.S. Supreme Court[12]—in part because there is a connection between the vaccinations and protection of the student himself/herself and others in the context of attending school.

Some incentives may be appropriate, whether directed at clinicians/physicians or at patients/families. For instance, it is important for physicians to be adequately compensated for providing vaccinations. Some other alternatives, variously called incentives or sanctions but verging on the latter, have been employed with some success but not without ethical difficulties.

Over a period of several years, the Community Preventive Services Task Force, an independent body appointed by the CDC, has provided evidence-based guidance about how best to increase the population's rate of vaccinations.[13] **Table 7.3** lists the interventions the Task Force has examined and indicates whether it recommended that intervention or found insufficient evidence in the relevant scientific literature to recommend it.

The first several interventions are grouped under "Enhancing Access to Vaccination Services." The Task Force found evidence to recommend several of these, including incorporating vaccination programs in the setting of the Special Supplemental Nutrition Program for Women, Infants and Children (WIC), a federally supported program, and in schools and organized childcare centers. Enhanced access interventions that involve home visits and reduce potential users' out-of-pocket costs were also recommended as

TABLE 7.3 Community Preventive Services Task Force Evaluation of Ways to Increase Vaccination Rates

Intervention	Finding
Enhancing Access to Vaccination Services	
Expanded Access in Healthcare Settings When Used Alone	Insufficient Evidence December 1997
Home Visits to Increase Vaccination Rates	Recommended March 2009
Reducing Client Out-of-Pocket Costs	Recommended October 2008
Vaccination Programs in Schools & Organized Child Care Centers	Recommended June 2009
Vaccination Programs in WIC Settings	Recommended March 2009
Increasing Community Demand for Vaccinations	
Client or Family Incentive Rewards	Recommended April 2011
Client Reminder & Recall Systems	Recommended February 2008
Client-Held Paper Immunization Records	Insufficient Evidence March 2010
Clinic-Based Education When Used Alone	Insufficient Evidence February 2011
Community-Wide Education When Used Alone	Insufficient Evidence March 2010
Monetary Sanction Policies	Insufficient Evidence April 2011
Vaccination Requirements for Child Care, School & College Attendance	Recommended June 2009
Provider- or System-Based Interventions	
Healthcare System-Based Interventions Implemented in Combination	Recommended December 2010
Immunization Information Systems	Recommended July 2010
Provider Assessment & Feedback	Recommended February 2008
Provider Education When Used Alone	Insufficient Evidence March 2010
Provider Reminders	Recommended June 2008
Standing Orders When Used Alone	Recommended June 2008
Community-Based Interventions Implemented in Combination	Recommended June 2010

Reproduced from the Guide to Community Preventive Services. Increasing appropriate vaccination: universally recommended vaccinations. www.thecommunityguide.org/vaccines/universally/index.html. Last updated January 3, 2011.

effective, based on the available evidence. The reduction of out-of-pocket costs to users can be viewed as a removal of a disincentive, or, in the language of the Nuffield Council on Bioethics Intervention Ladder[b], as enabling choice. This and the other recommended interventions under "Enhancing Access to Vaccination Services" do not raise any serious ethical concerns (though there are always important questions about allocating funds for different programs and interventions).

The Task Force's review of the evidence for "Increasing Community Demand for Vaccinations" and for "Provider- or System-Based Interventions" found several that were effective and some for which there was insufficient evidence to warrant a recommendation. It also found that combinations were effective. Under "Increasing Community Demand for Vaccinations," we have already noted requirements for school attendance, and that discussion will suffice for the intervention the Task Force labels "Vaccination Requirements for Child Care, School & College Attendance." Here, we will examine more closely two of the interventions that relate to the Intervention Ladder and pose some questions for closer examination: Client or family incentive rewards[14] and monetary sanctions.[15] The Task Force found sufficient evidence to support the former, but not the latter—and, as we will see, the latter raises special ethical concerns.

The Intervention Ladder distinguishes interventions that guide choices through incentives and those that guide choices through disincentives, proposing in general that it is more difficult to justify the latter than the former. We have already distinguished both of these from the removal of disincentives (what the Intervention Ladder labels *enabling choice*)—for instance, reducing the out-of-pocket costs of parents or guardians may reduce a disincentive to have their children vaccinated. (See our fuller analysis of the Intervention Ladder in Chapter 2.)

We will start with the creation of disincentives through the use of sanctions for parental or guardian failures to have their children vaccinated on schedule. One big problem is that the employment of certain sanctions creates coercive situations. That is a reason for caution. However, we do justifiably use nonmonetary sanctions such as not allowing school attendance if children lack certain vaccinations. (This may also have monetary effects, for instance, by inducing parents to engage in home schooling.) A related ethical concern is justice and fairness in the distribution of burdens and benefits as a result of the monetary sanctions; this will be evident in the studies to which we now turn.

One study evaluated the impact of an initiative that linked immunization to the distribution of food vouchers in the inner city. The intervention varied the frequency of the distribution of food vouchers to participants in the Special Supplemental Nutrition Program for Women, Infants, and Children (WIC), depending on the children's immunization status and their referral to an immunization provider. Parents of children whose immunizations were not up to date received only 1 month's supply of food vouchers rather than the usual 3 months' supply. This intervention led to a rapid increase in and maintenance of high rates of childhood immunization in an inner-city population—over 15 months, immunization rates increased from 56% to 89%.[16] Concerns arose, however, about possibly depriving these children and damaging their welfare by reducing the food available to them at any time: "the use of financial sanctions against families that are poor and often struggling to provide their children with basic necessities raises ethical and moral issues and should be undertaken only with great caution and careful monitoring for both positive and untoward outcomes."[17] Furthermore, screening, education, and referral, which were also part of the program, may have contributed to intervention's success.[17] Failure to immunize children may result from other social, institutional, and professional factors aside from lack of parental motivation.[18]

Similar concerns have arisen about another study that demonstrated a strong effect of a monetary sanction on the rates of immunization of children in families with dependent children. Following is the description of the intervention: "Families in the intervention group (n-1500) were informed that the receipt of the welfare benefit for any preschool-aged children was contingent on provision of proof of up-to-date immunization status at the beginning of welfare eligibility and, subsequently, semiannually or annually."[19] According to the researchers, these families faced "relatively little increased burden" in complying with the requirements, and the sanction had to be administered only 11 times. However, two commentators worry that such supposedly innovative policies could overestimate the long-term benefit of the sanctions and, at the same time, "underestimate worsening health status among eligible program beneficiaries."[20,c] Critics also fault these studies for not examining the potential negative effects of the sanctions used.

In addition, going back to the Intervention Ladder, we can quarrel with the researchers' description of these sanctions as incentives. An incentive can be characterized as any additional motivation beyond persuasion, but much depends

[b] Nuffield Council on Bioethics report, *Public Health: Ethical Issues* (London: Nuffield Council, November 2007) Available at: www.nuffieldbioethics.org. (accessed January 17, 2013).

[c] Davis and Lantos also challenge the granting of the waiver for research in the laboratory of experimentation in the states.[20]

on the baseline and on whether the intervention is positive or negative. Providing targeted money to families could remove a disincentive by covering the costs of travel, etc., for their children's immunization, or it could add increased funds to create a positive incentive, which can be useful.[21] However, starting with the baseline of eligibility for welfare benefits for preschool-aged children and then threatening to stop those benefits in an effort to motivate parental or guardian behavior is a sanction, rather than an incentive, and it is arguably unfair to the children as well as coercive to the parents. Even though such sanctions should not always be rejected, they should be used only as a last resort when persuasion, removal of disincentives, and provision of positive incentives fail to work.

The Community Preventive Services Task Force looked at studies that included the following types of positive incentives, which it calls "incentive rewards":

Government payments

- One time payment of $208 AUD [Australian dollars] and child care assistance (1 study: Australia)

Lottery prizes

- Grocery vouchers ($50)
- Monetary prizes ($175)

Gift cards

- Baby products ($10)

Food vouchers and baby products

- Combination of the above

The Task Force concludes that, on the basis of the studies it examined, there is sufficient evidence of effectiveness of such incentive rewards in increasing adult and children vaccination rates to warrant their recommendation either singly or in combination with other interventions.[14]

Concerns voiced about such incentive rewards include their potential "coercive" effects, but we do not find this concern cogent in light of our understanding of what constitutes coercion.[d] These incentive rewards may provide "undue" incentives, but they are not coercive—nor is it even clear that they are "undue." Another concern frequently registered is that such incentives do not improve, and may even damage, participants' character. They only generate short-term motivations, without changing the underlying motivational structure of the individuals or families involved. While this point is probably true, it does not necessarily constitute a reason not to use incentives, if they are shown to be effective and cost-effective, since, arguably, the major public health goal is—or should be—to secure the results sought, in this case increased vaccination rates, rather than primarily to alter or preserve the character of the participants in the program. One unresolved question is whether both aims can be achieved simultaneously.

Another negative incentive or disincentive comes from physicians, especially pediatricians, who refuse to care for unvaccinated children (and their families). Many members of the American Association of Pediatrics—as many as 7 out of 10—report a parental refusal of a childhood vaccination over a 12-month period.[22] In light of reports of physician dismissal of and refusal to care for unvaccinated children or their families,[23] the Committee on Bioethics of the American Association of Pediatrics argues for respecting parental refusals and continuing to provide care.[24] The Committee's statement—rightly, in our judgment—urges physicians to try to understand the parents' perspective, correct misinformation, and encourage parents to reconsider their stance while continuing to ensure the children's access to medical care and to create opportunities to promote vaccination. In the process, physicians may need to provide special accommodations, such as a separate waiting area, for unvaccinated children in order to protect other patients who may lack full immunity even though they have been vaccinated.

Targeted Vaccinations

We are focusing mainly on mass immunization programs in this chapter, but there are good reasons to consider targeted mandatory vaccinations in some contexts. These usually relate to situations where people are at particularly high risk because of certain health conditions, or where they conduct or fill social roles or functions that either would put others at serious risk through spreading an infection or would deprive the society of important goods or services if they came down with a particular vaccine-preventable disease.

CASE STUDY: ANNUAL INFLUENZA VACCINATION FOR NURSING HOME STAFF: MANDATORY OR VOLUNTARY?

Because of the risks of influenza, the director of a large nursing home has determined that it needs to implement a mandatory influenza vaccination program because only about 40% of the staff (in contrast to over 90% of the residents) receives the recommended influenza vaccinations each year. (This percentage of staff vaccination is similar to the national rates—see **Figure 7.1**.) Staff vaccinations can help protect

[d] As noted elsewhere, "coercion" has been misused in a variety of contexts. We take the position that coercion involves a threat that impels an individual toward a choice they would not otherwise normally make.

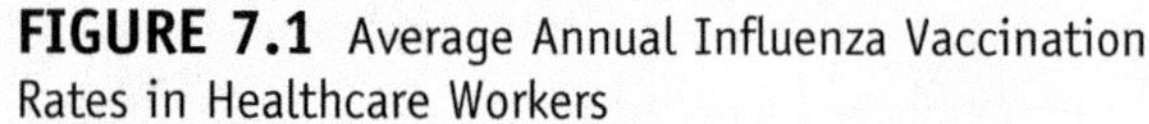

FIGURE 7.1 Average Annual Influenza Vaccination Rates in Healthcare Workers

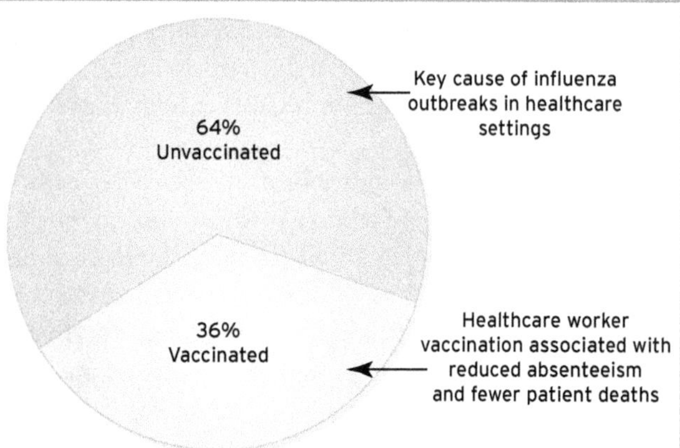

Modified from: the CDC. Prevention and Control of Influenza. Recommendations of the Advisory Committee On Immunization Practices (ACIP), Recomm Rep. 2003 S2 (R. R-8):1–44.

residents and reduce staffing problems caused by the spread of influenza among the employees. The nursing home director asks the local public health director for advice on the practical and ethical issues raised by the proposal to require the staff to be vaccinated.

There is widespread agreement about the ethical obligation of healthcare workers (HCWs), particularly those involved in direct patient care, to be vaccinated in order to protect patients and others with whom they work; this obligation is based on the principle of nonmaleficence, captured in the maxim "first of all, or at least, do no harm." The question being raised by the nursing home director is how to motivate these HCWs and others on the staff to live up to this obligation, which can be largely discharged by undergoing a safe and effective vaccination. Even though more than 90% of the nursing home residents are vaccinated each year, the effective immunization is less among this older population, and "ring vaccination" (i.e., vaccinating those around this population) is considered to be an important protective measure.

Studies have identified a number of barriers to annual influenza vaccination by HCWs. Many of them are similar to barriers for the general public: concerns about time involved and inconvenience, costs, worries about adverse reactions, perception of vaccine ineffectiveness, and so forth.[25, 26] In view of such barriers, the Advisory Committee on Immunization Practices (ACIP) recommends several strategies. These include educational and promotional campaigns stressing the influenza vaccination's benefits for providers and patients, modeling by senior providers and leaders, removal of any barriers such as costs (for instance, many on the staff may lack health insurance), providing vaccinations at convenient times and in readily accessible locations, and reporting vaccination rates to the staff.[25] Some hospitals and healthcare organizations use incentives and require individuals to sign declinations or refusals if they seek to opt out.

In short, these approaches incorporate removal of disincentives related to access, such as cost, as well as provision of incentives and nudges of various kinds, such as requiring an explicit, written declination of a vaccination. Some organizations have imposed stronger requirements for vaccination not only for healthcare providers with direct patient contact, but for others in the organization. These generally stop short of absolute mandates.

One argument in favor of mandatory influenza vaccination for all HCWs focuses on the irony that "influenza vaccination is still considered voluntary [for HCWs], although other, less effective infection control and healthcare practices are expected and enforced in healthcare facilities to protect patients."[26] Furthermore, there are other strong precedents in requiring healthcare workers to show immunity to rubella and measles and to be vaccinated for hepatitis B prior to employment in certain contexts. Hence, a coercive requirement of influenza vaccination could be ethically justifiable as well as effective; some evidence suggests that voluntary programs do not achieve influenza vaccination rates as high as mandatory programs.[27]

The arguments against an influenza vaccination mandate for HCWs stresses that the best voluntary programs—which embody several of the features noted above, including active declination or refusal—achieve rates of 75% or so. Even if a mandatory program would raise the rates higher, perhaps to 85% to 90%, opponents argue that this positive outcome is outweighed by the ethical price of authoritarian coercion, the costs in alienation of HCWs, potential legal battles, and the diversion of attention from a full range of infection control measures.[28]

EXEMPTIONS FROM MANDATORY VACCINATION PROGRAMS

Variations in State Exemptions

Even mass immunization programs are not universal in scope. School immunization laws in every state in the U.S. grant exemptions to children for medical reasons. These are available to children with medical or health conditions that are contraindications to vaccinations and are verified by a physician (or, in some states, other health professionals).

For instance, Virginia law has the following requirement for a medical exemption: "The parent or guardian presents a statement from a physician licensed to practice medicine in Virginia, a licensed nurse practitioner, or a local health department that states that the physical condition of the child is such that the administration of one or more of the required immunizing agents would be detrimental to the health of the child."[29]

Forty-eight states (and the District of Columbia) also grant exemptions to persons with religious objections to immunizations, including children whose parents or guardians object to immunizations. The two exceptions are Mississippi and West Virginia, which recognize only medical reasons for exemption. Moreover, in 19 states (as of December 2012), exemptions may be granted to persons (or to parents or guardians of minors) who object to immunizations for philosophical, personal, moral, or other beliefs (**Figure 7.2**).[30] (California allows religiously-based exemptions under the broad rubric of personal beliefs.) These exemptions spread in the wave of compulsory vaccination laws related to school attendance, dating from the 1960s and 1970s, in part under the impact of lobbying by Christian Scientists. Vaccination legislation dating back to the 19th century tended not to include these exemptions.[31 (p. 13)]

With these exemptions in place, the so-called mandatory or compulsory vaccination laws are hardly as strict as the language might suggest. The language of "quasi-mandatory" might be more accurate.[32] Furthermore, the effect is more coercive than, strictly speaking, compulsory. Individuals and children are not forcibly vaccinated, but are subjected to restrictions and penalties that tend to influence them to accept vaccinations—in particular, sanctions associated with the enforcement of the immunization requirements for school attendance. However, proponents of laws requiring vaccination for school attendance have tended to frame these laws as educational, symbolic, attention-getting, and persuasive prompts rather than as coercive mechanisms.[31] Nevertheless, the coercive sanctions remain an important component.

In many, if not all, states, the recognized exemptions may be denied or withheld in a declared emergency or epidemic.

FIGURE 7.2 Map of State Vaccination Exemptions 2011–2012

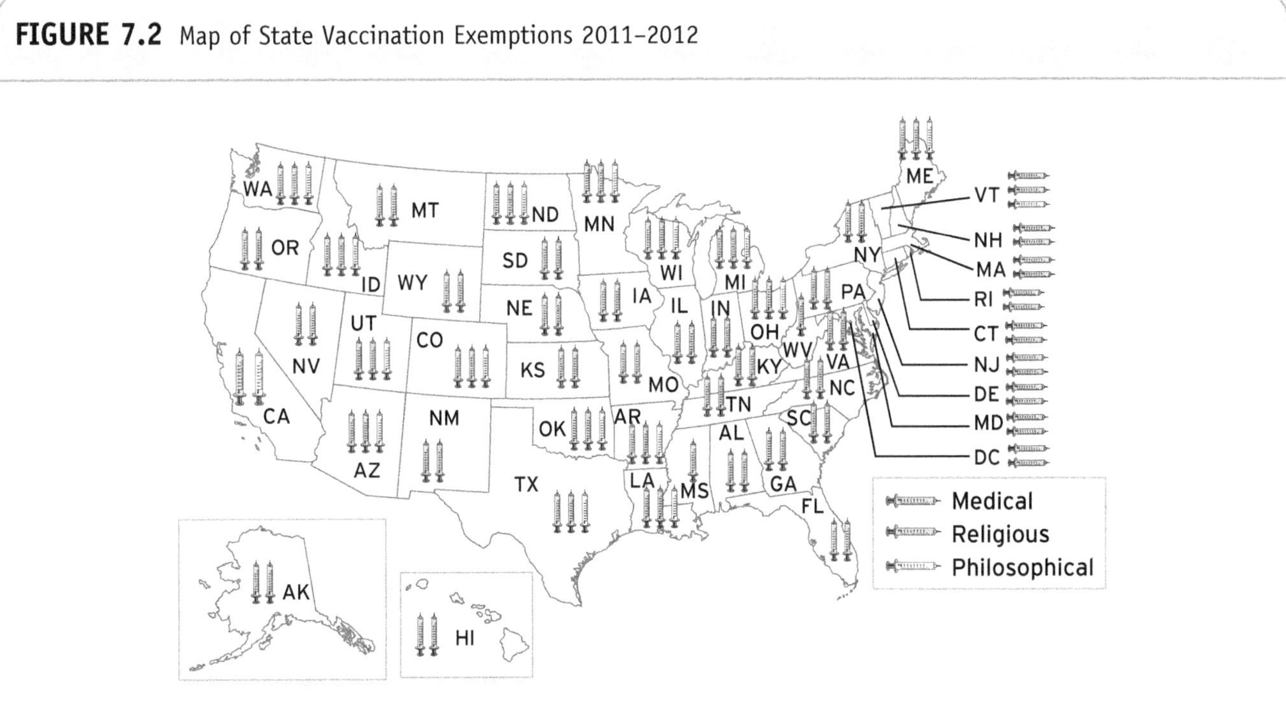

This map is reproduced with the permission of the National Vaccine Information Center (NVIC.org) and can be accessed at http://www.nvic.org/Vaccine-Laws/state-vaccine-requirements.aspx. Use of it in this book does not imply an NVIC endorsement of statements or opinions of the authors. NVIC is a charitable nonprofit organization founded in 1982 to prevent vaccine injuries and deaths through public education and advocates for the inclusion of informed consent protections in public health policies and laws.

For instance, Virginia's code indicates that the mandatory vaccination law will not apply if "[t]he parent or guardian of the child objects thereto on the grounds that the administration of immunizing agents conflicts with his religious tenets or practices, *unless an emergency or epidemic of disease has been declared by the Board* ..." (italics added).[29] As the italicized clause indicates, "an emergency or epidemic of disease" declared by the state Board of Health will allow public health officials to override the individual's or the parent's or guardian's religiously based objection. (The Virginia code includes a broader and less stringent basis of objection to the HPV vaccination, which we will discuss later in this chapter.)

Exemption of Conscientious Objectors

There are good reasons to exempt conscientious objectors—whether religious, philosophical, moral, or personal—from military service or from vaccination *if* the exemption will not compromise the societal defense against external enemies or against disease. Conscientious objection involves not only an appeal to personal autonomy or liberty but also a claim about the role, place, and significance of certain fundamental beliefs and values in a person's life. In general, in our public philosophy, the government should not force a person to violate those beliefs and values unless it is necessary to do so. These fundamental beliefs and values define a person's identity such that a violation would threaten that individual's personal integrity—who he or she is—and not only his or her bodily integrity.[33]

Courts have consistently recognized that both military and immunization exemptions are a matter of "legislative grace." Legislatures are not constitutionally bound to grant these exemptions, even though they have good reasons, in our public philosophy, for doing so. However, they may not grant these exemptions arbitrarily and capriciously to some groups but not to others. In the context of military conscription, a series of court cases largely eliminated the requirement that conscientious objection be religiously based or informed. This opened the door to philosophical and moral objections that are sincerely and deeply held and occupy a place in the life of the nonreligious objector parallel to the belief in God or the divine in the life of the traditional religious objector. Some court decisions on compulsory vaccination laws have also taken a similar direction, and, as a result, several state laws also include "philosophical" or "personal" beliefs of a secular nature.[30, 31]

In 2012, debates erupted in several state legislatures about the basis and scope of exemptions, about the procedures and processes for granting particular exemptions, and about the threat of such exemptions to the public's health, especially in the outbreak of pertussis (whooping cough) that at mid-year portended the worst epidemic in the last half-century.

CASE STUDY: SHOULD RELIGIOUSLY BASED AND PHILOSOPHICAL/PERSONAL OBJECTIONS TO VACCINATIONS BE RECOGNIZED AS BASES FOR EXEMPTION?

Religious Convictions

In 2012, a vigorous debate occurred in West Virginia—one of only two states without a religious exemption from mandatory vaccination—about a bill in the legislature to allow some nonmedical exemptions. Opposition to the lack of a religion-based exemption has surfaced before, for instance in court cases. Not surprisingly, religious objections to vaccination differ widely in scope. Some broadly object to all vaccines out of religious concerns for what is taken into the body, while others focus on the purpose of certain vaccines (e.g., to protect against diseases that are not transmitted via casual contact but are largely transmitted through the exchange of bodily fluids, as in sexual contact or drug use). Still others object to the source of biological materials used to create the vaccines.

Regarding the last, Lori Lee, a leader of the movement for recognition of religious exemptions, stressed the link between vaccines and abortions. At a public hearing in 2012 she stated: "Fourteen of the vaccines required by the state of West Virginia contain aborted fetal tissue, of over 150 babies, and their cell lines are aging. That bothers me as a Christian, that I have to choose between my faith in God and sending my children to public or private school."[34] In rebuttal, Dr. Raheel Khan, who teaches pediatrics at West Virginia University, stressed that this misstates the science involved. Some vaccines have been cultivated in cell cultures from fetuses that were aborted more than 40 years ago, but Khan emphasized, "No pregnancies were intentionally terminated to produce these vaccines. None of these vaccines contain any genetic material from the donor cells."[34]

Still another religious–moral argument focused on specific vaccines; this objection is also selective rather than universal. One parent objected to the requirement of a vaccine for hepatitis B, an infectious inflammatory disease that can damage the liver. This parent, an ophthalmologist, argued that since hepatitis B "is a sexually transmitted disease," his "toddlers are not at risk to develop a sexually transmitted disease. They are not sharing drug needles. They are not having promiscuous sex."[34] In response, Dr. Khan stressed the other ways hepatitis B can be transmitted through bodily fluids, which may be shared by drooling or biting.[34]

In testifying at the West Virginia hearing, Mary Holland, a research scholar at the New York University School of Law, made several arguments including, but going beyond, the ones just noted. First, she viewed vaccinations as the same as other medical interventions; hence, "individuals must have the right to prior, free and informed consent to vaccination as they have for all other medical interventions." This is what "modern ethical medicine" requires, and she does "not believe that even infectious disease risks justify deviation from this fundamental standard."[35] So whether public health interventions must be held to the same standard is a fundamental question, and we have argued throughout that there are important differences.

Holland also appealed to a virtue standard, a standard of good character, for the state. In light of the recognition of conscientious vaccination refusals in other states, she asked legislators, "What kind of state do you want West Virginia to be?" Everyone wants a state with healthy children, but exactly "how should West Virginia achieve this end—through compulsion to vaccinate, and criminalization for failure to comply, or through tolerance, education, and the requirement that unvaccinated children remain out of school during any disease outbreak?"[35] The latter requirement, she stressed, would partially rebut the charge of "free riding," because it would entail significant financial and other commitments by working families.[35]

Spokespersons for public health at the hearing warned that West Virginia already had a low average vaccination rate for immunizations, and that moving to nonmedical exemptions, whether religious and/or philosophical, would lead to even fewer vaccinations and increase the risk of outbreaks.[34] While many of the arguments in West Virginia focused on religious exemptions, perhaps because of the role of religious convictions in that state's public culture, several arguments had broader implications for, or explicitly called for, recognition of philosophical/personal objections that are broad enough to encompass a different risk-benefit calculus about vaccinations than applied by public health officials.

Philosophical and Personal Beliefs

The language of nonmedical, nonreligious exemptions varies. For instance, among the 19 states recognizing such exemptions, Maine recognizes "moral, philosophical or other personal beliefs," and California recognizes parents' personal beliefs, which may include religious beliefs, without specification. Vermont has granted exemptions to a person or minor's parent or guardian who has "religious or philosophical convictions opposed to immunization."

In 2012, however, efforts were made in Vermont to remove the philosophical exemption while retaining the religious exemption. Rep. George Till, MD, author of the House version of the bill, said it is important to act soon: "We don't want to wait until we're in the middle of a crisis. As elected officials, we have an obligation to protect the public health."[36] These efforts were supported by the Vermont Medical Society and the Vermont Chapter of the American Academy of Pediatrics, among other groups. The Vermont Senate voted to eliminate this exemption, but the House voted to retain it. A conference committee failed to adopt a proposal that would have authorized the Commissioner of Health to remove the philosophical exemption if rates of vaccination fell below a 90% threshold for combined measles, mumps, and rubella vaccines (MMR) as well as combination vaccines for diphtheria, tetanus, and pertussis (DTaP and Tdap).

However, the final legislation did include some "nudges" toward immunization. A person or, in the case of minors, a parent or guardian must submit a signed form each year, prepared by the Vermont Department of Health, to the school or child care facility, attesting to holding "religious or philosophical convictions opposed to immunization," and to understanding

- evidence-based educational material provided by the Department of Health regarding immunizations, including information about the risks of adverse reactions to immunization;
- that failure to complete the required vaccination schedule increases risk to the person and others of contracting or carrying a vaccine-preventable infectious disease; and
- that there are persons with special health needs attending schools and childcare facilities who are unable to be vaccinated or who are at heightened risk of contracting a vaccine-preventable communicable disease and for whom such a disease could be life-threatening.[37]

Free Choices or Hurdles and Nudges?

There are two levels of debate. One is whether nonmedical exemptions—based on religious or philosophical/personal beliefs and values—should be recognized, and the other, also evident in the debate and legislation in Vermont, is whether the requests for exemptions should be automatically granted or subjected to closer scrutiny and accompanied by further requirements. In the wake of a serious outbreak of pertussis, some states have tightened their standards and procedures for granting exemptions, and others are considering such measures.

The Vermont legislation built in some low but important hurdles so that those who claim religious and/or philosophical objections will have to take some action every year.

It rightly applies this to both religious and philosophical convictions, in contrast to some proposed hurdles only for the exercise of "secular personal beliefs." What is most important is not the *source* of the beliefs but whether they are conscientious objections that are firmly and sincerely held.[7] This is consistent with U.S. policies regarding the exemption of conscientious objectors from military service. According to the Pediatric Infectious Diseases Society, laws that recognize personal belief exemptions should contain provisions that are "intended to minimize use of exemptions as the 'path of least resistance' for children who are behind on immunizations (whereby it would be easier to obtain an exemption than to catch-up the child's immunizations)."[38 (p. 1)] The reality is that immunizations lag in the child's early years, and parents must catch up on immunization before the child can enroll in public schools (and, in some states, private schools). Hence, the claim of an exemption based on conscientious objection could be easier than catching up on immunizations.

The requirements implemented in Vermont constitute modest hurdles or nudges that keep a claim of religious or philosophical exemption from being so much easier than securing children's vaccinations. They slightly encumber, but do not preclude or even unduly burden, the exercise of conscientious objection. In our judgment, various hurdles and nudges can be ethically justified in order to increase vaccinations. As Salmon and Siegal note, the "ease of obtaining an exemption has been quantitatively associated with the frequency of exemptions."[7] Indeed, studies indicate that not only do states recognizing personal belief exemptions have higher rates of nonmedical exemption than states that recognize only religious exemptions—as would be reasonably expected since there are more bases for exemption—but also that states with easy exemption processes have both higher and increasing rates of exemption than those with medium and difficult exemption processes.[39] Furthermore, these increased and higher rates have been associated with a greater incidence of pertussis.[39]

CASE STUDY: DEBATING WHETHER THE HPV VACCINATION SHOULD BE MANDATORY

An important case study for testing the arguments for actual or proposed mandatory immunization programs is the debate over the human papillomavirus (HPV) vaccine, especially for young girls, and whether its administration, which needs to start before sexual activity occurs, should be voluntary, under parental control, or state mandated. James Colgrove and colleagues describe this as a "case study in public health lawmaking amid political and scientific controversy"[40 (p. 785)] and, we might add, amid conflicting ethical perspectives, norms, and arguments. Moreover, the two models for justifying mass immunization programs—societal self-defense and balancing principles—tend to come to different conclusions about mandating the HPV vaccine.

Background

HPV, a sexually transmitted disease, is very common among sexually active adults. It is, indeed, the most common sexually transmitted disease, and is linked to several health problems of wide-ranging severity. Several HPV strains are linked to less severe health problems such as genital warts, but some HPV strains cause the vast majority of cases of cervical cancer, approximately 90% of cases of anal cancer, and a smaller percentage of other cancers of vulva, vagina, and penis.[41] Currently, there are two vaccines approved for vaccination against cancer-inducing strains of HPV (HPV-16 and -18): Gardasil, manufactured by Merck, and Cervarix, manufactured by GlaxoSmithKline.

Following Gardasil's approval, the Advisory Committee on Immunization Practices in 2006 recommended that the vaccine be routinely administered to girls at age 11 or 12.[40] In this context, various laws, regulations, and policies have been considered as ways to increase the use of the HPV vaccine. Some measures involve educational campaigns, others public subsidies, and still others insurance mandates, but none of these has been as controversial as efforts to require the vaccine as a condition of school attendance for girls beginning with sixth grade. In 2007, 24 states in the United States considered legislation mandating HPV vaccination. To date, only Virginia and the District of Columbia have mandated HPV vaccination for girls. Vigorous debate has persisted, because the vaccine implicates numerous heated topics ranging from parental rights to sexual politics to resource allocation.[40]

Pro and Con Arguments About the HPV Vaccine

Table 7.4 lists several topics based on interviews by Colgrove and colleagues with a number of informants from six sample states that had actively debated policies and laws regarding the HPV vaccine. It lists three reasons frequently invoked for mandating the HPV vaccine for school attendance (for girls above a certain age), and then several factors that, according to respondents, stood in the way of such mandates and generally affected the policy debates. The first set of these countervailing factors is specific to the HPV vaccine, while the second set focuses on factors in vaccination policymaking, whatever the vaccine under consideration. We will briefly summarize these factors and then examine more closely a few of the most important ones in order to determine their strength.

TABLE 7.4 HPV Vaccine Mandate for Girls: Pro-Con Factors

Arguments in Favor of the Mandate
• Seriousness of cervical cancer
• Efficacy of vaccine
• Justice of ensuring that all girls are vaccinated
Against the Mandate: Factors Specific to the HPV Vaccine
• Newness of the vaccine
• Sexually transmitted nature of HPV
• Lack of transmissibility of HPV in the classroom setting
• Discomfort with the vaccine manufacturer's involvement
Against the Mandate: Factors Related to Vaccination Policymaking
• Antipathy toward governmental coercion
• Antivaccination activism
• Nature of the policymaking process
Data from: Colgrove J, Abiola S, and Mello MM. HPV Vaccination Mandates—Lawmaking amid Political and Scientific Controversy. The New England Journal of Medicine 2010; 363, No. 8 (August 19): 785–791. Table prepared by the authors of this volume.

According to this study, the major arguments offered for mandating HPV vaccination for girls are that (1) cervical cancer is a serious disease and (2) the vaccine is efficacious. A mandate would also promote justice by ensuring that all girls receive it, even if their parents lack the knowledge or will to encourage or obtain it.[40]

Among the factors reportedly standing in the way of HPV vaccine mandates, several in the policymaking process apply to vaccination generally, not simply to the HPV vaccine. One of these concerns the appropriate locus of policy making about vaccination (legislation, executive order, or public health regulation), while another is the strong resistance from anti-vaccination activists in several states, based in part on concerns about vaccine safety. We will examine more fully below arguments surrounding the other factor related to vaccination policy making, opposition to governmental coercion, which also has a basis in the ethical arguments in our public philosophy at least for setting (rebuttable) presumptions.

The factors specific to the HPV vaccine that function as arguments against its mandate include its newness and recent approval. The drive toward a mandate started a few months after the vaccine was approved, and thus well before the accumulation of long-term safety data as well as education of the public about the vaccine and its value. It was propelled in part by the vigorous efforts by Merck, Gardasil's manufacturer. These efforts helped to get the HPV mandate on the policymaking table but soon became a liability, as did the cost of Gardasil—which at $320 for a full course of three doses, was much more expensive than other mandated vaccines. This cost not only raised more suspicions about Merck's involvement in the policymaking process (as being motivated by profit rather than health concerns) but also negatively impacted cost-benefit and cost-effectiveness assessments and created issues for vaccine coverage.[40]

The sexually transmitted nature of HPV meant that casual contact in the classroom creates no risk of transmission, and mandating the vaccine would require parents of 11- or 12-year-old girls to have discussions about sex with their daughters at an earlier stage than they might consider appropriate. Additionally, there are concerns about whether a legal mandate for protection of teenagers against a sexually transmitted disease would subvert abstinence-based prevention messages.[40] We will further analyze and assess this last argument below.

As we noted earlier, the two main justifications for governmental mandates of vaccination do not appear to be very different on the surface: one weighs and balances different ethical principles, allowing utility to override liberty in some cases, while the other indicates that collective security can override the presumption in favor of liberty in some cases. Nevertheless, these can easily come out at very different places depending on assumptions about HPV and its transmission.

In line with *Jacobson*, Javitt and colleagues hold that "societal self-defense" does not justify mandating HPV vaccination.[6] Among other reasons, there is no "public health necessity" for this vaccine because HPV is neither highly contagious nor highly lethal (for instance, cervical cancer can be detected early via routine gynecological exams and usually is successfully treated when it is detected early).[6] Moreover, there is no "reasonable relationship" between this vaccination and school attendance, since no child can be infected simply by casual contact. Using the language set forth in the *Jacobson* decision, Javitt and colleagues contend that the state's ethical duties to provide collective security for its citizens through mandatory vaccination that compromises personal liberty are triggered only in the most extreme circumstances, where the disease appears deadly and the possibility of infection highly likely.[6] But even if self-defense is understood more loosely, and includes individuals (not merely the state), it is hard to justify mandating the HPV vaccine because individuals can readily avoid being infected and infecting others, since the virus is transmitted through sexual contact and the risk of transmission can be reduced, though not eliminated, through the use of condoms in sexual intercourse.

By contrast, an ethical analysis that balances various moral principles against each other to determine the best course of action may be more open to mandatory HPV vaccination. For instance, Balog, applying a principle-based approach to moral reasoning, concludes that the societal or individual self-defense standard for justification of mandatory vaccination is set too high:

> [T]he rightness or wrongness of a compulsory vaccination program should be determined from a public health perspective by assessing whether key ethical principles justify such action, whether the action reduces harm to individuals and society, and whether the action produces consequences that are at least as good as, if not better than, alternative actions that are present in society for preventing disease and death. Compulsory HPV vaccination meets this test.[42]

This approach sets a very low threshold for justified state coercion in compulsory mass immunization programs. It neglects—indeed, deliberately sets aside—the kinds of justificatory conditions that we have emphasized here. We have argued, for instance, that there is no justification for mandatory immunization programs if voluntary measures would be sufficient and if less coercive measures are available. This is a key difference between a presumptivist approach, and a mere balancing approach.[e]

For Females Only?

Another ethical question concerns who should be vaccinated—especially if the vaccine-preventable disease more seriously affects certain groups, such as females or males. Should the public health vaccination recommendation or mandate, if adopted, be limited to the gender primarily affected? This question is especially pointed in debates about the HPV vaccine, since many proposals suggest that only females (rather than both females and males) be required to receive the vaccine. Proponents of this view argue that this selective coercion is justified because the major public health risk from HPV infection is cervical cancer, and the vaccine is very costly—so giving it to males isn't cost-effective.

There are precedents for requiring vaccination of both males and females even when the most serious effects of the vaccine-preventable diseases fall mainly on one or the other, rather than both. For instance, rubella (sometimes called German measles) is not a serious problem for males, but it is for pregnant women (the fetuses they are carrying can develop serious abnormalities), while mumps is not a serious problem for females but is for males, approximately 20% of whom develop painful testicular inflammation that sometimes (though rarely) results in sterility.[32] In both cases, despite these differential effects, vaccination is mandated for both males and females in the U.S.

The Advisory Committee on Immunization Practices at first recommended HPV vaccination only for females, but in October 2011, it recommended the quadrivalent HPV vaccine for males as well as for females.[43] Even before that recommendation, questions had arisen about the acceptability of coercing citizens of only one gender to receive the HPV vaccine. Caseldine-Bracht, for instance, suggests that arguments in favor of single-gender immunization often overlook the obvious fact that if men were vaccinated against HPV, women will be less likely to be infected through sexual contact.[44] Others contend that the HPV vaccine can benefit men (by preventing certain forms of genital warts, for example), and that these benefits are sufficient to warrant mandating the vaccine for men as well as for women and the additional cost.[45] In addition, Zimet argues that our strong ethical preference for the principle of equality suggests that both men and women should bear the burden and potential risks of the HPV vaccination, at least in the U.S.[45] A further argument is that gender-based policies regarding the mandatory HPV vaccination may not survive legal challenges based on constitutional requirements of due process and equal protection.[6]

Cost

The HPV vaccine has a comparatively high cost, but cost does not appear to have been as influential as several other factors in most state decisions about the HPV vaccine.[40] However, it does pose an unavoidable question: Who will bear the cost of an expensive vaccine?

The Code of Virginia indicates that while parents or guardians may choose to have the mandated vaccinations administered by a physician or registered nurse, they may have the child vaccinated by the local health department "without charge."[29] Virginia has also mandated health

[e] According to Field and Caplan (Reference 8) who are proponents of the balancing approach, the argument for mandating vaccination becomes stronger in such a case if one probable benefit is population immunity.

insurance coverage for HPV vaccination. Furthermore, the federal Vaccines for Children (VFC) program has approved coverage for the HPV vaccine.

Studies suggesting that HPV infection affects a disproportionate number of black and Hispanic women add weight to a justice argument for government funding (and, some argue, for mandatory vaccination). Others contend, however, that government expenditures for the HPV vaccination represent a misuse of public funds, which ought to be allocated toward other public goods, in part, again, because of HPV's mode of transmission. At least in the HPV debate, the ethical questions surrounding mandating the vaccination cannot be separated from ethical questions surrounding allocation of government funds and resources—what is an efficacious, efficient, and fair allocation of funds for and within public health activities and services?

Symbolic Significance of Legal Mandates

Legal mandates, backed by sanctions, not only coerce behavior but they are also symbolically important. They communicate messages about the behavior's importance—for instance, the societal value of mandated vaccinations. However, symbolic communication through public policies is often fraught with ambiguities, as is evident in the debate about state mandates of HPV vaccination. The messages conveyed and received may be quite mixed.

Much of the ethical debate surrounding HPV vaccine laws and policies has focused on concerns about the government's supposed endorsement of sexual promiscuity and the effect this might have on adolescent sexual activity.[46] The concern is that by mandating (or even encouraging and providing) a vaccination for young girls to prevent a sexually transmitted disease, the state is tacitly endorsing premarital sex and a sexually active lifestyle among adolescents. Some critics even labeled the HPV vaccine as the "promiscuity vaccine." Over against this concern, Albala calls for better communication about public health, in part by framing the HPV vaccine as a vaccine against cancer.[46] Of course, HPV vaccines do not offer direct protection against cancer, but rather against certain strains of HPV that commonly cause cancer, especially cervical cancer. This point suggests the vital role that description plays in any debate over the ethical justifications for mandatory vaccination. If the HPV vaccine is viewed as cancer prevention, there is a weighty justification for state coercion; if it is viewed primarily as preventing a sexually transmitted disease, it is harder to justify state coercion. Hence, descriptions of the vaccine matter in the ethical justification of state-mandated vaccination and in the message(s) communicated by such a mandate.

Exemption from HPV Mandates

Virginia mandates HPV vaccination for girls as a condition for school attendance after fifth grade. Its statutory code requires the State Board of Health's regulations to mandate "three doses of properly spaced human papillomavirus (HPV) vaccine for females," the first dose to "be administered before the child enters the sixth grade."[29] However, this measure is less demanding and stringent than the statutory context and language of this requirement might suggest. Parents or guardians may decline to have a female child vaccinated for HPV at their "sole discretion" without offering any religious or other reasons for their decision; the only requirement is that they review health board-approved materials on HPV's link with cervical cancer. The rationale in the law for distinguishing HPV vaccination from other mandated vaccinations for which there is only a medical or religiously-based exemption is HPV's mode of transmission—it "is not communicable in a school setting, but is transmitted sexually."[29]

With an exemption this broad, it is appropriate to ask whether HPV vaccination is, in fact, practically mandated in Virginia even though the HPV vaccine mandate is on the books. The mandate may be more symbolic than practically coercive.

JUSTICE, FAIRNESS, AND COMPENSATION FOR VACCINE-RELATED INJURIES

We have emphasized justice and fairness in the distribution of benefits and burdens of public health programs, and, more specifically, Vermeij and Dawson stress in their fifth principle: "Collective vaccination programs should involve a just distribution of benefits and burdens."[10] One important implication is compensation for vaccine-related injuries. There are real risks associated with vaccines, even though they have been greatly exaggerated by anti-vaccine activists, particularly those claiming a causal connection between MMR and autism.[2]

In 1986, Congress instituted the National Vaccine Injury Compensation Program (NVICP), a mandatory no-fault alternative to tort lawsuits against healthcare providers and drug companies for vaccine-related injuries or death. This program protects drug manufacturers from liability, and provides an alternative system in which those seeking compensation for vaccine-related injuries pursue their claims through an established federal process. To be eligible for compensation, a claim must "(1) be made within the 'relevant timeframe,' (2) establish that the vaccine caused the injury, or (3) show the vaccine aggravated a preexisting condition."[47]

Claims are paid out of the Vaccine Injury Compensation Trust Fund, a fund created by taxation of the purchase of each dose of a vaccine. The CDC reports roughly 30,000 reports of vaccination-related complications each year to the Vaccine Adverse Event Reporting System.[47]

Without examining the specifics and adequacy of the Vaccine Injury Compensation Trust Fund, we will briefly note the ethical rationale for such a program of compensation for vaccine-related injuries. First, injured participants in immunization programs deserve just or fair compensation for those injuries. Since the government is mandating, for public health reasons, mass immunization programs, it is a matter of justice and fairness for the government to compensate those injured in the war against disease, just as it compensates those injured in the war against external enemies. Some focus on whether the immunization was mandated or voluntary, but in a mass immunization program, that difference should be minimized, just as it is in the compensation of military personnel for injuries sustained in combat. It does not—and should not—matter whether these military personnel were volunteers or conscripts—either way, they assumed a position of risk on behalf of the society.

Nevertheless, the case in public health may be stronger when the vaccination is mandatory; if citizens are coerced to be vaccinated, we tend to believe that we ought to mitigate any collateral harm that results from such coercion.[48] The concept of solidarity, so emphasized in European bioethics and public health ethics, is also relevant: Because we all benefit from vaccination policies, we have some obligation to care for those adversely affected by these policies.[48] Furthermore, it is a limited and reasonable burden to contribute to a low-cost insurance plan for the societal benefit of immunization (the VICP involves a tax of $0.75 per vaccination). Hence, these several moral considerations, embedded in our public philosophy, support a vaccine-injury compensation program.

Another argument is based on utility—provision of compensation for vaccine-related injuries will encourage people to be vaccinated. This is an empirical argument, but some find little empirical support for the claim that the assurance of compensation encourages vaccination—often, the key concern over vaccination is linked to perception of risk, rather than to the possibility of compensation if the harm does occur.[48]

ALLOCATING SCARCE VACCINES: UTILITY AND FAIRNESS

To this point, we have concentrated on the ethics of mass immunization programs. More specifically, we have considered the ethical criteria for justifiably mandating some vaccinations, if voluntary measures do not suffice to establish the needed level of herd or population immunity, and the ethical conditions for granting some exemptions, including those based on religious and philosophical convictions. Now we turn to seasonal influenza, where there is a strong public health rationale for recommending, but not mandating, widespread immunization.

CASE STUDY: ALLOCATING INFLUENZA VACCINE IN A SERIOUS SHORTAGE: THE 2004–2005 "CRISIS"

In the United States, influenza and its complications lead each year, on average, to more than 200,000 hospitalizations and more than 36,000 deaths, mainly in at-risk persons over 65 years of age. When there is a shortage of vaccine in a given influenza season, how should public health officials and other health professionals, as well as the government and various social institutions, address this shortage?

In 2004–2005, such a shortage occurred, creating numerous uncertainties, requiring difficult decisions, and provoking vigorous debates about appropriate criteria and methods of allocating a vaccine in limited supply. For many analysts, this experience demonstrated the inadequacy of our current preparations, not only for seasonal influenza outbreaks marked by vaccine shortage, but, more importantly, for pandemic influenza which could wreak havoc on the order of the 1918–1919 pandemic influenza that killed more people than died in all of World War I and perhaps as many as 50 million world wide.[f]

Background

Seasonal influenza, symptoms of which often include a cough, fever, and headache, has variable severity. Recovery for most people occurs within a week or two. However, serious and life-threatening complications, including pneumonia, can sometimes develop, leading to the large number of hospitalizations and deaths already noted. These severe medical problems emerge more often in certain populations at risk, including persons 65 and older, children under age 2, anyone with chronic medical conditions, and women who are pregnant.[49]

---

[f] Epidemic is often defined as the occurrence in a particular population of a substantially higher number of cases of a disease than expected on the basis of past experience; a pandemic is generally considered to be more widespread, with a larger number of cases and usually covering a larger geographical area. For an examination of the 2009 H1N1 pandemic, see The 2009 H1N1 Pandemic: Summary Highlights, April 2009–April 2010 (updated June 2010), available at http://www.cdc.gov/h1n1flu/cdcresponse.htm. (accessed March 23, 2013).

Vaccination is the main protection against seasonal influenza, but other recommended measures include social distancing and hand washing. Unfortunately, the influenza vaccine must be reformulated each year in order to match, as closely as possible, the strains that emerge late in the flu season and are likely to be prevalent the next season, which usually starts in October and ends in April, with a peak in January or February. The process of creating the vaccine, which takes at least 6 months, needs to be modernized, but for now it involves cultivating the influenza virus in millions of fertilized chicken eggs. The two types of influenza vaccines that are recommended in the United States are an injectable inactivated virus vaccine, by far the most widely used (over 95%), and a nasal spray live-virus vaccine, which is recommended for use only in people who are between 2 and 49 years old, are healthy, and are not pregnant.

As the 2004–2005 influenza season approached, the CDC recommended vaccination of approximately 188 million Americans, a recommendation that was reiterated as late as September 24, 2004.[50] This number included approximately 85 million who were considered to be at high risk of serious complications and a variety of others, including persons who would be in close contact with high-risk persons—for instance, those engaged in providing care to nursing home residents. Assuming the availability of vaccine, the CDC also suggested vaccination for those wanting to reduce their chances of contracting influenza, those providing important community services, and those in institutional settings, such as students. The amount of vaccine ordered that season in both the public and the private sectors was 100 million doses, well below the 188 million vaccinations recommended. However, this lower amount seemed sufficient. After all, the previous high number of doses distributed was about 83 million, because many at-risk persons do not get an annual flu shot.

On September 28, 2004, before the severity of the shortage of vaccine was confirmed for that season, the U.S. Government Accountability Office (GAO) offered a prescient observation: "there is no system in place to ensure that seniors and others at high risk for complications receive flu vaccinations first when vaccine is in short supply."[49 (p. 11)] This observation was confirmed by what transpired less than 2 weeks later, when it was discovered that the overall available vaccine supply in the U.S. would be reduced by approximately half as a result of serious contamination problems at one of the manufacturing companies.

Public Health Decisions About Vaccine Allocation

Under such circumstances, who should receive the scarce vaccine? Several criteria and methods for allocating vaccine were developed at the federal, state, and local levels in 2004–2005; we will examine them, along with their implicit and explicit justifications. As is usually the case, the relevant laws left considerable room for public health officials, at different levels, to make difficult choices, which they had to justify publicly, most prominently in this case, by the ethical principles of utility and justice or fairness.

Defining the Public Health Problem and Setting Goals

One important question was how to define the public health problem and to set (or reset) the public health goals as the situation evolved. Not surprisingly, the public health problem was defined as a shortage of influenza vaccine, and the proposed solution, at least for the time being, was to formulate criteria and methods for allocating this scarce resource. While understandable and defensible, this approach to defining the public health problem and setting the public health goals was problematic for several reasons.

First, the demand for the influenza vaccine was created to a great extent by public health media campaigns over several years as part of an effort to reduce the risk that many individuals will experience considerable discomfort and will be relatively unproductive for several days, and to reduce the risk of serious morbidity and morality among more vulnerable individuals. In some sense, the problem, at least in its intensity, was "an artificial crisis," as some put it.

Secondly, the media viewed the public health problem almost exclusively as a shortage of a single technology, a vaccine that to a great extent (but not universally) immunizes individuals against influenza. However, the reduction of the risk of contracting influenza involves other strategies as well. Some public health officials distinguish an influenza *vaccination* program from an influenza *prevention* program, recognizing that the latter can and should include vaccination as an important component, along with other measures such as hand washing and social distancing. The public health goal could have been defined as a risk-reduction program, and this is how many public health officials viewed it.

By contrast, in the public view, the question became one of who, given the shortage of vaccine, should be vaccinated immediately or within a short period. As has been noted elsewhere, different terms have been used to describe the provision of a vaccine and other resources to some rather others when the supply is limited: distribution, (micro)allocation, selection, triage, rationing, prioritization, etc. Even though each term may denote a similar process, their somewhat different connotations bear on public communication and justification. Some terms appear to invoke different interpretations of the situation and different values. Here we will mainly use distribution and rationing.

CDC Priority Groups

Once it became clear that the supply of vaccine was going to be severely limited, reduced by as much as half, the CDC revised its recommendations on October 5, 2004 and issued "interim recommendations" that identified "priority groups" for the influenza vaccination (**Table 7.5**).[51] (In this discussion, "influenza vaccine" without a qualifier will refer to the injectable inactivated influenza vaccination.) These recommendations sidestepped many of the hard questions that would arise if the supply of flu vaccine proved to be insufficient to meet the demand within and among those priority groups.[g] Instead, the CDC viewed all the "priority groups" as being of "equal importance."

TABLE 7.5 CDC "Priority Groups" for Influenza Vaccine October 5, 2004e

AT RISK INDIVIDUALS
1. All children aged 6–23
2. Adults aged 65 years and older
3. Persons aged 2–64 with underlying chronic medical conditions
4. All women who will be pregnant during the influenza season
5. Residents of nursing homes and long-term care facilities
6. Children aged 6 months–18 years on chronic aspirin therapy
INDIVIDUALS IN SOCIAL ROLES THAT PUT OTHERS AT RISK
7. Healthcare workers involved in direct patient care
8. Out-of-home caregivers and household contacts of children aged < 6 months

Modified from: Centers for Disease Control and Prevention. Interim Influenza Vaccination Recommendations—2004–05 Influenza Season. Morbidity and Mortality Weekly Report (MMWR) 2004 (October 8);53:923–924. Available at: http://www.cdc.gov/mmwr/preview/mmwrhtml/mm5339a6.htm (accessed August 5, 2013).

It is possible to justify assigning priority to those at greatest risk from influenza and its complications—those in categories 1–6 in Table 7.5—on grounds of the effective and efficient use of scarce resources. This expresses the ethical principle of utility—of doing the greatest good overall. However, this principle receives at least two major interpretations and specifications in the context of the allocation of scarce medical or public health resources: (1) medical/health utility, and (2) social utility. Medical or health utility focuses on the greatest medical or health good for persons at risk of ill health, disability, or death, while social utility focuses on the greatest good for the society including but going beyond judgments of medical or health utility.

Risk has two dimensions: the probability of a negative event and the seriousness of that event. Hence, being "at risk"—or as most elaborations of the CDC criteria indicate, at high (or higher or highest) risk—may include (1) the probability that individuals within certain categories will contract influenza in the absence of a vaccine because of special vulnerabilities and susceptibilities, and/or (2) the probability that they will become very sick or even die from influenza and its complications because of their conditions. Both interpretations are important, but the second—the probable severity of the outcome—has been central in identifying risk groups.

While inevitably value-laden, risk judgments must be scientifically grounded. Priorities based on level or degree of risks need as much rigorous scientific evidence as possible. The CDC apparently went as far in its risk-based prioritization as it believed it could at the time, in light of the available scientific evidence. Its recommendations appeared to be based on statistical risks of morbidity and mortality, without further quantitative specification in terms—for instance, of loss of life-years, or quality-adjusted life-years, or the like. However, if both children on the one hand, and elderly persons on the other, have identical risk factors, it is not implausible to argue that priority should go to the young, which would be warranted if the public health goal is to maximize the number of life-years or quality-adjusted life-years saved, rather than individual lives saved. Even though this debate does not appear to have occurred around the initial CDC's formulation of its priority groups, it certainly emerged later and was a subject for the ethics subcommittee established in October 2004 to report to the Advisory Committee to the Director of the CDC.[52]

In addition to the groups at risk because of special vulnerabilities, the CDC assigned equal priority to two groups labeled in Table 7.5 as "Individuals in Social Roles that Put Others at Risk." These two groups are (7) healthcare workers involved in direct patient care, and (8) out-of-home

[g] For an excellent discussion of the legal context of these decisions about allocation and distribution of influenza vaccine, see Hodge JG, O'Connell JP. The legal environment underlying influenza vaccine allocation and distribution strategies. *Journal of Public Health Management Practices*, 2006;12:340–348.

caregivers and household contacts of children aged < 6 months. The risk-based concern is that, if unvaccinated, these individuals will get influenza and then infect high-risk patients or children under 6 months of age. The public health goal is to protect the individuals in these social roles in (7) and (8) in order to better protect high-risk persons under their care or in close household contact.

Because of the severe vaccine shortage in the fall of 2004, it was not possible for all the individuals in the CDC's several, equally important "priority groups" to receive the influenza vaccine in a timely fashion. Furthermore, not all of the supply was available at one time. Rather than proposing further prioritization, the "interim recommendations" suggested the use of the first-come, first-served criterion within and among priority groups. After indicating that doses should not be held in reserve for children who might need a second dose, the CDC recommended: "Instead, available vaccine should be used to vaccinate persons in priority groups on a first-come, first-serve basis."[51] In another effort to reduce the pressure on the scarce supply, the CDC asked persons not in one of the priority groups "to forego or defer vaccination."[51]

Other Criteria and Methods of Rationing Vaccine

Some state and local health departments attempted to further prioritize within and across the CDC's priority groups, with particular attention to the populations in their jurisdictions. This was difficult because of scientific uncertainties about risk prioritization or sub-prioritization, and some simply turned to physicians for their assessments of particular individuals at risk. Others adopted first-come, first-served as a method, as suggested by the CDC, while still others—sometimes after trying first-come, first-served—turned to lotteries. In short, public health officials used a variety of criteria and methods for rationing within and among the priority groups. **Table 7.6** shows options that were used in some contexts, often in combination.

TABLE 7.6 Criteria and Methods in Influenza Vaccine Rationing in 2004-2005

1. Priority based on risk a. Risk to the individual b. Risk the individual may create for others
2. First-come, first-served
3. Lottery
4. Priority based on social function

Each of these criteria and methods had an explicit or implicit ethical justification in the discourse surrounding the policies developed in different public health jurisdictions. These ethical justifications included principles of utility, with attention to the most effective and efficient reduction of risks to those at highest risk, and of justice or fairness, especially an egalitarian notion of equal opportunity. A review of the major newspaper articles at the height of the perceived crisis in the fall of 2004 shows the pervasiveness of the language of fairness, even though different conceptions of fairness emerged. Also evident in the justifications were other factors, including feasibility, costs, and medical and public cooperation based on transparency and on trust.

The Use of First-Come, First-Served and Lotteries

The methods of first-come, first-served—or queuing, as it is often called in the U.K.—and lotteries are both often viewed as forms of "random selection." In both, impersonal, even random factors determine the outcome, rather than criteria based on medical/health utility or social utility. They represent ways to realize egalitarian justice insofar as they treat each person as an equal and provide equality of opportunity.[53, 33] As in this case, medical/health utility may establish the basic pools from which individuals will be selected if not everyone at risk can be vaccinated.

Some jurisdictions that started to use first-come, first-served to address the overflow in priority groups soon encountered serious difficulties. This approach placed heavy burdens on some elderly and otherwise frail persons—while waiting in long lines for vaccination, some of them became very ill, some had to be hospitalized, and at least one died. As a result, some health departments went to first-*call*, first-served, while others abandoned queues in favor of lotteries—eligible people could call in or submit forms to enter the lottery for the vaccine. For instance, the Portland, Maine health department had a small supply of vaccine, which it had obtained prior to the announced shortage, and it was able to supplement that supply by several hundred additional doses donated by a medical center in the area and by the state health department. It proceeded to use a lottery to distribute its vaccine. People who wanted to enter the lottery had to provide a note from their healthcare provider indicating that they belonged to one of the priority groups.[54 (p. 19)] The city's director of public health proposed the lottery when "it became clear it really is a fair—probably the fairest—way to administer flu vaccine." In Montgomery Country, Maryland, the health department also established a lottery and received 19,000 entries from eligible persons in that county for its 800 remaining doses. A computer randomly selected the recipients.[55]

A lottery is attractive because, as Goodwin notes, it reflects "the moral judgment that people should be treated as absolutely equal where basic life chances (chance of life or survival) are involved."[56] In the vaccine distribution in 2004–2005, a lottery was used as part of a mixed system, its application being limited to those in priority groups. This combination reflected both judgments of medical/health utility—these judgments established the pool of persons eligible for the lottery—and considerations of equal opportunity—everyone at risk who entered the pool had an equal chance at getting the vaccine. However, both queuing and lotteries raise difficult questions of background justice and injustice: Who has the resources to enter the pool and when? Problems in transportation, telephone access, and the like, are all important limiting factors that affect the justice of the final outcome.

Valuable Social Functions

The fourth criterion in Table 7.6 above is "priority based on social function." Arguably, in Table 7.5, those categorized as "1B"—that is, individuals in roles that could put others at risk—also gain priority based on social function. As represented in Table 7.5, (7) and (8) include healthcare workers with direct patient contact and other caregivers of young children at risk. Their valuable social function (their social utility, narrowly conceived) is based on medical/health utility and social utility. However, some other social roles and functions also received priority for the influenza vaccination; persons in those roles received vaccinations independently of the CDC and its priority list.

The Department of Defense, after the influenza vaccine shortage became evident, anticipated "that all of our high-risk beneficiaries and all of our operationally employed service members will be vaccinated on time this flu season."[57, 58] A memorandum from the Assistant Secretary of Defense on October 13, 2004, stated the priorities somewhat differently, with first priority to operational forces in the Global War on Terror. The Department of Defense

> will provide influenza immunization to those critical operational forces who are conducting the Global War on Terror. Our top priorities are to immunize forces that are forward deployed in Operations Enduring Freedom and Iraqi Freedom, as well as forces who are preparing to deploy in the near future. We will also immunize those other forces that are designated as critical to our nation's defense. ...[59]

After noting a request for an expedited review of and guidance for these further priority groups, the Assistant Secretary indicated, "[Department of Defense] will administer the remainder of our limited flu vaccine supply in strict accordance with ...[CDC] recommendations. ..."[59] Less than 2 weeks later, the Department of Defense priorities were further specified in "Final Policy Guidance for the Use of Flu Vaccine for the 2004–2005 Season, with first group being "Critical Operational Forces as specified by Service Headquarters and Combatant Commands."[60]

This prioritization can be justified on the basis of (narrow) social utility, here understood in terms of a limited, important social function rather than individuals' broad overall worth or value. Outrage erupted when media reports mistakenly indicated that the Chicago Bears football team and members of Congress had been vaccinated. These did not appear to meet the publicly justifiable standards of important social functions required by the principle of utility. In fact, two members of the Chicago Bears who had severe asthma—and hence were at high risk from influenza—received vaccinations, and not all members of Congress received a vaccine.[61] In a major pandemic that seriously threatens the society, certain social functions—perhaps even congressional membership—will justifiably receive priority for vaccination (and antiviral treatments) based on the principle of social utility or, in its stronger version, the principle of national self-defense. However, some medical treatments may not be warranted on these social utility grounds. For instance, ventilator treatment would probably not restore patients to functional capacity in the course of the pandemic; hence, the distribution of ventilators should be based only on medical/health utility and justice/fairness, not on social function.[62, 63]

Lessons Learned, Questions Raised for a Possible Influenza Pandemic

Successful Allocation Strategies?

The sudden and unexpected shortage of seasonal influenza vaccine in October 2004 forced the CDC, state and local health departments, and many other institutions and healthcare providers to quickly develop and implement criteria and methods of allocation in a rapidly changing environment. Following is the overall assessment offered by the U.S. Government Accountability Office (GAO): "efforts to mitigate the sudden and unexpected shortage of influenza vaccine for the 2004–05 season were largely successful. ..."[54 (p. 32)]

These mitigation efforts were aided by the fact that the 2004–2005 influenza season was not as serious as many had feared, in part because the influenza strain turned out less virulent than had been predicted. However, there were problems, including ones we have noted in setting and implementing criteria and methods for rationing the vaccine. Many in high-priority groups chose not even to try to get vaccinated because of the shortage, while many others tried unsuccessfully. Indeed, a CDC survey determined that 37% of seniors (aged > 65 years) and 54% of adults who had chronic illnesses were not successful in getting the vaccine when they sought it, at least in the early part of the flu season.[64, 65] Nevertheless, CDC data indicate that vaccination rates for certain high-risk groups, such as older persons and young children, were close to the norm for the season.[54] High-risk priority groups received the majority of the influenza vaccine in 2004–2005. The CDC attributed this in part to "17 million healthy Americans stepping aside"[66]—although from another standpoint, we could say that they were pushed aside insofar as they were excluded from the priority groups.

As the GAO and others have noted, the lack of advance planning hampered the mitigation efforts in 2004–2005. This experience underlined the need for better preparation for sudden, unexpected crises, including not only short-term shortages of seasonal influenza vaccine but also shortages of resources to address a rapidly emerging influenza pandemic. Considerable progress has been made since this "artificial crisis," but whether it is sufficient will be unknown until a crisis occurs.

Difficult background questions remain, especially for the federal government, about how best to facilitate the modernization of vaccine production so that less time is required for production of a particular vaccine and it will be easier to respond to emergent crises. These questions also concern how much money should be allocated for these resources both in general and for a particular influenza season—or in preparation for a possible outbreak of pandemic influenza—since funds used for vaccines for public health will not be available for other public health needs.

Consistency and Variation

Clearly, there were many different players in the allocation of influenza vaccine in this scenario. The CDC played an active role in ensuring an equitable distribution of vaccine across different states. It allocated its supply in proportion to the needs and available supplies in different areas; some state and local health departments had their own (though inadequate) supplies that they had ordered directly.

We have focused on the criteria and methods of distribution and their justifications. While state and local public health departments generally distribute vaccines according to their own criteria and methods, as do healthcare institutions and providers, in this case, the CDC gave strong guidance by recommending against vaccination of any outside the priority groups it set. However, the state and local health departments had some discretion—as long as their policies and practices retained these priority groupings—to allocate their supply in accord with needs in their communities (e.g., a heavily elderly community with a number of nursing homes) and operative standards of fairness. They and others often had to improvise, but in a context that required public justification with attention to both utility (meeting greatest needs) and fairness. One big question, especially in a possible future influenza pandemic, is how much variation can be tolerated, especially among institutions and providers in close proximity.

Public/Private Collaboration

A significant portion of the supply of vaccine in 2004–2005 was not under the direct control of the public health infrastructure. Many healthcare providers, both institutions and individuals, had ordered and received supplies of vaccine before the shortage became evident. In a declared public health emergency, government at different levels has the authority, within limits, to commandeer private resources, including vaccines. Some states, including California and Florida, issued emergency public health directives requiring healthcare providers to offer the vaccine to, and only to, persons in the priority groups. Directives in some jurisdictions, including the District of Columbia and Michigan, indicated that the failure to comply could result in fines or imprisonment or other penalties. Although the data are not comprehensive, there is evidence that healthcare providers in many states, Minnesota being a prime example, voluntarily complied with the CDC's guidelines for distributing the vaccine.[54]

Studies of public attitudes related to the 2004–2005 influenza vaccine shortage suggest that the public was generally more confident in individual doctors and nurses than in a government agency making decisions about who should receive the scarce vaccine: Only 14% were very confident that "government agencies, together with the vaccine industry" would ensure a fair distribution of the limited supply of vaccine, and two-thirds thought that wealthy or influential persons would obtain a vaccine even if they were not in a high-risk group.[65 (p. 825)]

The need for clear, consistent, and well-grounded communication was evident throughout. CDC was urging vaccinations for large numbers and assuring the public of the sufficiency of the supply just a few weeks before the perceived crisis hit. Then, in part because of unclear, inconsistent, and rapidly changing public health messages, the media helped to generate the perception of a crisis. So one lesson is the need for clear and consistent communication.[54] This also connects with the need for transparency as well as the active and proactive engagement of various stakeholders.

Public Justification and Engagement

Not only did the CDC set up an ethics committee for some guidance in the wake of the 2004–2005 vaccine shortage crisis, but policies and practices of public engagement became common around the country. These have continued in part because the problems of the 2004–2005 influenza season would be greatly multiplied in an influenza pandemic, and criteria and methods of allocation, as well as other issues, need advance attention. Some ethicists appear to dismiss public engagement in favor of more academic philosophical theories. In defending their argument about how to set priorities for the allocation of vaccine in the context of pandemic influenza, Emanuel and Wertheimer, perhaps unintentionally, seem to downplay public engagement when they say that it is "unlikely that this is an issue that can be fruitfully resolved by a referendum or public opinion poll, and so although we would welcome a lively debate, we think that policy makers must assume the responsibility of producing the principles that are most ethically defensible."[67, 68] This could be viewed as question-begging; it is important to produce principles "most ethically defensible" *to whom*? The criteria and methods of allocation need to be "ethically defensible" not only to ethical theorists, but to relevant stakeholders, including the public, public health and healthcare professionals, and the institutions whose cooperation is essential to the development and maintenance of a just, fair, equitable system. Of course, what is called for is not an unreflective "referendum or public opinion poll"—these have limited value—but rather vigorous and rigorous engagement with the relevant stakeholders, along the lines we suggested earlier.[63 (pp. 18–19), 69 (p. 3), 70]

In making tragic choices in an influenza pandemic—about who will live and who will die—public health officials and other policy makers need to develop policies and practices that can engender and maintain the public's trust. In making these choices, where fundamental values in our public philosophy are at stake, decision makers must "attempt to make allocations in ways that preserve the moral foundations of social collaboration."[71]

CONCLUSIONS

Vaccines have made a tremendous contribution to public health in the 20th and the 21st centuries, both within the U.S. and around the world. As beneficial as they are, ethical questions still arise about whether particular vaccinations, such as for HPV, should be approved; whether they should be mandated or only recommended; and whether, if mandated or recommended, they should be for everyone or only for people with certain risks. In general, in mass immunization programs, noncoercive means of gaining widespread acceptance of needed vaccinations have ethical priority, but building on *Jacobson*, there are strong reasons to mandate vaccinations in some circumstances. Gaining compliance with recommended vaccinations may involve several measures, many of which may raise ethical issues—e.g., the use of incentive rewards or monetary sanctions. Another complex set of ethical issues surrounds whether and to what extent to recognize medical, religious, philosophical, and personal objections as bases for exemption from mandatory immunizations. While much of this chapter has considered how to gain compliance with mandated or recommended vaccinations, in some contexts the demand may be greater than the supply, as occurred in the perceived "crisis" caused by the shortage of influenza vaccine in 2004–2005. Then it is necessary to determine how ethically to distribute and allocate the scarce supply.

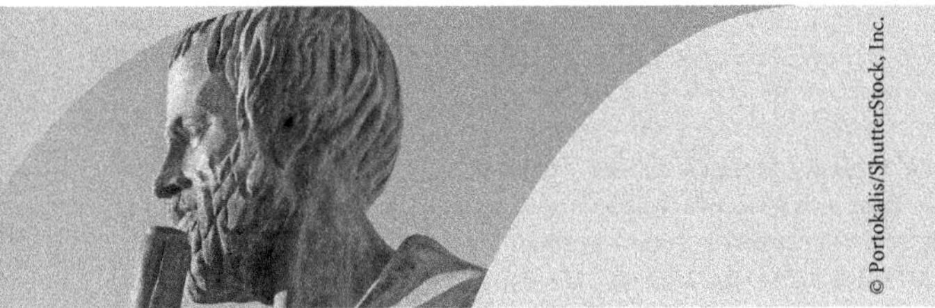

Discussion Questions

1. When is it ethically justifiable to mandate a vaccination? What conditions need to be met?
2. Is it ethically justifiable to mandate the HPV vaccination at this time? Why or why not? If yes, should it be mandated for females only or also for males?
3. Should we grant any nonmedical exemptions from mandated vaccinations? Why or why not?
4. If nonmedical exemptions are granted, should they be limited to religiously-based objections, or should we also include philosophical, personal, and moral objections? What are the pros and cons?
5. If we grant some nonmedical exemptions, should we erect some hurdles such as requiring the completion of an annual request for exemption in order to weed out objectors who are simply taking the easiest option?
6. Should healthcare workers in a hospital or nursing home be required to get an annual influenza vaccination? Why or why not?
7. Of the different criteria and methods used to allocate the scarce influenza vaccine during the perceived "crisis" of 2004–2005, which, if any, do you consider to be ethically justifiable? Are these the criteria and methods you would also use in an influenza pandemic with a high rate of infection and a high rate of mortality? Why or why not?

REFERENCES

1. National Immunization Program, Center for Disease Control. Achievements in Public Health, 1900–1999. *Morbidity and Mortality Weekly Report*, 1999;48:243–248.

2. Colgrove J. *State of Immunity: The Politics of Vaccination in Twentieth-Century America*. Berkeley, CA: University of California Press; New York: Milbank Memorial Fund, 2006.

3. Ten Great Public Health Achievements—United States, 1900–1999. *Morbidity and Mortality Weekly Report*, 1999;48:241–243.

4. *Jacobson v. Massachusetts*, 197 U.S. 11 (1905). Available at http://supreme.justia.com/cases/federal/us/197/11/ (accessed August 14 2013).

5. Mill JS. *On Liberty*. Ed. Spitz D. New York: W.W. Norton & Company, Inc. 1975.

6. Javitt G, Berkowitz D, Gostin LO. Assessing mandatory HPV vaccination: Who should call the shots? *Journal of Law, Medicine, and Ethics*, 2008;38:384–395.

7. Salmon DA, Siegel AW. Religious and philosophical exemptions from vaccination requirements and lessons learned from conscientious objectors from conscription. *Public Health Reports*, 2001;116:289–295.

8. Field R, Caplan A. A proposed ethical framework for vaccine mandates: competing values and the case of HPV. *Kennedy Institute of Ethics Journal*, 2008;18:111–124.

9. Gostin LO, de Angelis C. Mandatory HPV vaccination: public health vs. private wealth. *JAMA*, 2007;297:1921–1923.

10. Verweij M, Dawson A. Ethical principles for collective immunization programmes. *Vaccine*, 2004;22:3122–3126.

11. Vaccines for Children Program (VFC). Centers for Disease Control and Prevention. Available at http://www.cdc.gov/vaccines/programs/vfc/index.html (accessed March 22, 2013).

12. *Zucht v. King*, 260 U.S. 174 (1922) Available at http://supreme.justia.com/cases/federal/us/260/174/case.html (accessed August 14, 2013).

13. Community Preventive Services Task Force. *Guide to Community Preventive Services. Vaccinations to Prevent Diseases: Universally Recommended Vaccinations*. Available at www.thecommunityguide.org/vaccines/universally/index.html (accessed August 5, 2012).

14. Community Preventive Services Task Force. *The Community Guide: Universally Recommended Vaccinations: Client or Family Incentive Rewards*. Review completed April 2011. Available at http://www.thecommunityguide.org/vaccines/universally/IncentiveRewards.html (accessed August 6, 2012).

15. Community Preventive Services Task Force. *The Community Guide: Universally Recommended Vaccinations: Monetary Sanction Policies*. Review completed April 2011. Available at http://www.thecommunityguide.org/vaccines/universally/MonetarySanctions.html (accessed August 6, 2012).

16. Hoekstra EJ, LeBaron CW, Megaloeconomou Y, et al. Impact of a large-scale immunization initiative in the Special Supplemental Nutrition Program for Women, Infants, and Children (WIC). *JAMA*, 1998;280:1143–1147.

17. Wood D, Halfon N. Reconfiguring child health services in the inner city. *JAMA*, 1998;280:1182–1183.

18. Minkovitz CS, Guyer B. Effects and ethics of sanctions on childhood immunization rates, *JAMA*, 2000;284:2056.

19. Kerpelman LC, Connell DB, Gun WJ. Effect of a monetary sanction on immunization rates of recipients of aid to families with dependent children. *JAMA*, 2000;284:53–59.

20. Davis MM, Lantos JD. Ethical considerations in the public policy laboratory. *JAMA*, 2000;284:85–87.

21. Belluck P. For forgetful, cash helps the medicine go down. *The New York Times*, June 13, 2010. Available at http://www.nytimes.com/2010/06/14/health/14meds.html (accessed August 14, 2013).

22. American Academy of Pediatrics, Division of Health Policy Research. *Periodic Survey of Fellows No. 48: Immunization Administration Practices*. Elk Grove Village, IL: American Academy of Pediatrics, 2001.

23. Flanagan-Klygis EA, Sharp L, Frader JE. Dismissing the family who refuses vaccines: A study of pediatrician attitudes. *Archives of Pediatric and Adolescent Medicine*, 2005;159:929–934.

24. Diekema DS, and the Committee on Bioethics. Responding to parental refusals of immunizations. *Pediatrics*, 2005;115:1428–1431

25. Immunization of Health-Care Personnel. Recommendations of the Advisory Committee on Immunization Practices (ACIP). *Morbidity and Mortality Weekly Report*, 2011;60 (RRO7):1–45.

26. Backer H. Counterpoint: In favor of mandatory influenza vaccine for all health care workers. *Clinical Infectious Diseases*, 2006;42:1144–1146.

27. Association for Professionals in Infection Control and Epidemiology (APIC). *APIC Position Paper: Influenza Vaccination Should Be a Condition of Employment for Healthcare Personnel, Unless Medically Indicated*. January 27, 2011. Available at http://www.apic.org/Advocacy/Position-Statements (accessed March 22, 2013).

28. Finch M. Point: Mandatory influenza vaccination for all health care workers? Seven reasons to say 'no.' *Clinical Infectious Diseases*, 2006;42:1141–1143.

29. Code of Virginia 32.1-46 http://leg1.state.va.us/cgi-bin/legp504.exe?000+cod+32.1-46 (accessed August 5, 2012).

30. The National Conference of State Legislatures. *States with Religious and Philosophical Exemptions from School Immunization Requirements*. http://www.ncsl.org/issues-research/health/school-immunization-exemption-state-laws.aspx (accessed March 22, 2013.)

31. Colgrove, J. The coercive hand, the beneficent hand: What the history of compulsory vaccination can tell us about HPV vaccine mandates. In Wailoo K, Livingston J, Epstein S, Aronowitz R (eds). *Three Shots at Prevention: The HPV Vaccine and the Politics of Medicine's Simple Solutions*. Baltimore, MD: The Johns Hopkins University Press, 2010.

32. Nuffield Council on Bioethics. *Public Health: Ethical Issues*. London: Nuffield Council on Bioethics; November 2007. Available at: www.nuffieldbioethics.org (accessed January 17, 2013).

33. Beauchamp TL; Childress JF. *Principles of Biomedical Ethics*, 7th edition. New York: Oxford University Press, 2013.

34. Messina L [Associated Press]. Parents seek more exemptions for WV vaccinations. *West Virginia Gazette*, July 8, 2012. Available at http://www.wvgazette.com/News/201207080019 (accessed August 14, 2013).

35. Holland M. *Mary Holland's Testimony at West Virginia Vaccine Exemption Hearing*. Elizabeth Birt Center for Autism, Law, & Advocacy. Available at http://www.ebcala.org/areas-of-law/vaccine-law/mary-hollands-testimony-at-west-virginia-vaccine-exemption-hearing (posted July 16, 2012; accessed August 14, 2013).

36. O'Reilly KB. California, Vermont consider tougher vaccine-exemption laws. *American Medical News*, April 9, 2012 http://www.ama-assn.org/amednews/2012/04/09/prsa0409.htm (accessed July 19, 2012).

37. Vermont Legislature. *Act No. 157 An act relating to immunization exemptions and the immunization pilot program*. Available at http://www.leg.state.vt.us/database/status/summary.cfm?Bill=S.0199&Session=2012 (accessed August 9, 2012.)

38. Pediatric Infectious Diseases Society. *A Statement Regarding Personal Belief Exemption from Immunization Mandates*. March 2011. http://www.pids.org/news/238-pids-position-statement-on-pbes.html (accessed March 22, 2013).

39. Omer SB, Pan WKY, Halsey NA, et al. Nonmedical exemptions to school immunization requirements: secular trends and association of state policies with pertussis incidence. *JAMA*, 2006;296:1757–1763.

40. Colgrove J, Abiola S, Melo MM. HPV vaccination mandates—lawmaking amid political and scientific controversy. *The New England Journal of Medicine*, 2010;363:785–791.

41. Kim JJ. The role of cost-effectiveness in U.S. vaccination policy. *The New England Journal of Medicine*, 2011;365:1760–1761.

42. Balog JE. The moral justification for a compulsory human papillomavirus vaccination program. *American Journal of Public Health*, 2009;99:616–622.

43. Advisory Committee on Immunization Practices, Vaccines for Children Program. *Resolution No. 010/11-1: Vaccines to Prevent Human Papillomavirus, October 25, 2011.* Available at http://www.cdc.gov/vaccines/programs/vfc/downloads/resolutions/1011-1-hpv.pdf (accessed August 14, 2013).

44. Caseldine-Bracht J. The HPV vaccine controversy: Where are the women? Where are the men? Where is the money? *International Journal of Feminist Approaches to Bioethics*, 2010;3:99–112.

45. Zimet GD. Potential barriers to HPV immunization: From public health to personal choice. *American Journal of Law and Medicine*, 2009;35:389–399.

46. Albala I. Mandatory HPV vaccination: Is there a happy medium? *University of Pennsylvania Journal of Law and Social Change*, 2008;12;221–248.

47. Staats CES, Hamme JM. The greater good: rethinking risks and benefits of childhood vaccination programs. *Journal of Health and Life Sciences Law*, 2009;3:164–196.

48. Melo MM. Rationalizing vaccine injury compensation. *Bioethics*, 2008;22:32–42.

49. United States Government Accountability Office. *Infectious Disease Preparedness: Federal Challenges in Responding to Influenza Outbreaks.* Testimony before the Special Committee on Aging. U.S. Senate. September 28, 2004. Available at http://www.gao.gov/products/GAO-04-1100T (accessed July 24, 2012).

50. Centers for Disease Control and Prevention. Notice to Readers: Supplemental Recommendations about the Timing of Influenza Vaccination—2004–05 Influenza Season. *Morbidity and Mortality Weekly Report*, 2004 (September 24);53:878–879 http://www.cdc.gov/mmwr/preview/mmwrhtml/mm5337a7.htm (accessed March 23, 2013).

51. Centers for Disease Control and Prevention. Interim Influenza Vaccination Recommendations—2004–05 Influenza Season. *Morbidity and Mortality Weekly Report*, 2004 (October 8);53:923–924. Available at: http://www.cdc.gov/mmwr/preview/mmwrhtml/mm5339a6.htm (accessed March 23, 2013).

52. Harris G. U.S. creates ethics panel on priority for flu shots. *The New York Times.* October 28, 2004. Available at: http://www.nytimes.com/2004/10/28/health/28vaccine.html?ex=1130644800&en=4d4abf6aacf56603&ei=5070 (accessed August 5, 2012).

53. Peterson M. The moral importance of selecting people randomly. *Bioethics*, 2008;22:321–327.

54. United States Government Accountability Office. *Influenza Vaccine: Shortages in 2004–2005 Season Underscore Need for Better Preparation.* Report to Congressional Committees, September 2005. Available at http://www.gao.gov/products/GAO-05-984 (accessed July 24, 2012).

55. More than 19,000 entries in flu shot lottery. *WJLA/NewChannel 8*, Rockville, Md., October 25, 2004.

56. Goodwin B. *Justice by Lottery*. Chicago: University of Chicago Press, 1992.

57. U.S. Department of Defense. *DoD Influenza Vaccine Program—2004/05.* Available at fhp.osd.mil/vso_mso/2004/fluvaccine.pdf (accessed March 23, 2013).

58. Donna Miles. Defense Department expands flu vaccine. *U.S. Department of Defense News.* December 23, 2004. Available at http://www.defense.gov/News/NewsArticle.aspx?ID=24504. (accessed March 23, 2013).

59. Assistant Secretary of Defense (Health Affairs). *Memorandum: Interim Policy Guidance for the Use of Influenza Vaccine for the 2004–2005 Flu Season.* HA Policy: 04-024. Oct 13, 2004. http://mhs.osd.mil/About_MHS/HA_Policies_Guidelines.aspx?policyYear=2004 (accessed August 5, 2012).

60. Assistant Secretary of Defense (Health Affairs). *Memorandum: Final Policy Guidance for the Use of Flu Vaccine for the 2004–2005 Season, Oct 25, 2004.* http://mhs.osd.mil/libraries/HA_Policies_and_Guidelines/04-025.pdf (accessed March 23, 2013).

61. Vaccine for Congress and the Bears (Editorial). *The New York Times*, October 23, 2004. Available at http://www.nytimes.com/2004/10/23/opinion/23sat2.html (accessed July 27, 2012).

62. Childress JF. Triage in response to a bioterrorist attack. In Moreno, JR (ed.) *In the Wake of Terror: Medicine and Morality in a Time of Crisis.* Cambridge, MA: The MIT Press, 2003.

63. Ventilator Document Workgroup, Ethics Subcommittee of the Advisory Committee to the Director, Centers for Disease Control and Prevention. *Ethical Considerations Regarding Allocation of Mechanical Ventilators during a Severe Influenza Pandemic or Other Public Health Emergency*, July 1, 2011. Available at http://www.cdc.gov/od/science/integrity/phethics/ESdocuments.htm (accessed July 28, 2012).

64. Centers for Disease Control. Experiences with obtaining influenza vaccination among persons in priority groups during a vaccine shortage—United States, October–November, 2004. *Morbidity and Mortality Weekly Report*, 2004 (December 17);53(49):1153–1155.

65. DesRoches CM, Blendon RJ, Benson JM. Americans' responses to the 2004 influenza vaccine shortage. *Health Affairs*, 2005;24:822–831.

66. Centers for Disease Control and Prevention. *Targeting and Collaborations a Big Success: Priority Groups Received Majority of 2004–05 Influenza Vaccine Thanks to 17 Million Healthy Americans Stepping Aside.* March 31, 2005. Available at: http://www.cdc.gov/media/pressrel/r050331.htm (accessed March 23, 2013).

67. Emanuel EJ, Wertheimer A. Letter to Editor: Response. *Science*, 2008;314:1539–1540.

68. Emanuel EJ, Wertheimer A. Who should get influenza vaccine when not all can. *Science*, 2006;312:854–855.

69. *Ethical Guidelines in Pandemic Influenza* – Recommendations of the Ethics Subcommittee of the Advisory Committee to the Director, Centers for Disease Control and Prevention, February 15, 2007. Available at http://www.cdc.gov/od/science/integrity/phethics/panFlu_Ethic_Guidelines.pdf (accessed August 5, 2012).

70. Bailey TM, Haines C, Rosychuk, RJ, et al. Public engagement on ethical principles in allocating scarce resources during an influenza pandemic. *Vaccine*, 2011;29:3111–3117.

71. Calabresi G, Bobbitt P. *Tragic Choices.* New York: W. W. Norton and Company, 1978.

© Portokalis/ShutterStock, Inc.

CHAPTER 8

Containing Communicable Diseases: Personal Control Measures

by Alan L. Melnick

Learning Objectives

By the end of this chapter, the reader will be able to

- Distinguish quarantine and isolation
- Identify and assess the ethical trade offs involved in voluntary and mandatory quarantine
- Understand the ethical issues involved in selecting among the following types of quarantine: home, facility, and working
- Distinguish latent from active tuberculosis
- Understand the ethical issues surrounding Directly Observed Therapy (DOT) for multiple drug resistant tuberculosis
- Distinguish active from passive monitoring and identify the ethical issues associated with each

INTRODUCTION

The nature of governmental public health work, including activities involving communicable disease control, requires that public health officials make trade-offs between individual rights and community benefits virtually every day.[1] When responding to communicable disease threats, as in other areas of public health, governmental public health officials have many interventions at their disposal. These are indicated on the Nuffield Council on Bioethics' Intervention Ladder[a], which describes interventions that range from providing health education to constraining individual liberties, such as isolating someone with a communicable disease (isolation), restricting the movements of healthy people exposed to a communicable disease such as severe acute respiratory syndrome (quarantine), and excluding children from school until they obtain immunizations. All of these decisions, which invoke the state police powers available to public health officials, involve balancing individual liberties with community benefits.

Often it is possible to persuade individuals and families to comply with the recommended protective measures, but sometimes it is necessary to move up the Intervention Ladder to achieve compliance. Using sanctions to require compliance raises concerns about paternalism and the trade-offs between individual liberty and community benefit, and public health officials must provide justifications for these actions. As has been discussed elsewhere, public health law tells public health officials what they *can* do, but it rarely offers clear and sufficient guidance to public health officials regarding what they *should* do in specific situations, especially when officials must balance community concerns against individual liberties and property rights. In addition, public health law varies by state, and decision making based on legal authority thus differs across jurisdictions. In many situations, legal authority may be ambiguous, leaving public health officials without clear guidance regarding actions they should take and requiring them to offer ethical justifications and reasons for their actions.

When implementing interventions that may place individual liberties, privacy, and other interests at odds with community benefits, public health officials should consider three factors:

- Whether the proposed intervention is the least restrictive of individual rights consistent with realizing the public health goal;

[a] Nuffield Council on Bioethics report, *Public Health: Ethical Issues* (London: Nuffield Council, November 2007) Available at: www.nuffieldbioethics.org (accessed January 17, 2013).

- Whether public health officials have attempted to reduce any negative effects of these restrictions, such as providing food and water for quarantined individuals, or providing directly observed therapy for tuberculosis in a confidential location and, on the Intervention Ladder, using incentives rather than coercion;
- Whether the burdens involved do not disproportionately affect a minority or otherwise vulnerable population.

Decisions about controlling communicable diseases that are based solely on epidemiology or on legal authority might not always have the best outcomes. As in medicine, there is often uncertainty about the effectiveness of specific public health interventions. Public health officials should always question whether a given action is necessary, whether there are less restrictive alternatives, and whether they can justify their actions to their community constituents. Ethical deliberations using a variety of tools, including the Public Health Code of Ethics, can provide systematic ways to balance trade-offs between individual and community interests as well as systematic guidance for justifying public health interventions on the basis of what is good and right for health and social welfare. The use of ethical principles in guiding decision making recognizes that processes—"doing things right"—are as important as outcomes—that is, "doing the right things." In addition, the use of ethical principles recognizes that public health officials are accountable to the communities they serve, that the law alone does not justify specific actions, and that public health officials cannot perform their work adequately without the public's trust.[1]

In this chapter, we will present two case studies illustrating the use of ethical analysis in helping public health officials make better decisions regarding communicable disease control. The discussion will focus on debates about whether, which, and when public health interventions that restrict civil liberties, such as mandated treatment, quarantine, and isolation, are necessary to control communicable disease; what public health officials should consider when contemplating restrictive measures; and what processes they should use to justify their decisions and promote trust. The chapter will also address how officials can recognize whether less-restrictive alternative measures are available, whether proposed measures disproportionately affect specific and vulnerable populations, and how they can include relevant stakeholders in their decision-making process. This ethical analysis can also help public health officials determine when and which laws and regulations are ethically justifiable for communicable disease control.

DIRECTLY OBSERVED THERAPY FOR MULTIPLE DRUG-RESISTANT TUBERCULOSIS

Background

Tuberculosis (TB) remains one of the world's deadliest diseases. In 2010, nearly 9 million people developed active TB, and 1.4 million died from it. In the United States, where public health efforts to prevent, identify, and treat active TB are robust, TB incidence has declined, especially among persons born in the United States. The 11,182 cases reported in the United States in 2010 was the lowest recorded number since reporting began in 1953. Among reported cases in the United States, 60% occurred in foreign-born persons. The case rate among foreign-born persons (18.1 cases per 100,000) in 2010 was approximately 11 times higher than among U.S.-born persons (1.6 cases per 100,000).

Since 1993, when the Centers for Disease Control and Prevention (CDC) expanded the TB surveillance system to include drug-susceptibility results, multiple drug-resistant TB (MDR TB) cases have decreased in the United States.[2] Like TB infection in general, MDR TB is more common in foreign-born persons. Since 1998, of the total number of reported primary MDR TB cases, the proportion occurring in foreign-born persons increased from 25.3% (103 of 407) in 1993, to 82% (72 of 88) in 2010.[3] MDR TB is especially concerning because of limited options for treatment and because failure to treat it appropriately can lead to even more deadly forms of TB, including extremely drug-resistant TB (XDR TB).

Fortunately, most people who become infected do not develop active infection. With active infection, the bacteria multiply and cause symptomatic illness. Although active disease can involve virtually any part of the body, active lung infection, known as pulmonary tuberculosis, is most common. Tuberculosis infection spreads from person to person through the air, when people with active pulmonary tuberculosis expel droplets by coughing, talking, singing, or sneezing. Successful transmission depends on the environment in which exposure occurs. Prolonged exposures in indoor environments are more likely to result in transmission.[7] Studies have demonstrated that successful transmission has occurred in homes, ships, trains, office buildings and healthcare facilities.[4, 8–11]

About 90% of people who become infected develop a condition known as latent TB infection (LTBI), in which a small number of bacteria live in the body without replicating or causing illness. People with LTBI are not contagious. However, individuals with LTBI have about a 5% to 10% risk of developing active TB over their lifetime, with the risk highest in the first 2 years after becoming infected.[4, 5] Immigrants from high-incidence countries are at highest risk of developing active disease within the first 5 years after arrival in the United States.[6] Daily treatment with one oral antibiotic, isoniazid, for 9 months can eliminate the infection and prevent the development of active disease. On the other hand, once active disease develops, those affected require a minimum of several drugs for 6 months, while those with active MDR TB can require up to 2 years of treatment with multiple drugs, many with significant side effects.

Within the United States, populations most likely to suffer from active tuberculosis include the poor, the homeless, immigrants from developing countries, people living with HIV, substance abusers, and prisoners. Consequently, TB is a highly stigmatized illness, and issues of social justice/injustice surround its transmission because of these background conditions of vulnerability. These issues of justice/injustice also arise in the diagnosis and treatment of TB, because those most often affected have the most limited access to appropriate treatment and other resources.

CASE 1: ORDERING DIRECTLY OBSERVED THERAPY FOR MDR TB

Background

Several months ago, a family adopted several children from a developing country with a high TB prevalence, including MDR TB. The children range in age from 5–13 years. On arrival in the United States, the children received screening for communicable disease, including TB. At that time, the evaluation revealed that although the children were infected, they did not have active disease. Instead, they had LTBI and consequently were not contagious to others. Current recommendations for new arrivals with LTBI are for them to receive antibiotics to treat the LTBI and prevent the development of active disease. The family has strong religious beliefs about medical care, believing that prayer will cure most health issues. Accordingly, the family has refused LTBI treatment, immunizations, and other preventive care for their children. The parents have home-schooled the children, but the children travel into the community for other activities. Health officials who conducted the entry evaluation discussed TB with the parents, including what to watch for, and instructed them to seek medical care if any of the children developed symptoms.

Soon after arrival, one of the adopted children, a teenager, developed a cough, night sweats, and weight loss, symptoms typical for TB. The family did not immediately seek medical care. However, after several months of continued symptoms, the parents took the child to a local pediatrician who, after obtaining a chest x-ray and sputum samples, diagnosed the child's condition as active pulmonary TB. The physician, as required by law, notified the local health department. The sputum samples were positive by smear (staining) and culture, revealing that the child's infection was contagious. The physician and public health officials were concerned because transmission of TB is more frequent where there is prolonged, close contact, such as between family members in a home.

After several weeks, cultures revealed multiple drug resistance, including resistance to the commonly used drugs isoniazid and rifampin. The child's pediatrician referred the case to a pediatric infectious disease/TB specialist. Treatment of TB sensitive to all drugs requires several drugs taken over at least 6 months; for MDR TB, treatment can take up to 18–24 months. If a TB patient does not take the full course of treatment, relapse with an infection resistant to additional medications, including extremely drug-resistant TB (XDR TB), can develop. Therefore, inadequate treatment can be worse than no treatment at all. The most common reason that patients do not receive the appropriate treatment is failure to take the entire regimen. This is not surprising, given the long course of treatment, the need to take multiple medications, and the potential side effects. In addition, patients develop significant relief from their symptoms within weeks to months, making it more difficult for them to comply with long treatment regimens. This is a particular problem for patients with MDR TB, given that they require up to 2 years of treatment.

Because of the risks associated with incomplete compliance and concomitant treatment failure, the Centers for Disease Control and Prevention and the World Health Organization (WHO) recommend Directly Observed Therapy (DOT). DOT involves giving the TB medications directly to patients and observing them swallow the medications. Priority cases for DOT include patients with contagious TB (pulmonary disease with positive sputum smears), patients with drug-resistant TB, and children. Besides ensuring treatment adequacy, DOT helps physicians treating the patient to follow their progress. With DOT, the treating physician knows that the patient has received all the appropriate medications. Therefore, the physician can be aware that lack of clinical improvement is likely due to additional drug resistance or failure to absorb the medication rather than not taking the medication. DOT is part of the general standard of care for active TB within the United States, though questions remain about exactly what counts as adequate DOT—for instance, videophone or in-person DOT—and how to secure compliance with recommended or required DOT—for instance, through persuasion or incentives.

When the case began treatment, a health department nurse visited the family's home to administer DOT.

The regimen of second-line drugs the child was taking for MDR TB required twice daily dosing. The parents objected to having the home visit, stating that DOT was an invasion of their privacy and parental rights. The parents especially did not like having the nurse interrupt their breakfast at home. They assured the nurse that they cared about their child and that they could be trusted to give the medication. Concerned about the risk from inadequately treated MDR TB, the health department offered to administer DOT at an alternative time and setting acceptable to the family. The family refused, but questioned whether videophone DOT would be possible.

Although videophone DOT was a potential alternative, given that the child was contagious with MDR TB, the pediatric TB specialist supported in-person DOT for at least the morning dosages of the medication, with videophone-observed administration in the evening. Consequently, the family's relationship with the specialist deteriorated, and the parents refused to let the specialist treat the child.

The health officer agreed with the pediatric TB specialist and informed the family that in-person DOT, at least for the morning dose, was necessary to protect the child and the community. At first the family agreed, but became increasingly reluctant to have the nurse visit, and eventually refused in-person DOT, although they insisted that they would treat the child themselves for the full 18 months or longer. The health officer had the statutory authority to require in-person DOT, and even impose isolation of the case and removal from the family if deemed necessary to protect the public health. The statutes also provided due process for the family. Although the statutes stated what the health officer *could* do, it is not clear what the health officer *should* do faced with this situation.

Ethical Analysis and Assessment of this Case

The public health ethics framework uses ethical considerations to provoke deliberation that will help the health officer and the Health Department decide how to approach this case. The framework includes three steps: (1) analyze the ethical issues; (2) evaluate the ethical dimensions of the choices available to the health officer; (3) justify a particular decision/action. Each step includes several questions that public health officials and their partners can ponder when making decisions. Depending on the features of the particular case, one or several of the questions might become the primary focus of the analysis.[1, 12–16]

Step 1: Analyze the Ethical Issues

The analysis includes the considerations identified in **Table 8.1**.

As a first step, the local health officer and the health department will need to clarify the harms and risks of concern in the situation, as well as the goal of public health action. While answers to these questions often seem obvious, careful analyses may reveal separable concerns or unclear goals that limit good decision making and cloud justification. In this example, is the primary public health goal primarily to control the spread of TB, to prevent XDR TB, or to provide appropriate care for the child? The purpose of this question is not to challenge any one goal, but rather to clarify each goal that may provide justification for public health decisions.

TABLE 8.1 Analyzing Ethical Issues in Public Health

What public health problems, needs, concerns are at issue?
What are appropriate public health goals in this context?
What is the source and scope of legal authority, if any, and which laws and regulations are relevant?
What are the relevant norms and claims of stakeholders in the situation and how strong or weighty are they?
Are there relevant precedent legal and ethical cases?
Which features of the social-cultural-historical context are relevant?
Do professional codes of ethics provide guidance?

Data from: Bernheim RG, Nieburg P, Bonnie RJ. Ethics and the Practice of Public Health. In: Goodman RA (ed) *Law in Public Health Practice*, 2nd edn. New York: Oxford University Press, 2007.

As in most settings involving active TB, the public health goals are to prevent transmission of TB—including in this case, MDR TB—and to ensure that the child receives the appropriate curative care. Requiring in-person DOT creates risks for the child as well as for the community. The risks for the child from requiring in-person DOT include the side effects of treatment and social/behavioral harms associated with isolation and loss of privacy during visits. Requiring in-person DOT may harm the community by driving potential cases "underground," leading to delayed identification and treatment of persons with TB. For example, if other families in similar situations perceive that they could face similar sanctions, they may be reluctant to have their children evaluated, increasing the risk of TB exposure in the community. On the other hand, the decision to allow the parents to administer the full course of treatment without observation or even via videophone DOT with limited resolution has risks for both the child and the community. Without in-person DOT, physicians caring for the child would be unable to determine definitely whether failure to improve clinically was due to insufficient dosing or some other reasons, such as increased resistance of the infection or malabsorption of the medication. This, in turn, could lead to inappropriate medical decisions that could adversely affect the child's health. In addition, without in-person DOT, the child faces an increased risk of treatment insufficiency, leading to continued infectiousness or relapse with an equally or more resistant infection, perhaps even extremely drug-resistant TB, which would put the community, as well as the child and other family members, at greater risk.

The analysis also poses questions to elucidate the moral claims of the various stakeholders drawing an approach to ethical analysis called "stakeholder theory." This approach has particular relevance for public health ethics since it implicitly focuses attention on the fundamental partnership of public health professionals with individuals and groups in the community in assessing the value-laden benefits and harms of particular public health actions. Although it emphasizes utility—the greatest overall good—it makes explicit the costs and benefits for different groups, thus raising questions of distributive justice—who bears the burdens and who gains the benefits—while recognizing the complex ongoing nature of the human relationships involved.

In this case, there are several stakeholders: the child, the child's family (including not only the parents but also several siblings), and the public, which expects the health department to protect the community from TB. Regarding moral claims, the child has some expectations of freedom of movement, and privacy; the family has similar expectations regarding privacy, respect for parental rights, and the freedom to administer medications to their child at a convenient time and place. However, these claims are not absolute, and competing moral claims can outweigh them. The child has a moral claim that could compete with her parent's claim, specifically, that receiving DOT will reduce the risk of inappropriate treatment and relapse compared to having her parents administer the medications. In addition, the public has a moral claim based on two expectations: (1) that the health department will protect the community from TB, and (2) that people contagious for TB and other infectious diseases will protect others by behaving in an appropriate manner, including staying home when contagious and cooperating with treatment recommendations. This is especially concerning in this case because the immigration health officials had discussed the risks with the parents, warning them to seek treatment as soon as the child developed symptoms, yet the parents waited several months before taking the child to a pediatrician.

The ethical framework also invites consideration of previous cases. An analysis of a new situation's relevant similarities to and differences from paradigm or precedent cases—cases that have gained a relatively settled moral consensus—often provides an important starting point or presumption in deliberation. Because ethical reflection on any public policy issue takes place within a particular community with a unique history and culture, the framework specifically asks that public health officials and other stakeholders clarify the conflicting ethical tensions in the political–social context, since ethical norms and tensions can vary from community to community. What may be morally acceptable in some communities, for example, needle-exchange programs to prevent HIV transmission, may not be in others.

In this particular case, given state statute, the health officer's scope of authority is clearly not in question. State statute directly addresses health officer authority to control TB (**Exhibit 8.1**).[17]

In addition, the state clinical guidelines strongly recommend treating all TB patients with DOT, as does the CDC.[4, 18]

EXHIBIT 8.1 Local Health Officers

Health Officials, Broad Powers to Protect Public Health

(1) TB has been and continues to be a threat to the public's health in the state.

(2) While it is important to respect the rights of individuals, the legitimate public interest in protecting the public health and welfare from the spread of a deadly infectious disease outweighs incidental curtailment of individual rights that may occur in implementing effective testing, treatment, and infection control strategies.

(3) To protect the public's health, it is the intent of the legislature that local health officials provide culturally sensitive and medically appropriate early diagnosis, treatment, education, and follow-up to prevent TB. Further, it is imperative that public health officials and their staff have the necessary authority and discretion to take actions as are necessary to protect the health and welfare of the public, subject to the constitutional protection required under the federal and state constitutions. Nothing in this chapter shall be construed as in any way limiting the broad powers of health officials to act as necessary to protect the public health.

(Continued)

EXHIBIT 8.1 Local Health Officers (*Continued*)

Powers and Duties of Health Officers

Each health officer is hereby directed to use every available means to ascertain the existence of, and immediately to investigate, all reported or suspected cases of TB in the infectious stages within his or her jurisdiction and to ascertain the sources of such infections. In carrying out such investigations, each health officer is hereby invested with full powers of inspection, examination, treatment, and quarantine or isolation of all persons known to be infected with TB in an infectious stage or persons who have been previously diagnosed as having TB and who are under medical orders for treatment or periodic follow-up examinations and is hereby directed:

(a) To make such examinations as are deemed necessary of persons reasonably suspected of having TB in an infectious stage and to isolate and treat or isolate, treat, and quarantine such persons, whenever deemed necessary for the protection of the public health.

(b) To make such examinations as deemed necessary of persons who have been previously diagnosed as having TB and who are under medical orders for periodic follow-up examinations.

(c) Follow local rules and regulations regarding examinations, treatment, quarantine, or isolation, and all rules, regulations, and orders of the state board and of the department in carrying out such examination, treatment, quarantine, or isolation.

(d) Whenever the health officer shall determine on reasonable grounds that an examination or treatment of any person is necessary for the preservation and protection of the public health, he or she shall make an examination order in writing, setting forth the name of the person to be examined, the time and place of the examination, the treatment, and such other terms and conditions as may be necessary to protect the public health. Nothing contained in this subdivision shall be construed to prevent any person whom the health officer determines should have an examination or treatment for infectious TB from having such an examination or treatment made by a physician of his or her own choice who is licensed to practice osteopathic medicine and surgery under chapter 18.57 RCW or medicine and surgery under chapter 18.71 RCW under such terms and conditions as the health officer shall determine on reasonable grounds to be necessary to protect the public health.

(e) Whenever the health officer shall determine that quarantine, treatment, or isolation in a particular case is necessary for the preservation and protection of the public health, he or she shall make an order to that effect in writing, setting forth the name of the person, the period of time during which the order shall remain effective, the place of treatment, isolation, or quarantine, and such other terms and conditions as may be necessary to protect the public health.

(f) Upon the making of an examination, treatment, isolation, or quarantine order as provided in this section, a copy of such order shall be served upon the person named in such order.

(g) Upon the receipt of information that any examination, treatment, quarantine, or isolation order, made and served as herein provided, has been violated, the health officer shall advise the prosecuting attorney of the county in which such violation has occurred, in writing, and shall submit to such prosecuting attorney the information in his or her possession relating to the subject matter of such examination, treatment, isolation, or quarantine order, and of such violation or violations thereof.

(h) Any and all orders authorized under this section shall be made by the health officer or his or her TB control officer.

(i) Nothing in this chapter shall be construed to abridge the right of any person to rely exclusively on spiritual means alone through prayer to treat TB in accordance with the tenets and practice of any well-recognized church or religious denomination, nor shall anything in this chapter be deemed to prohibit a person who is inflicted with TB from being isolated or quarantined in a private place of his own choice, provided, it is approved by the local health officer, and all laws, rules and regulations governing control, sanitation, isolation, and quarantine are complied with.

Data from Washington State Legislature, Administrative Code of Washington, Chapter 246-100-036, Responsibilities and duties—Local health officers, http://apps.leg.wa.gov/WAC/default.aspx?cite=246-100-036 (accessed 6/20/13).

However, statutes and guidelines vary from state to state, and the authority to order DOT might be less clear elsewhere. While state statutes address the health officer's authority to order DOT, specifically stating what the health officer can do, the Public Health Code of Ethics provides some guidance for deliberation about what the health officer should do.[19] Several of the 12 principles in the Code (Principles 1, 2, 4, 5, 6, 8, 10, 12) are particularly relevant to the decision to order the family to comply with DOT, and are relevant for Step 2 and Step 3 of the framework.[19]

TABLE 8.2 Principles of the Ethical Practice of Public Health (Public Health Leadership Society)

1	Public health should address principally the fundamental causes of disease and requirements for health, aiming to prevent adverse health outcomes.
2	Public health should achieve community health in a way that respects the rights of individuals in the community.
3	Public health policies, programs, and priorities should be developed/evaluated with community members' input.
4	Public health should advocate and work for the empowerment of disenfranchised community members, aiming to ensure that the basic resources and conditions necessary for health are accessible to all.
5	Public health should seek the information needed to implement effective policies and programs that protect and promote health.
6	Public health institutions should provide communities with the information they have that is needed for decisions on policies or programs and should obtain the community's consent for their implementation.
7	Public health institutions should act in a timely manner on the information they have within the resources and the mandate given to them by the public.
8	Public health programs and policies should incorporate a variety of approaches that anticipate and respect diverse values, beliefs, and cultures in the community.
9	Public health programs/policies should be implemented in manner that most enhances the physical and social environment.
10	Public health institutions should protect the confidentiality of information that can bring harm to an individual or community if made public. Exceptions must be justified based on the high likelihood of significant harm to the individual or others.
11	Public health institutions should ensure their employees' professional competence.
12	Public health institutions and their employees should engage in collaborations and affiliations in ways that build the public's trust and the institution's effectiveness.

Reproduced from: Public Health Leadership Society (2002). Principles of the ethical practice of public health version 2.2. New Orleans, LA. PHLS.

Step 2: Assess the Ethical Dimensions of the Public Health Options

The case evaluation, directed at determining whether one or more public health decisions/actions are more justifiable ethically than other decisions, includes the following considerations (**Table 8.3**).

As noted above, the state statutes permit, but do not require, the health officer to order the family to comply with DOT for the child. Given the risk to the child and the community from inadequately treated MDR TB, and given the parents' earlier delay in seeking treatment for the child, is there any justification for *not* requiring DOT? On the other hand, the family's perspective is that requiring them to comply with DOT violates their parental rights, autonomy, and privacy. Given that the parents believe and state strongly that their primary goal is appropriate treatment for the child, is there any justification for *not* allowing the parents to administer the treatment themselves?

When deciding whether to require compliance with DOT, the health officer might focus his or her deliberation on the following questions the framework raises, specifically,

1. Will requiring in-person DOT probably produce a net balance of benefits over harms and other costs?
2. Will it distribute benefits and burdens fairly?[12]

TABLE 8.3 Ethical Considerations

Utility: Does a particular public health option produce a balance of benefits over harms?
Justice: Are the benefits and burdens distributed fairly (distributive justice), and do legitimate representatives of affected groups have the opportunity to participate in making decision (procedural justice)?
Respect for liberty: Does the public health action respect individual choices and interests (autonomy, liberty, privacy)?
Respect for legitimate public institutions: Does the public health action respect professional and civic roles and values, such as transparency, honesty, trustworthiness, promise-keeping, protecting confidentiality, and protecting vulnerable individuals and communities from undue stigmatization?

The answers to these questions would depend in part on the values and relationships in the particular context, such as the degree of trust and cooperation between the family and the public health workers, including the staff visiting the home for in-person DOT. Certainly, health officials have an obligation to ensure that the nurse or healthcare worker implementing DOT is competent and professional. As mentioned earlier, the family agreed to those visits at first, but over a few weeks, the level of trust and cooperation deteriorated, and the family eventually refused in-person DOT.

In the United States, in both law and public philosophy, there is a tentative priority or presumption for liberty over coercion in public health measures. If so, to justify the order for in-person DOT, the health officer would have the burden of showing that the public health value in this circumstance (perhaps because the potential public health risk and harm from MDR TB are great) overrides the liberty interest of the family and the burdens imposed on them. In addition, this is particularly salient because this case involves a family that considers themselves members of a vulnerable religious community and distrusts government. It might be possible to demonstrate that both in-person DOT and videophone DOT are ethically defensible options. The question then becomes, how does one choose and justify one option over another? Part 3 of the framework poses questions to help public health decision makers justify a particular option.

Step 3: Provide Justification for One Particular Public Health Action

Justifying the final decision when several options are available includes addressing the following questions, to determine if the relevant justificatory conditions have been met (**Table 8.4**).

TABLE 8.4 Justificatory Conditions

Questions
Effectiveness: Is the action likely to accomplish the public health goal?
Necessity: Is it necessary to override the conflicting ethical claims to achieve the public health goal?
Least infringement: Is the action the least restrictive and least intrusive?
Proportionality: Will the probable benefits of the action outweigh the infringed moral considerations and any negative effects?
Impartiality: Are the burdens and benefits of the action distributed fairly?
Public justification: Can public health officials offer public justification that citizens, and in particular those most affected, could find acceptable in principle?

Data from Childress JF, Faden RR, Gaare RD, et al. Public health ethics: Mapping the terrain. *Journal of Law, Medicine*, & Ethics, 2002;30(2):169–177, at 172.

Choosing one option often means that one value, such as public health benefit, overrides another value, such as individual liberty. When overriding a significant value, it is important that an action address the conditions underlying these questions. (Lawyers will recognize that these conditions are analogous to those that the state must meet to justify restrictions on constitutionally protected liberties.)

In public health, as in medicine, there is often uncertainty about the effectiveness of interventions. DOT is no exception. We know that failure to complete appropriate treatment for TB is the primary cause of drug resistance and relapse and is the reason why the CDC and the WHO strongly recommend DOT. However, questions have been raised about the evidence citing the effectiveness of DOT compared to self-administration in ensuring treatment adequacy and completion. One question relates to the strength of evidence, particularly the availability of randomized clinical trials in demonstrating DOT effectiveness. For example, one review questioned a WHO study for using mathematical modeling rather than relying only on evidence from randomized clinical trials.[20] A Texas study frequently cited as evidence for DOT used a pre- and post-intervention design, a relatively weak study design, to demonstrate that implementing DOT for all active TB cases resulted in a significant reduction in drug resistance and relapse.[21] Unfortunately, however, randomized clinical trial evidence is limited, probably because of the difficulty getting approval for such study designs given problems related to compliance and the risk related to the potential of inadequately treated TB in control groups. A recent Cochrane review of a limited number of randomized and quasi-randomized clinical trials found no significant difference between DOT and self-administration using "cure" as an outcome.[22] However, the methodologies and outcome measures used varied across studies, and the definition of cure was questionable, especially in a disease such as TB, where relapse is possible years after treatment ends. In addition, when the review grouped trials by the location of DOT, there was a small yet significant improvement in outcome for delivering DOT in a home setting compared with self-administration. Home delivery of DOT, as frequently practiced in the United States, might be effective by reducing the barriers for patients who have to travel at least 2 and up to 5 days a week for clinic-administered DOT.

The comparison between home-administered and clinic-administered DOT provides insight into questions about proportionality, necessity, and least infringement. Certainly, requiring this family to bring their child to a clinic twice daily for DOT for MDR TB provides a greater infringement on liberty compared to home administration and would tip the scales towards the moral concerns of the parents related to autonomy and fairness. In this case, the health officer and the health department were willing to visit the family twice daily. In addition, the health department was willing to observe the family set up and begin the intravenous infusion of the evening medication and have the parents initial the intravenous infusion bag in the morning after the infusion, rather than have health department staff wait at the home until the infusion was completed. Because the parents objected to having the public health staff interrupt their breakfast, the health department offered to meet the child with one of the parents at an alternative time and/or location for the morning dose.

The family asked the health officer to consider two less intrusive interventions: (1) using a videophone to observe all doses and/or (2) requiring DOT for only the first several months of treatment while the child's infection could still be contagious, rather than the full 18 months. One commentator has argued that after several months of treatment, once a case is noninfectious, the original purpose of the DOT (protecting the public) no longer applies and the reduced risk of self-administration is acceptable.[23] In addition, populations at risk for bearing the burdens of DOT, such as low-income populations, prisoners, and those with HIV infection, often lack access to preventive health care that might reduce their risk of developing active TB.[23] In this case, the health officer consulted with the TB specialist who recommended against use of the videophone because of technological limitations (particularly, the lack of resolution), and the concern that any medication administration error in this child with MDR TB (of which there are only around 90 cases in the U.S. each year) could lead to XDR TB, with consequences for the public. In addition, after consultation with the state Department of Health TB program, and given the evidence, albeit limited, for DOT's greater effectiveness and concerns about the risk of relapse with XDR TB, the health officer and the TB specialist both recommended DOT for the full 18 months.

Explicitly addressing these questions is essential in explaining public health decisions to affected individuals and to the public. Public health officials should justify actions and policies with rhetorical strategies that build not only community support and trust, but also build support and trust from the individuals and families directly affected. Certainly, even in-person DOT requires patient cooperation, since public health officials do not have the right to force people to take medication.[24] In justifying their decisions, health officials might appeal to principles, rights, and duties, and by acknowledging that while a particular action overrides important values, the action is likely to be effective and involves the least restrictive infringement, given the situation.[12]

PERSONAL AND COMMUNITY CONTROL MEASURES IN RESPONSE TO OUTBREAK OF SEVERE RESPIRATORY ILLNESS

Background

SARS (Severe Acute Respiratory Syndrome) is a severe viral respiratory illness caused by the SARS-associated coronavirus (SARS-CoV). SARS-CoV first appeared in the winter of 2002–2003, when it caused over 8,000 cases and nearly 800 deaths in 26 countries.[25,26] Patients generally present with nonspecific symptoms, such as fever, muscle aches and pains (myalgias), malaise, and chills, making it difficult for clinicians and public health officials to differentiate SARS from other respiratory illnesses, such as influenza or community-acquired pneumonias. Patients frequently develop a cough, shortness of breath, and chest pain. Affected elderly are less likely to have fever or any other specific symptoms other than malaise and diminished appetite.[26] The prognosis is poor. Although one-third of patients improve with resolution of their pneumonia, the rest continue to have fever and increased shortness of breath, with 20–30% requiring intensive care, most on ventilators. Death is generally secondary to severe respiratory failure, multiple organ failure, superimposed bacterial sepsis, or due to complications such as myocardial infarction. The mortality rate in the elderly is 50%, whereas children, especially those under 12, are likely to recover completely.[26]

SARS–CoV transmission occurs primarily through the respiratory route through direct and indirect contact of mucous membranes of the eyes, nose, or mouth with infectious respiratory droplets or fomites. Epidemiologic studies reveal that SARS-CoV is moderately transmissible, with an average of two to four secondary cases resulting from each index case. Transmission has occurred mostly in healthcare and inpatient settings,[26–28] possibly facilitated through procedures that generate aerosols, such as endotracheal intubation, bronchoscopies, and treatment with aerosolized medications.[26, 27, 29–31] Although transmission to casual and social contacts rarely occurs, documented transmission has occurred occasionally after close contact in the workplace, on airplanes, and in taxis.[26] On the other hand, studies have revealed some so-called super-spreading events, in which a few infected persons transmitted the infection to a disproportionate number of contacts. Consequently, public health authorities believe that SARS-CoV is capable of causing large epidemics but can be controlled through public health measures, such as isolation, quarantine, and other forms of social distancing.[26, 27] Most countries have reported a median incubation period of 4–5 days, and a mean of 4–6 days, with a maximum of 14 days.[27] Although mild infections are rare, infected persons with mild symptoms are less likely to transmit the infection. Studies have failed to document transmission from asymptomatic patients or before symptom onset.[26]

Monitoring: Active and Passive

One important and indispensable public health response to such outbreaks is monitoring. This involves either the public health department or its designee contacting exposed persons by phone or in person at least daily to determine whether the exposed person has developed symptoms of the disease. The purpose is to identify symptoms early, thereby providing an opportunity for health officials to reduce the time between onset of symptoms, during which the person becomes contagious, and the institution of precautions, including isolation.

Monitoring activities can be passive or active, and health officials can monitor individuals and/or populations.[32] With both types of monitoring, the first step health officials must take is to identify individuals, such as family members exposed to a case, or populations that might share common exposure. By interviewing individual ill cases or family members of ill cases, health officials can identify household members, close friends, or individual classmates who might have suffered exposure. Health officials can also identify populations sharing common exposure, such as people who have attended a public event, airline passengers, schoolmates, faculty workers,[33] or, in the case we will present below, students living in an international dormitory.

Passive monitoring, the less invasive form of monitoring, involves notifying exposed individuals or populations and asking them to assess themselves (for SARS, at least twice daily) and to notify health officials immediately if they develop respiratory symptoms or fever. The CDC recommends passive monitoring for situations in which the exposure and subsequent illness risks are low and the risk to contacts from delayed disease recognition is low.[32] Here, the potential harms apply to the exposed individuals, exposed populations, and the general community. The risks for the exposed individuals from passive monitoring include the social-behavioral harms associated with potential invasion of privacy as well as stigmatization. Monitoring specific populations, such as students and other people living in an international dorm, also presents potential risks and harms from invasion of privacy as well as stigmatization of the international student community, particularly the international students and their families. As in the MDR TB case, the attendant loss of privacy and stigmatization from notification could create community risks by driving potential cases underground, leading to delayed identification and isolation of contagious cases. On the other hand, passive monitoring involves minimal constraints on individual freedoms compared to the more restrictive options and it is less expensive. Because passive monitoring relies on exposed persons to perform self-assessment and notify health officials as soon as they develop symptoms, failure to comply could harm the community due to an increased risk of exposure.

Compared to passive monitoring, active monitoring is more restrictive, in that it requires healthcare or public health staff to contact exposed individuals regularly (at minimum, once daily) by phone or in person to evaluate whether the individual is developing symptoms or signs of severe respiratory illness, such as SARS-CoV. The CDC recommends active monitoring for situations in which the exposure and subsequent illness risks are moderate to high, resources are available to contact and evaluate individuals, and the risk to contacts from delayed disease recognition is low to moderate.[32] In addition, health officials must have contingency plans in place for dealing with individuals who fail to comply. Failure to comply can lead to additional restrictions on individual freedoms. For example, health officials could ask law enforcement to confine or otherwise restrict activities of noncompliant individuals.[32] Active monitoring presents similar risks to exposed individuals as passive monitoring, but additional restrictions can increase the potential harms from loss of privacy and stigmatization. However, the additional restrictions for noncompliant individuals increase the potential harms from loss of privacy and stigmatization of individuals and their particular communities as well as the potential loss of income, especially for noncompliant individuals. Moreover, active monitoring is more expensive and the potential restrictions may drive some exposed individuals underground. On the other hand, compared to passive monitoring, active monitoring more likely reduces the risk of disease transmission for the broader community.

Types of Quarantine

Voluntary and Mandatory

Like monitoring, quarantine is an action health officials impose on exposed people who are not ill. However, quarantine goes beyond monitoring in that it adds separating and restricting the movement or activities of those monitored.[32, 33] The purpose of quarantine is to reduce disease transmission by separating exposed persons from others, limiting their movements, monitoring them for symptoms, and instituting appropriate infection control precautions, including isolation, as soon as monitoring activities detect symptoms.[32] Quarantine can be either voluntary or mandatory, and public health officials can apply quarantine to individuals or groups of people.[32, 33] Even under voluntary quarantine, however, public health officials have the authority to enforce restrictions for groups or individuals who fail to comply.[32] These restrictions include, but are not limited to, posting guards outside of homes, using electronic forms of monitoring, and using guarded facilities.[32]

Home, Facility, and Working Quarantine

Public health officials have three options for quarantining exposed people: home quarantine, quarantine in specific facilities, or working quarantine.[32] Based on previous experience with SARS-CoV, these restrictions could remain in place for up to 10 days or longer.[32]

Home quarantine, the least intrusive quarantine measure, requires that those quarantined are capable of monitoring their own symptoms or have a caregiver present who can monitor their symptoms. In addition, restrictions for those quarantined within the home should be adequate to protect other household members from potential exposure. Typical restrictions that minimize interactions with housemates might include sleeping and eating in a separate room, using a separate bathroom, and wearing surgical masks when in common areas.[32] Although health officials can monitor those quarantined for symptoms passively or actively, the CDC suggests that active monitoring is more likely to prevent delays in recognizing symptom onset. Household members of the quarantined individuals do not face restrictions and may continue to travel to work or school in the community unless or until the quarantined individual develops symptoms. At that time, health officials can (and probably will) order restrictions, including quarantine, for the newly exposed household contacts.[32]

Health officials might choose to use specific quarantine facilities for housing-exposed persons who do not have a home environment conducive to protecting other occupants from potential exposure. Exposed persons who might meet these criteria include travelers, the homeless, and persons living in dormitories. Working quarantine measures apply to exposed persons who work in essential occupations, such as law enforcement officers and firefighters, and exposed healthcare workers who might need to continue working, especially during outbreaks when human resources are scarce. During off-duty hours, those under work quarantine remain in quarantine at home or in designated facilities. During work hours, health officials require those under work quarantine to minimize contact and use personal protective equipment, such as masks, while traveling to and from work and while working.[32]

Burdens and Risks of Quarantine

Each form of quarantine infringes some personal values and creates potential harms for the quarantined individuals and the community. Quarantined individuals face restrictions on their personal freedom and mobility, and they often experience feelings of isolation. Those quarantined at home might feel isolated from friends and coworkers, while those quarantined in designated facilities might feel isolated from family as well. Quarantine at home or in designated facilities could lead to loss of income or employment. In addition, quarantined individuals with chronic health problems, especially those with mental health conditions, risk complications from their illness. Health officials can reduce the occurrence and magnitude of these harms and increase compliance by ensuring those quarantined receive essential goods and services, including food, medical care and supplies, mental health, and other social support services.[32, 33] This is an expression of community solidarity rather than the mere imposition of communal norms. (See our discussion of this distinction in Chapter 3).

Quarantine, especially group quarantine, presents an additional risk related to stigmatization of a particular population. As with other restrictive measures, the threat of quarantine could create community risks by driving potential cases underground, leading to delayed identification and isolation of contagious cases. Furthermore, the costs associated with quarantine, including the costs of monitoring, the costs of designated quarantine facilities, and the cost of providing essential services to quarantined individuals and groups could present quite a significant burden for the community.

Focused and Community-Wide Measures to Create Social Distance: Benefit-Risk Analysis

Public health measures to increase social distance may be focused or community-wide. Focused measures might be effective in reducing disease transmission among groups or populations public health officials consider at particular risk of exposure, including those living or working at specific sites or buildings. And it is usually reasonable to start with focused measures. However, as the outbreak evolves, a number of new cases may lack epidemiological links with existing cases. At this stage, public health officials may consider applying social distancing measures to an entire community, but the boundaries of the relevant community may vary. Community-wide measures public health officials could consider include cancellation of all public gatherings, community-wide furlough days ("snow days"), reducing mass transportation schedules, closing bridges and tunnels, and closing schools and worksites throughout the community.[32, 33] The final, most restrictive option available to local public health officials is community-wide quarantine, also known as *cordon sanitaire* (sanitary barrier). Community-wide quarantine restricts movement of large groups of people into and out of a specific area.[33]

Each of these measures creates burdens and risks for the affected groups and the community. Measures applied to specific populations can compromise personal freedoms and increase the risk of stigmatization. Other harms may include interrupted education, loss of recreational options, loss of business, loss of employment/income, and loss of access to essential goods and services, such as food, medical supplies, medical appointments, mental health, and other social services. If the measure applies to an entire community, it could affect contiguous jurisdictions that rely on workforce from the restricted area. Health officials and their partners can reduce some risks by ensuring that essential services and support and alternative arrangements for employment and education, such as telecommuting or online curricula, are available. In addition, public health officials should endure that adequate mental health and other psychological support services are available for individuals with mental health conditions and for other individuals subject to increased stress and stigmatization.[32] Additional potential harms for the community stem from the requirement to enforce community-wide measures. Although some measures, such as cancellation of public events or scaling back of mass transit services, require no enforcement, other measures, such as community-wide quarantine, will require use of physical measures ranging from physical barriers to law enforcement checkpoints.[32]

There are debates about the effectiveness of nonpharmaceutical restrictive and social distancing measures. One recent study of 43 cities involved in the 1918–1919 influenza pandemic, long before influenza vaccines or antiviral drugs were available, revealed that a variety of nonpharmaceutical restrictive measures, including isolation, quarantine, and other social distancing measures were effective in mitigating the consequences of the pandemic, which is estimated to have killed 550,000 individuals in the U.S. and approximately 40 million individuals worldwide.[34] During that pandemic, multiple interventions, such as school closures and suspensions of public events, were more effective than single interventions in reducing excess death rates from pneumonia and influenza. In addition, early implementation of these measures was more effective than implementing them after morbidity and mortality rates began to rise. Recognizing this, the CDC released its Interim Pre-pandemic Planning Guidance: Community Strategy for Pandemic Influenza Mitigation in the United States. The guidance recommends implementing these nonpharmaceutical interventions as soon as public health officials confirm that an outbreak due to a pandemic virus strain is occurring in a state or metropolitan area.[35] On the other hand, however, there is some uncertainty about these recommendations. During the 1918–1919 influenza pandemic, strategies effective in some cities were not as effective in others, and some cities experienced better outcomes with public health responses that were less robust compared to others.[34]

More recently, during the 2003 SARS epidemic, several countries successfully implemented isolation and mass quarantine measures, most of which were socially acceptable.[33, 36] Strategies included isolation at home and in general hospitals, although some countries considered constructing special infectious disease hospitals.[36] Health authorities in Canada and Asia implemented social distancing by closing congregate settings, such as schools, hospitals, factories, hotels, restaurants, and entertainment venues.[36] In the United States, local health officials quarantined a foreign tourist in a hospital and kept an incoming flight on the tarmac while investigating a potential case.[36] Although most quarantine orders were voluntary, some countries used measures that were more restrictive. For example, Singapore officials used thermal scanners, Web cameras, and electronic bracelets, and Hong Kong used a police electronic tracking system to enforce mass quarantines.[36]

CASE 2: CONTROLLING SEVERE RESPIRATORY ILLNESS OF UNKNOWN ETIOLOGY AT A MAJOR UNIVERSITY

The following case scenario requires an ethical analysis at several stages of an outbreak of a severe respiratory illness at a major university. It is complicated, as many real-life cases are, by its context, by uncertainties at various stages, particularly regarding the etiology of the severe respiratory illness, and by the comparative effectiveness and potential negative effects of different public health measures for this particular illness.

Background

Stage 1: Index Case

During the first 2 weeks of classes in December, a graduate student who had recently arrived in the U.S. was admitted to the hospital with severe respiratory illness. Before entering the U.S., the student had visited his elderly father in a hospital in Vietnam. One week before admission, several days after entering the U.S., the student developed upper respiratory symptoms, rapidly progressing to pneumonia and respiratory failure. The student gradually recovered without incident. Meanwhile, the WHO was reporting a number of respiratory failure cases of concern, including several casualties, in Vietnam. According to the WHO, these cases appeared to represent a particularly virulent form of severe acute respiratory syndrome (SARS) or avian influenza. Fortunately, at this time, there is no evidence of sustained person-to-person transmission.

Laboratory tests performed on the student, more than 1 week after onset, are negative for seasonal influenza, SARS-CoV, and avian influenza. Nevertheless, the infectious disease specialist, aware of the situation in Vietnam and the student's possible exposure, reports the case to the local public health department. At this point, public health officials and treating physicians have been unable to identify a specific etiological agent. The possibilities include, but are not limited to, infection with SARS-CoV or infection with a novel avian influenza virus. No vaccine is available, and there is no evidence that antiviral treatment would be effective. Therefore, health officials have only nonpharmacologic interventions at their disposal. Actions public health officials could currently consider for preventing transmission include:[26]

- Notifying students and parents that anyone who visited the campus during the first 2 weeks of classes might have been exposed to a serious respiratory illness
- Notifying university staff, including faculty, administrative, and support staff, that they may have been exposed to a serious respiratory illness
- Identification, then passive and active monitoring (surveillance) of patient contacts
- Quarantine of exposed contacts at home or in designated facilities combined with surveillance
- Working quarantine
- Closing the university and surrounding business, canceling events
- Community-wide measures to increase social distance, such as furloughs or "snow days"
- Quarantine of the entire university community

Stage 2: Cluster of Secondary Cases

Within the following week at the university, 20 other students who live in the same "international" dorm develop respiratory symptoms. Ten of them have tests for seasonal influenza A, and all are negative. Most of the students have not received seasonal influenza vaccination. Two children among the international student families are admitted to the ICU with respiratory failure, with one death. Most student victims appear to be relatively stable, although they are not responding to antiviral medications or antibiotics. Tests for avian influenza, specifically H5N1, and SARS-CoV are pending.

Stage 3: Wider Outbreak with Person-to-Person Transmission

Several days later, the respiratory illness appears to be spreading rapidly. Both the ER and the ICU have a growing number of their staff calling in sick, apparently with influenza-like symptoms. Student health and the hospital ER also report increases in the number of patients with respiratory symptoms. They have sent many of these patients home with the usual recommendations for fluids, antipyretics, etc. In addition, the hospital has admitted 10 more students and university staff members with severe respiratory illness. Of these, five have been admitted to the ICU, and one more death has occurred (a 2-year-old child whose parent works at the university). The hospital epidemiologist and nursing staff, working with university student health, have collected information on all patients and hospital staff who have had respiratory symptoms. Laboratory results are positive for SARS-CoV for several of the students. Student health employees have reported the cases to the local health department, and the health department has conducted an epidemiologic analysis that suggests person-to-person spread of infection. After reviewing the results of clinical and epidemiologic analysis, you are concerned that a SARS-CoV outbreak threatens your community.

Ethical Framework

Step 1: Analyze the Ethical Issues

Following the steps identified in Table 8.1 above, the first step local public health officials should take, as in the MDR TB case, is to clarify the risks of concern in the situation, as well as the goal of public health action. Again, careful analysis may reveal different concerns or goals that might or might not be compatible. In this example, is the primary public health goal primarily to prevent the transmission of this unknown respiratory illness—especially at stage 1, when there is no evidence that this particular case is transmissible—or to ensure that the student receives appropriate care? Public health officials will need to address these questions to provide justification for any interventions they choose.

As in most settings involving an illness that is potentially transmissible, the public health goals are to prevent transmission while supporting efforts to ensure that the student receives appropriate care. At stage 1, any type of public notification has creates risks for the student as well as the community. The risks for the student include social-behavioral harms associated with potential invasion of privacy as well as stigmatization. In addition, as in the MDR TB case, the attendant loss of privacy and stigmatization from notification could harm the community by driving potential cases underground, leading to delayed identification and isolation of contagious cases. On the other hand, failure to notify potential contacts has risks for the student's contacts, including local family members, friends, colleagues and healthcare providers, who might delay taking appropriate measures, such as staying home when sick (voluntary isolation) or seeking appropriate treatment at the onset of symptoms. Late notification could damage the public health system, by eroding health officials' trust and credibility because they withheld information,[37–41] particularly information from minority populations who often are already wary of the public health system.[42]

By stage 2, and certainly by stage 3, when it becomes clear that the disease is transmissible, preventing further transmission might become the primary public health goal, and health officials might contemplate several actions ranging from less to more restrictive. Given the rapid development of the outbreak, it is unlikely that a vaccine or effective antiviral treatment would be available. Public health officials can apply the additional nonpharmacologic actions individually, specifically to exposed individuals or communities that share common exposure risks.[32] All these options, which involve varying degrees of monitoring, or quarantine, have varying degrees of effectiveness in different situations, impose a variety of burdens and costs, and create sundry risks identified above.

As the scenario progresses to stage 2 and stage 3, public health officials become aware of increased transmission and fewer epidemiological links between individual and subsequent cases. It thus becomes obvious that measures they had targeted at individuals and groups, such as quarantine, are becoming less effective. In this situation, health officials might consider population-based measures to reduce transmission by increasing social distance.

Focused population-based measures (as distinguished from community-wide measures) seek to reduce disease transmission among groups or populations at particular risk of exposure. Such groups or populations include those living or working at specific sites or buildings, such as students in the international dorm. Actions could include closing the university theatre, suspending classes, closing the entire university, and shuttering nearby businesses the students frequent.

Health officials could consider community-wide measures of social distancing as the outbreak spreads and the new cases lack epidemiologic links to existing cases. These could include closing schools and worksites throughout the entire community or even, in the most extreme situation, the most restrictive measure of all: a community-wide quarantine that limits the movement of large groups of people in and out of specific areas, such as a dormitory, university, or even a whole city.

We noted above the various burdens, costs, and potential harms associated with these different measures, and stressed that health officials should consider them only when the options are severely limited and the disease in question cannot be adequately controlled by those options. Even then, health officials should undertake efforts to reduce those burdens, costs, and potential harms, as experienced by different stakeholders.

In this case, a number of stakeholders have moral claims: the ill student, the ill student's family members, other university students, including Southeast Asian students, university faculty, staff, and administration, healthcare providers who have cared for the student, local businesses, as well the public that expects the health department to protect the community from respiratory illness. The student has some expectations for privacy. Likewise, the Southeast Asian students and their families have some expectations regarding privacy. Furthermore, several of these measures could mark them as being at risk for the disease and lead to their stigmatization. All stakeholders, especially if specific measures affect their movement, have expectations related to freedom to travel unrestricted, access to food and necessary services, access to work, and freedom to attend community events and recreational activities. All local businesses have expectations that they should have the freedom to set their hours of operation, serve their customers safely, and remain free from unnecessary restrictions on their activities.

However, these claims are not absolute, and competing moral claims can override them in some circumstances. The public has a moral claim based on three expectations: (1) that the health department will protect the community from epidemics, (2) that people contagious for severe respiratory illness and other infectious diseases will protect others by behaving in an appropriate manner, and (3) that public health officials will use scarce resources judiciously.

Consequently, public health officials should use scientific evidence and epidemiology to select the least restrictive alternative, compatible with realizing the public health goal. When doing so, they should consider the level of community cooperation and the available healthcare and public health resources.[32] For example, when health officials obtain evidence that the outbreak is waning, as soon as appropriate, they should discontinue the community-wide measures, withdrawing the most restrictive measures, such as geographic, mass transit, and travel restrictions first.[32]

In this particular case, as in the MDR TB case, given the statute in Washington State (as in many other states), the health officer's basis and scope of authority are clearly not in question. For example, the Washington State statute directly addresses the health officer's authority to control communicable disease. Specifically, the statute gives the health officer the authority to "take such action as is necessary to maintain health and sanitation supervision over the territory within his or her jurisdiction" and "control and prevent the spread of any dangerous, contagious or infectious diseases that may occur within his or her jurisdiction."[17] In addition, Washington State administrative code states that "local health officers shall, when necessary, conduct investigations and institute disease control and contamination control measures, including medical examination, testing, counseling, treatment, vaccination, decontamination of persons or animals, isolation, quarantine, vector control, condemnation of food supplies, and inspection and closure of facilities, consistent with those indicated in the 17th edition, 2000 of the *Control of Communicable Disease Manual*, published by the American Public Health Association, or other measures he or she deems necessary based on his or her professional judgment, current standards of practice and the best available medical and scientific information."[43]

Because the authority to order isolation and quarantine in the United States is a state power, delegated to the local level, the authority of local public health officials to restrict movement might not be clear in some states. Before the World Trade Center and anthrax events of 2001, many states relied on old statutes lacking clarity about the scope of state and local public health officials' authority. Subsequently, and in response to concerns about natural or man-made biologic disasters, many states updated their statutes to reflect the Model State Emergency Health Powers Act to address this problem.[44] Therefore, when addressing questions about scope and authority, public health officials should check their relevant state statutes.

In this case, as in the MDR TB case, state statutes state what health officials can do but do not necessarily or always indicate what they should do in given situations. Similar points apply to past precedents in both legal interpretations and health officials' actions—they may be relevant and instructive but indeterminate for the current situation.

Step 2: Assess the Ethical Dimensions of the Public Health Options

In responding to the respiratory illness outbreak case, public health officials certainly have several options available at each stage of the outbreak, ranging from isolation and notification to mass quarantine. State statutes might permit, but do not require, the health officer to implement any of these measures. Given the risk to the community from a disease outbreak, at stage 1, is there any justification for *not* notifying students, the university, or the public, or for *not* taking more restrictive actions, such as surveillance, social distancing measures, or quarantine? On the other hand, the perspective of the student, his family, and perhaps the Southeast Asian student community is that these efforts would infringe their liberty and could lead to a loss of privacy and could stigmatize the community. In addition, other students and community businesses could suffer from missing classes, lost business, and loss of freedom to travel and engage in recreational activities. From these perspectives, the question would be whether any justification existed for taking restrictive measures, or even for merely notifying the public.

When deciding on actions on the Intervention Ladder, ranging from less to more restrictive, public health officials should evaluate the ethical dimensions of their choices by using the considerations listed in **Table 8.3**. As with the MDR TB case, this evaluation can help officials determine whether one or more public health decisions/actions are more ethically justifiable than other decisions/actions. When deciding whether to implement isolation, social distancing, or quarantine orders, health officials might focus their deliberation on the following questions the framework raises: (1) whether a particular option will probably produce a balance of benefits over harms, and (2) whether it will distribute benefits and burdens fairly.[12]

The answers to these questions would depend in part on the values and relationships in the particular context, including the degree of trust and cooperation between health officials and each of the stakeholders in this situation. Among the stakeholders are the ill student, the ill student's family, the Southeast Asian community, the university, local businesses, and the public. Similar to the earlier MDR TB case, this respiratory illness case involves a minority population vulnerable to stigmatization and other forms of discrimination, including potential violence.

When considering restrictive actions, health officials could mitigate potential harms and promote justice in several ways. If time permits, they could meet with stakeholder representatives, such as organizations representing Southeast Asian students and their families and organizations representing local businesses, listen to their concerns, and consider their input. Throughout the course of the outbreak, health officials could have a liaison representative meet with stakeholder representatives, listen to their input, and keep them informed of developments. In addition, health officials should ensure that anyone subject to quarantine receives adequate supplies and support.[33] In meeting with stakeholders and the public, health officials should clarify that they are imposing quarantine not to punish individuals or populations, but to protect the health of those quarantined as well as that of the public.[36] Consequently, health officials should consider home quarantine rather than mass quarantine when possible, because voluntary home quarantine is generally less restrictive and more acceptable. On the other hand, home quarantine measures can be discriminatory, since they are only available to those with homes.[36] In this case, home quarantine might not be available to the Southeast Asian students, subjecting them to possible additional stigmatization.

When imposing mass quarantine, health officials must mitigate harm by ensuring that the quarantine facilities are clean, safe, comfortable, and not degrading (e.g., a cell in a county jail used to isolate exposed persons may provide a clean, safe, and even [physically] comfortable location, but its use for quarantine may evoke feelings of humiliation, anger, and fear in quarantined individuals).[36] Because those quarantined are potentially exposed and at risk for illness, health officials must have monitoring systems in place to recognize and immediately remove ill persons from quarantine facilities to avoid additional exposure of those who are still well. In addition, health officials imposing quarantine must ensure that decent food—both from a nutritional and a culturally appropriate standpoint—clothing, schooling, medical supplies, medical care, and mental health services are available for those quarantined, and that they provide ways for those quarantined to communicate with family, friends, and legal representatives.[33, 36]

During the 2003 global SARS outbreak, very few of the large number of individuals quarantined ever developed clinical illness.[45] Clearly, these noninfected individuals suffered a disproportionate burden of the response to the outbreak. Depending on when public health officials impose quarantine or other restrictive measures, they should do whatever they can to ensure that they impose these measures as fairly as possible, and that, if possible, the entire community should bear the financial burden equitably. For example, for extended quarantine, health officials could mitigate harm by ensuring that those quarantined can use sick time or continue to receive income, that they have a way to pay bills, and that closed businesses receive some financial support to compensate for lost business income.[33, 36]

Because of the tentative priority or presumption for liberty over coercion in public health measures in the United States, health officials will bear the burden of showing that the public health utility of any of their decisions overrides the affected population's interests in liberty, privacy, etc., and outweighs the burdens imposed on them or created by these measures, such as stigmatization. Whether officials impose home quarantine or mass quarantine, they will need to ensure that those quarantined have the right to due process, specifically the right to be heard by an independent tribunal.[36]

At stage 1, it might be possible to demonstrate that notification and perhaps passive or active surveillance are ethically defensible options. When moving to stages 2 and 3, the more restrictive options become more defensible. The question then becomes, "how does one choose and justify one option over another?" Part 3 of the framework poses questions to help public health decision makers justify a particular option.

Step 3: Justify One Particular Public Health Action

Justifying the final decision when several options are available includes satisfying the justificatory conditions in Table 8.4 above. A fundamental theme in public health ethics is that choosing one option often means that one value, such as public health benefit—in this case, reducing disease transmission—overrides another value, such as individual liberty—in this case, freedom of movement. When overriding such an important value, it is important that an action address the conditions underlying the questions in Table 8.4. As noted in the previous case, these conditions are analogous to those that the state must meet to justify restrictions on constitutionally protected liberties.

Although the nonpharmacologic strategies available to public health officials, including monitoring, isolation, and quarantine, are fundamental measures historically used to control communicable disease transmission, there is some uncertainty about the effectiveness of these strategies.[32, 35] In addition, even when studies have found that individual measures, such as isolation, are effective, there remains uncertainty about whether adding additional strategies, such as quarantine, would have improved effectiveness. For example, in evaluating the effectiveness of strategies health officials used in combating the 2003 SARS outbreak, researchers still question which of the two strategies—isolation or quarantine—was more effective and whether using both rather than one was necessary.[45] Concerns about proportionality are critical given that, historically, only a very small percentage of individuals quarantined during outbreaks such as SARS were actually infected.[45]

When deciding whether to impose restrictive measures, such as quarantine, health officials should consider all possible factors that influence their effectiveness, and health officials should use the fewest and least restrictive measures necessary. For example, if isolating ill cases is effective in controlling transmission, it is unlikely that quarantining exposed, well contacts would provide any additional benefit.[46] On the other hand, if health officials discover that isolation of ill patients is insufficient in preventing transmission, they should consider other potential mitigating factors before imposing measures that are more restrictive. The effectiveness of isolation and quarantine will vary by disease, and, depending on the disease, quarantine might not be necessary or helpful. Studies have shown that quarantine can reduce transmission only if the cases can transmit the disease while asymptomatic, and only if the time during which cases are asymptomatic is not very long or very short.[46] For short asymptomatic periods, a characteristic of influenza, health officials will not have enough time to identify and quarantine exposed people before they develop symptoms. For diseases with long asymptomatic periods, health officials might have difficulty identifying exposed individuals, since infected cases would have had enough time to have many contacts while still asymptomatic. In addition, diseases with long asymptomatic periods would necessitate correspondingly long quarantine periods, making quarantine more onerous, lengthy, costly, and more difficult for health officials to implement overall.[46]

Timing is another factor health officials should consider in determining whether and when to impose restrictive actions such as quarantine. Health officials must implement restrictions early enough to prevent the initial rapid increase in cases and long enough to prevent transmission during the peak of the outbreak. In general, later interventions are less effective than early interventions; depending on the course of the outbreak, sustained and possibly combined interventions are more effective than interventions removed too early.[34, 35] On the other hand, implementing restrictive measures too soon might cause economic and social hardship without benefit, and implementing measures for too long might cause "intervention fatigue," reduce compliance, and erode public trust.[35]

In addition to uncertainty surrounding the effectiveness of restrictive measures, such as isolation and quarantine, there are uncertainties related to the effectiveness of other social distancing methods, such as personal protective equipment, cancellation of congregate activities, and furlough days. Although officials recommended the use of surgical masks in the 1918 influenza pandemic and during the SARS outbreak, there are no controlled studies proving their effectiveness.[46] In addition, studies demonstrating mask effectiveness in a controlled environment might not predict effectiveness in actual situations in which people must use properly fitted masks reliably and consistently throughout the course of the outbreak.[35, 46]

Even though authorities have used closure of congregate activities, such as closure of schools, childcare centers, workplaces, and mass transit and cancellation of public events, such as sports events, arts events, and conferences, it is possible that these closures were unnecessary, since ill and exposed persons, as well as fearful citizens, might have avoided such settings voluntarily.[46] On the other hand, some evidence suggests that school closures can interrupt influenza transmission. For example, when Israel closed schools during an influenza outbreak, influenza diagnoses, physician visits, emergency department visits, and medication purchases decreased significantly. In New York City, routine school furloughs, such as winter break, led to reduced emergency room visits for febrile illness of school-aged children beginning 2–3 days after the break began. These visits remained low for the duration of the break and increased within several days after school resumed. On the other hand, the furlough had no effect on emergency room utilization for ill adults with a fever.[35]

Although closing schools might prevent transmission, one consequence that could significantly reduce this benefit is that children who are not in school could re-congregate at alternative settings. Therefore, when health officials use school closure to prevent transmission, they should consider adding other congregate activity restrictions, such as cancellation of events, as part of a "bundled" strategy.[35] In general, implementing multiple social distancing strategies simultaneously might improve effectiveness by preventing people restricted from one congregate activity from engaging in alternative congregate activities.[35] One other factor that could reduce the effectiveness of social distancing methods relates to their geographical extent. Suppose that one community effectively achieves compliance with such interventions, while neighboring communities fail to do so; in such a case, infected individuals from neighboring communities could continue to introduce infections into the compliant community.[47]

At stage 1, public health officials might be able to justify public notification and perhaps passive or active monitoring. As the outbreak moves to stages 2 and 3, the more restrictive options become defensible. However, as in the TB case, the process health officials use to justify their actions, including answering the questions in Table 8.1, is as essential as the actions themselves. To control communicable disease outbreaks, health officials will need to build support from affected individuals, their families, and the entire community. Even the most restrictive actions require cooperation, especially for prolonged outbreaks, since it is much easier, less costly, and more effective to achieve voluntary compliance compared to using law enforcement. Clearly, health officials cannot achieve their goals without the public's trust. Those who use a principled process to justify communicable disease control decisions are more likely to achieve success because, in doing so, they demonstrate that they are accountable to the communities they serve, and that protecting the public's health is both an individual and a community responsibility.

CONCLUSIONS

In responding to communicable disease threats, governmental public health officials have many interventions at their disposal, each with ethical implications. Communicable disease control interventions include, but are not limited to: educational messages; surveillance activities, which involve gathering personal health information from individuals either passively or actively; isolating individuals with communicable disease; restricting the movements of healthy people exposed to communicable diseases; requiring individuals to comply with medication administration; and imposing social distancing measures, such as closures of businesses or events. All of these interventions, based on public health police powers, require balancing individual liberties with community benefits. When choosing among interventions, health officials must consider their goals; whether the interventions they propose to achieve those goals are the least restrictive of individual rights; whether they have attempted to mitigate any negative effects of any proposed restrictions; and whether the burdens their interventions impose affect minority or vulnerable populations disproportionately. Conducting a step-by-step ethical analysis, which involves analyzing the ethical issues and assessing the ethical dimensions of the intervention options, can help public health officials ensure that they have heard the moral claims of potentially affected stakeholders and that they have identified the least restrictive options necessary to achieve their goals. Ethical codes, such as the Public Health Code of Ethics, are tools that can help officials systematically and transparently balance tensions between individual and community interests, as well as guide them in justifying their ultimate decisions. By using ethical principles as guidance, public health officials can demonstrate that the process they use in making decisions, particularly those that restrict individual liberties, are at least as important as the outcomes, and that they cannot work effectively without individual and community consent and participation. In making decisions based on what they should do, rather than on what they can do, public health officials can build community trust, thereby increasing their effectiveness.

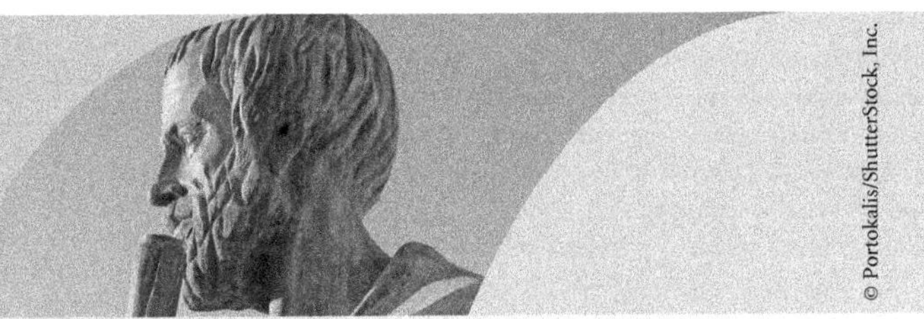

Discussion Questions

1. What can health officials do to increase the likelihood of voluntary compliance with Directly Observed Therapy (DOT) for tuberculosis?
2. When is it ethically justifiable to mandate DOT? What conditions need to be met? If they do mandate DOT, what can health officials do to reduce any imposed burdens?
3. What additional considerations are involved when the TB case is a child? When the case has Multiple Drug-Resistant TB (MDR TB)? When the case has Extremely Drug-Resistant TB (XDR TB)?
4. Should health officials ever grant exceptions for DOT and allow self-administration? If so, when and why should they do so?
5. During a communicable disease outbreak, what can health officials do to increase the likelihood of voluntary compliance with control measures, such as passive monitoring, isolation, and quarantine?
6. During a communicable disease outbreak, what should health officials consider before mandating interventions that restrict individual liberties, such as quarantine? What process should health officials use to justify their chosen interventions? What can health officials do to mitigate the negative consequences of any restrictive interventions?
7. How can public health officials use professional codes of ethics, such as the Public Health Code of Ethics, in guiding their decision making related to communicable disease control and prevention?

REFERENCES

1. Bernheim RG, Melnick A. Principled leadership in public health: integrating ethics into practice and management. *Journal of Public Health Management and Practice*, 2008;14(4):358–366.

2. Centers for Disease Control and Prevention. *Trends in Tuberculosis 2010*, Content updated October 2011. http://www.cdc.gov/tb/publications/factsheets/statistics/Trends.pdf (accessed February 5, 2012).

3. Centers for Disease Control and Prevention. *Multidrug-Resistant tuberculosis (MDR TB)*, April 2010. http://www.cdc.gov/tb/publications/factsheets/drtb/MDRTB.pdf (accessed February 5, 2012).

4. Centers for Disease Control and Prevention. Controlling Tuberculosis in the United States. *Morbidity & Mortality Weekly Report*, 2005;54 (November 4): No. RR-12. Available at http://www.cdc.gov/mmwr/indrr_2005.html (accessed August 22, 2013).

5. American Thoracic Society. Targeted tuberculin testing and treatment of latent tuberculosis infection. *American Journal of Respiratory and Critical Care Medicine*, 2000;161(4 Pt 2):S221–S247.

6. Centers for Disease Control and Prevention. Targeted tuberculin testing and treatment of latent tuberculosis infection. *Morbidity & Mortality Weekly Report*, 2000;49(June 9): No. RR-6. Available at http://www.cdc.gov/mmwr/indrr_2000.html (accessed August 22, 2013).

7. Bailey WC, Gerald LB, Kimerling ME, et al. Predictive model to identify positive tuberculosis skin test results during contact investigations. *JAMA*, 2002;287:996–1002.

8. Rieder HL. Risk of travel-associated tuberculosis. *Clinical Infectious Disease*, 2001;33:1393–1396.

9. Houk VN, Baker JH, Sorensen K, Kent DC. The epidemiology of tuberculosis infection in a closed environment. *Archives of Environmental Health*, 1968;16:26–35.

10. Houk VH, Kent DC, Baker JH, Sorensen K, Hanzel GD. The Byrd study. In-depth analysis of a micro-outbreak of tuberculosis in a closed environment. *Archives of Environmental Health*, 1968;16:4–6.

11. Suzuki S, Nakabayashi K, Ohkouchi H, et al. Tuberculosis in the crew of a submarine. *Nihon Kyobu Shikkan Gakkai Zasshi*, 1997;35:61–66.

12. Bernheim RG, Nieburg P, Bonnie RJ. Ethics and the practice of public health. In: Goodman RA, ed. *Law in Public Health Practice*, 2d edition. Oxford, U.K.: Oxford University Press, 2007.

13. Childress JF, Faden RR, Gaare RD, et al. Public health ethics: mapping the terrain. *Journal of Law, Medicine & Ethics*, 2002;30:170–178.

14. Childress JF, Bernheim RG. Beyond the liberal and communitarian impasse: a framework and vision for public health. *Florida Law Review*, 2003;55:1191–1219.

15. Kass NE. An ethics framework for public health. *American Journal of Public Health*, 2001;91:1776–1782.

16. Beauchamp TL, Childress JF. *Principles of Biomedical Ethics*, 7th edition. New York: Oxford University Press, 2013.

17. Washington State Legislature. Revised Code of Washington, Chapter 70.05 Local health departments, boards, officers—regulations. Available at http://apps.leg.wa.gov/rcw/default.aspx?cite=70.05 (accessed February 5, 2012).

18. Washington State Department of Health Tuberculosis Guidelines, March 2012. Available at http://www.doh.wa.gov/Portals/1/Documents/5000/150-Tuberculosis.pdf (accessed April 20, 2013).

19. Public Health Leadership Society. *Principles of the Ethical Practice of Public Health*. New Orleans, LA: PHLS, 2002. Available at http://phls.org/CMSuploads/Principles-of-the-Ethical-Practice-of-PH-Version-2.2-68496.pdf (accessed February 5, 2012).

20. Vermal G, Upshur REG, Rea E, Benatar SR. Critical reflections on evidence, ethics and effectiveness in the management of tuberculosis: public health and global perspectives. *BMC Medical Ethics*, 2004;5:2.

21. Weis SE, Slocum PC, Blais FX, King B, Nunn M, Matney GB, Gomez E, Foresman BH. The effect of directly observed therapy on the rates of drug resistance and relapse in tuberculosis. *New England Journal of Medicine*, 1994;330(17):1179–1184.

22. Volmink J, Garner P. Directly observed therapy for treating tuberculosis. Cochrane Database Systematic Reviews, 2007:CD003343.

23. Coker R. Tuberculosis, non-compliance and detention for the public health. *Journal of Medical Ethics*, 2000;26:157–159.

24. Campion EW. Liberty and the control of tuberculosis. *New England Journal of Medicine*, 1999;340:385–6.

25. Centers for Disease Control and Prevention. *Clinical Guidance on the Identification and Evaluation of Possible SARS-CoV Disease among Persons Presenting with Community-Acquired Illness*, version 2. Uploaded January 8, 2004. Available at http://www.cdc.gov/sars/clinical/guidance.html (accessed August 22, 2013).

26. Peiris JSM, Yuen KY, Osterhaus ADME, Stöhr K. The severe acute respiratory syndrome. *New England Journal of Medicine*, 2003;349:2431–2441.

27. World Health Organization Severe Acute Respiratory Syndrome (SARS) Epidemiology Working Group. *Consensus Document on the Epidemiology of Severe Acute Respiratory Syndrome (SARS)* WHO/CDS/CSR/GAR/2003.11. Geneva: World Health Organization, 2003. Available at http://www.who.int/csr/sars/en/WHOconsensus.pdf (accessed August 22, 2013).

28. Donnelly CA, Ghani AC, Leung GM, et al. Epidemiological determinants of spread of causal agent of severe acute respiratory syndrome in Hong Kong. *Lancet*, 2003;361:1761–1766. [Erratum, *Lancet* 2003;361:1832.]

29. Lee N, Hui D, Wu A, et al. A major outbreak of severe acute respiratory syndrome in Hong Kong. *New England Journal of Medicine*, 2003;348:1986–1994.

30. Varia M, Wilson S, Sarwal S, et al. Investigation of a nosocomial outbreak of severe acute respiratory syndrome (SARS) in Toronto, Canada. *Canadian Medical Association Journal*, 2003;169:285–292.

31. Scales DC, Green K, Chan AK, et al. Illness in intensive care staff after brief exposure to severe acute respiratory syndrome. *Emerging Infectious Diseases*, 2003;9:1205–1210.

32. Wray RJ, Becker SM, Henderson N, et al. Communicating with the public about emerging health threats: lessons from the pre-event message development project. *American Journal of Public Health*, 2008;98(12):2214–2222.

33. Golan K. Surviving a public health crisis: tips for communicators. *Journal of Health Communication*, 2003;8(S1):126–127.

34. Shore DA. Communicating in times of uncertainty: the need for trust. *Journal of Health Communication*, 2003;8(S1):13–14.

35. Covello V. Best practices in public health risk and crisis communication. *Journal of Health Communication*, 2003;8(S1):5–8.

36. Koplan JP. Communication during public health emergencies. *Journal of Health Communication*, 2003;8(S1):144–145.

37. Meredith LS, Eisenman DP, Rhodes H, Ryan G, Long A. Trust influences response to public health messages during a bioterrorist event. *Journal of Health Communication*, 2007;12:217–232.

38. Washington State Legislature. Administrative Code of Washington, Chapter 246-100-036, Responsibilities and duties—Local health officers. Available at http://apps.leg.wa.gov/WAC/default.aspx?cite=246-100-036 (accessed April 20, 2013).

39. Centers for Disease Control and Prevention. *Public Health Guidance for Community-Level Preparedness and Response to Severe Acute Respiratory Syndrome (SARS)*, version 2. Supplement D: Community Containment Measures, Including Non-Hospital Isolation and Quarantine. Uploaded January 8, 2004. Available at http://www.cdc.gov/sars/guidance/D-quarantine/downloads/D-quarantine-full.pdf (accessed January 21, 2012).

40. Cetron M, Landwirth J. Public health, ethics, and quarantine. *Yale Journal of Biology and Medicine*, 2005;78:325–330.

41. Gostin L. Public health strategies for pandemic influenza. Ethics and the law. *JAMA*, 2006;295(14):1700–1704.

42. Gostin LO, Sapsin JW, Teret SP, et al. The Model State Emergency Health Powers Act: planning and response to bioterrorism and naturally occurring infectious diseases. *JAMA*, 2002;288:622–628.

43. Markel H, Lipman HB, Navarro JA, Sloan A, Michalsen JR, Stern AM, Cetron MS. Nonpharmaceutical interventions implemented by US cities during the 1918-1919 influenza pandemic. *JAMA*, 2007;298(6):644–654.

44. Day T, Park A, Madras N, et al. When is quarantine a useful control strategy for emerging infectious diseases? *American Journal of Epidemiology*, 2006;163:479–485.

45. Centers for Disease Control and Prevention. *Interim Pre-Pandemic Planning Guidance: Community Strategy for Pandemic Influenza Mitigation in the United States: Early, Targeted, Layered Use of Nonpharmaceutical Interventions.* Atlanta, GA: CDC, 2007. Available at http://healthvermont.gov/panflu/documents/0207interimguidance.pdf (accessed January 18, 2012).

46. Gostin LO, Bayer R, Fairchild AL. Ethical and legal challenges posed by Severe Acute Respiratory Syndrome: implications for the control of severe infectious disease threats. *JAMA*, 2003;290:3229–3237.

47. Glass RJ, Glass LM, Beyeler WE, Min HJ. Targeted social distancing design for pandemic influenza. *Emerging Infectious Diseases*, 2006;12(11):1671–1681.

© Portokalis/ShutterStock, Inc.

CHAPTER 9

Health Communication

by Ruth Gaare Bernheim and Richard J. Bonnie

Learning Objectives

By the end of this chapter, the reader will be able to:

- Describe different government health communication strategies to change individual behaviors and social norms, the ethical values that underlie these health promotion strategies, and potential ethical tensions, including threats to individual autonomous choices and harms, that may arise in practice
- Address the question, are some government communications aimed at health promotion inescapably paternalistic, and if so, are they justifiable?
- Identify the moral claims that arise in health communication campaigns about the extent to which an individual should be held responsible for their health, including for a decision to engage in "unhealthy" lifestyle choices
- Understand the legal and moral justifications for and First Amendment constraints on government activity in the information environment, including delivering, regulating, and compelling speech

INTRODUCTION

Creating, delivering, and regulating health-related information and messages are increasingly important interventions in public health, particularly when linked with other health-promotion strategies that aim to motivate individuals to change unhealthy behaviors and lifestyles. The health challenges of obesity and tobacco, for example, have been declared "winnable battles" by the Centers for Disease Control and Prevention (CDC)[1]; addressing them involves large-scale media efforts and the use of images, as well as words, in the public information environment to shape community and social influences and promote healthy choices by individuals.

Public health professionals have a long history of providing health education and information. An emphasis by public health officials in recent years on health marketing and the use of advances in communication science and technology recognizes that too often in the past, there has been "the gap between relevant research on health and its availability to the public,"[2] as well as its impact on population health. Thus, public health communication now features not only mass media campaigns, but also other innovative message delivery technologies, such as mobile devices, streaming media and web-based communications. In addition, public health is using health marketing techniques, drawing on the social and behavioral sciences and the scientific fields of social marketing and risk communication. The stated goal is to ensure that health information and interventions are "people-centered" and delivered "in ways that inspire people to want to make good health choices and share their enthusiasm with others."[2]

Health communication activities often are part of multicomponent efforts in health promotion, and in this chapter we will explore some of the ethical dimensions of health promotion in general. The World Health Organization (WHO) defines health promotion as "the process of enabling people to increase control over, and to improve, their health. It moves beyond a focus on individual behavior towards a wide range of social and environmental interventions."[3] Thus, health promotion, understood broadly, includes a wide range of planned activities, from community-based efforts undertaken by voluntary organizations, such as those aimed at reducing driving under the influence of alcohol or encouraging safe sex practices, to more liberty-limiting government strategies that, for example, tax or restrict the sale and promotion of products such as tobacco or alcohol or require people to behave safely, such as mandated seat belt use. Key in this definition of health promotion is the emphasis in the first sentence on empowering people, in order to increase their control over their health.

In this chapter, we will focus in particular on health promotion activities in the information environment, including education, communication, and mass media campaigns, all of which are generally considered to be less restrictive of individual liberty than many laws and regulations. We take as our starting point two presumptions: (1) that it is legitimate for government to engage in health communication and to be active in the marketplace of ideas about a healthy lifestyle in order to reduce *individual behaviors* that increase the risk of individual mortality/morbidity and that reduce population health when aggregated; and (2) that specific health promotion activities, such as education and mass media campaigns, are ethically justifiable in so far as they are *liberty-enhancing* for individuals.

Ethical concerns can arise, however, about particular media campaigns or communication strategies a government may undertake that might, in fact, undermine individual autonomous choices and actions, such as messages that may be misunderstood or experienced by some to be manipulative or coercive, or that may cause harm by stigmatizing, embarrassing and shaming, or inducing undue fear.

Consider, for example, the following ad that is part of a media campaign on childhood obesity in Australia. A mother approaches a kitchen table where her young child is seated quietly doing artwork. There is a dark mood and ominous background music. The mother reaches into a brown bag, unwraps a substance wrapped in foil, heats it up on a spoon, pulls out a large syringe needle, and then wraps and ties a band around the child's arm as if about to inject the child. The camera then zooms in on the child, and the mother puts a napkin under the child's chin. Then the camera zooms back out to picture the same mother and child seated next to each other, each taking a bite out of a burger. Words flash on the screen: "You wouldn't inject your children with junk. So why are you feeding it to them? Childhood obesity. Break the habit."[4]

The video obviously compares food intake to drug abuse and targets parents in order to get their attention about the harm of eating junk food, perhaps even suggesting that parents may be responsible or to blame for "addicting" the child—in short, the message is that parents harm their children by providing unhealthy food. Would it be ethically appropriate for government to use or support the use of such ads in a media campaign for obesity in children? What, if any, are the ethical considerations, and how would a decision about whether to use or sponsor such an ad be ethically justified? Would the media campaign be more justifiable if it were being undertaken to counter specific advertising campaigns by companies encouraging parents to buy the particular "unhealthy" products for their children? Would it be more justifiable for government to regulate and limit the marketing by companies that advertise "unhealthy" products, rather than target parents through mass media campaigns? Or more justifiable to require that companies post large warnings or even unattractive pictures on the product packaging of the unhealthy products to provide the messages to parents at the point of sale? And, as with other public health tools, does the government have the authority to regulate advertising or require that words and/or images be included on product packaging?

This chapter will examine the legal and ethical justifications for, and constraints on, using communication strategies as tools for protecting and promoting public health. In Part 1, the chapter presents an historical overview of the ways in which governments has used channels of communication to promote healthy and safe behavior and of the possible justifications for doing so. Part 2 provides a brief overview of the constraints imposed by the First Amendment—which prohibits government officials from "abridging the freedom of speech"—because these constitutional principles play such a dominant role in our national discourse about the legitimacy and limits of the government's health promotion efforts. Because aggressive measures to discourage tobacco use have tested the boundaries of the First Amendment, tobacco control is used as an intensive case study in Part 3. Finally, Part 4 explores ethical perspectives on health communication in general and on particular health communication campaigns.

GOVERNMENT'S ROLE IN USING AND REGULATING MASS COMMUNICATION

Early Government Health Education Efforts

Public health has a long history of activity in education and health communication. The roots of modern-day efforts in the United States are traceable to health education campaigns in the late 19th and early 20th centuries, when two social ideas at that time influenced public health: a reformist movement in American politics that focused public health efforts on self-improvement and education rather than on the coercive force of law, and a growth in consumerism that led public health to engage in efforts to "sell" healthy behavior and to draw on advertising techniques, using such emotional appeals as fear, guilt, and social conformity.[5] Noting the reformers' belief in the "moral uplift" of education and the new bacteriological understanding of disease that located its source within individuals, reformers sought to help individuals protect themselves from disease. Colgrove uses the example of a statewide campaign in New York in the 1920s to encourage childhood diphtheria immunization to illustrate how public health embraced a new health education ideology focusing on behavior change and persuasion. Health educators focused not only on information, but also on the presentation of such messages through techniques designed to be "dramatic, entertaining, and carefully planned."[5] Essentially launching a widespread advertising campaign that included films and posters, public health professionals aimed to persuade parents and sell the public on diphtheria immunization.

In contrast to the coercive strategies used a few years earlier for smallpox immunization—when physicians and vaccinating squads went door-to-door, supported by vaccination law requirements—diphtheria immunization efforts highlighted mothers' responsibility in immunizing children and featured images of happy mothers and children. These approaches to health education were framed "as a uniquely American innovation—reflecting strong traditions of liberty, autonomy, and freedom from government interference."[5] The new American approach to health education differed from European approaches at the time, and Colgrove quotes Charles Bolduan, the health education director for New York City, who commented that in contrast to the German, who seemed to like to be bossed, the American "preferred to act based on an understanding of the value of various interventions." Europeans themselves took note of America's different approach to health education at the time, and Colgrove quotes British public health officials who, after reviewing the U.S. anti-diphtheria initiatives, observed that the American methods were "altogether more intensive and more spectacular than our sober-minded ideas. ... We in this country are apt to look askance at the flamboyant methods of propaganda used by our brethren on the American continent ... Our respectability rebels and our insular pride stands aloof from importing into our professional problems the methods of the marketplace and the habit of mind of the huckster."[5]

The diphtheria "education" campaign in the early 20th century suggests a number of ethical and legal issues that presage current public health communication strategies. One is the appropriate goal of government-sponsored campaigns and a shift in emphasis from educating the public to persuading the public. While education aims to inform individuals about health risks and interventions to help them make better choices, persuasion aims not only to inform, but also to influence choices and induce individuals to act in particular ways. Another, more specific issue arises about particular communication techniques, such as social marketing.[6] For example, persuasion that employs advertising techniques may even suggest blame or include guilt- and fear-inducing messages that are potentially harmful to some individuals. Colgrove points out that much of the rhetoric in the diphtheria messages had "strong undercurrents of parental culpability for the sickness of unprotected children" and even suggested that noncompliant parents might be guilty of criminal negligence, and he calls such messages "quasi-coercive rhetoric."[5] And yet another issue is whether there are constraints—either legal or ethical—on government activity in the health information environment. Is government regulation and restriction of the "harmful" messages of others—for example, of tobacco advertising—more justifiable and a less restrictive strategy than government's own use of marketing strategies that target and perhaps induce guilt or shame?

Possible Aims and Justifications

We turn now to an overview of the ways in which governments regulate channels of communication to curtail undesirable messages and propagate desirable ones, as well as the ways in which governments and private organizations use these channels of communication to promote healthy and safe behavior. The First Amendment—which prohibits government officials from "abridging the freedom of speech"—plays a dominant role in our national discourse about the legitimacy of these efforts. For this reason, key First Amendment concepts are used to organize the first part of this chapter, although ethical principles are introduced when room is left for them to operate within the constraints of the First Amendment. Tobacco control is used as the main case study.

Disseminating and shaping information through mass communication is an essential feature of virtually all public health action. Two common types of health communication seem uncontroversial. First, government routinely aims to *promote and facilitate informed individual choice* by disseminating information, mandating disclosure of material information to consumers of goods and services, and curtailing dissemination of false and misleading information. Second, and similarly, the government routinely (largely without controversy) aims to prevent and control disease and injury by providing information and instruction to *enable people to protect themselves* by avoiding exposure to germs, toxins, or other risks to health or safety (**Figure 9.1**). Third, some government health communications aim to *persuade people to engage in healthy behaviors and to discourage unhealthy behaviors*, and other policies may aim to *promote healthy social norms.* While disseminating healthy messages, the government might also

FIGURE 9.1 Message Picturing Injury-prevention Behavior

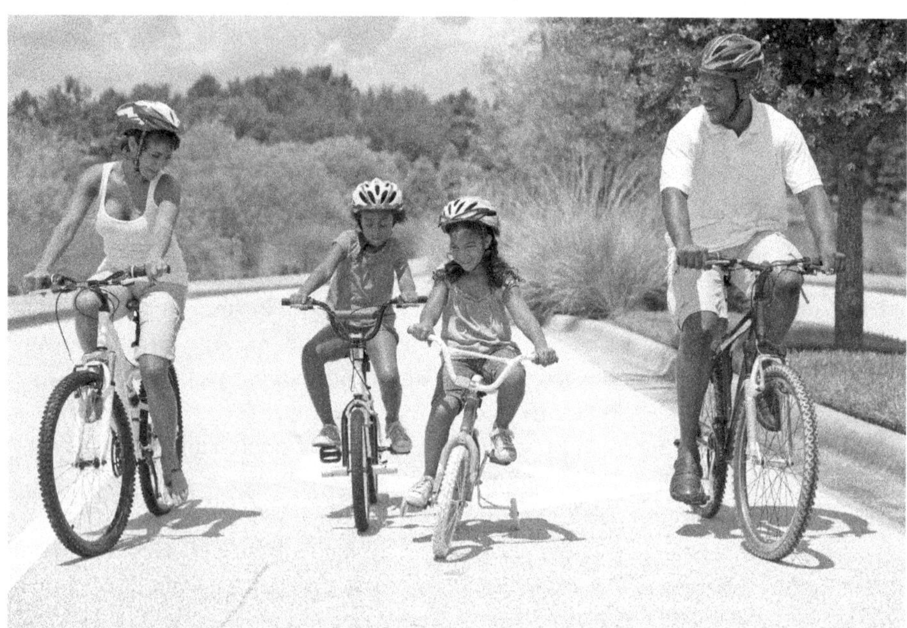

attempt to counteract "harmful" cultural influences (e.g., depictions in entertainment media, unhealthy marketing and advertising of alcohol, tobacco, unhealthy food).

These last two types of government action involve explicit efforts to influence behavior, and they therefore raise concerns about paternalism or government overreaching, sometimes popularly referred to as government becoming a nanny state. As public health policies become more aggressive in promoting, supporting, and reinforcing "healthy" social norms, they will also be contesting commercial and cultural influences that tend to promote and sustain "unhealthy" norms and behaviors. What constitutional boundaries constrain or limit policies aiming to suppress, regulate, or counteract messages in entertainment or commercial media that are thought to be inimical to the public health?

OVERVIEW OF FIRST AMENDMENT CONSTRAINTS

The First Amendment declares that "Congress shall make no law ... abridging the freedom of speech or of the press ..." Although the language technically is directed at lawmaking by the Congress of the United States, it is understood to refer to action by any official of the federal government. Moreover, because the protections of the First Amendment have been "incorporated" into the due process clause of the Fourteenth Amendment (which bars the states from curtailing "liberty" without an adequate justification), the First Amendment applies to government action at all levels of government, including city councils, local school boards, and health commissioners.

Principles and Concepts

The first point to understand about modern First Amendment jurisprudence is that not all "speech" or expression is protected by the constitution. The "freedom of speech" protected against abridgement does not include categories of expression that have traditionally been prohibited under Anglo-American common law, including "obscenity," "defamation," "fighting words," soliciting someone to commit crime, or inciting other people to engage in "imminent lawless action" (e.g., rioting, looting). Second, the protection afforded by the First Amendment is not "absolute." Even within the sphere of "protected categories of speech," the degree of protection varies according to "constitutional value" of the particular type of expression. Thus, as will be discussed later on, "commercial" speech is not as strongly protected as "political" or "religious" speech, and explicit but nonobscene depictions of sexual conduct are protected even less. This means that the government has more leeway to suppress these categories of speech. To use the Supreme Court's terminology, the "level of judicial scrutiny" is more or less demanding, depending on the category of speech under consideration. One good example of the more lenient rules that apply to commercial speech is that the FDA has traditionally reviewed advertising and labeling of drugs in advance to make sure the companies' claims are accurate; however, the government is virtually never allowed to restrain publication of political or artistic speech in advance. A famous example was the Supreme Court's refusal[7] to enjoin *The New York Times* from publishing the so-called "Pentagon Papers" in the face of the government's claims that the information was classified, had been illegally disclosed to the *Times*, and that its publication would be detrimental to national security. As will be seen, members of the Supreme Court are sharply divided on the evidence that is needed to justify a restriction on commercial advertising thought to be inimical to the public health.

A third principle of modern First Amendment jurisprudence is that unprotected speech must sometimes be protected in order to give ample "breathing room" to protected speech; a good example of this idea is that "false" speech about a person or organization obviously has no social value on its own and can cause harm, such as giving the liar a competitive edge or injuring the defamed victim's reputation. However, the Supreme Court ruled in *New York Times v. Sullivan* in 1961 that "public figures" (e.g., politicians, celebrities, or other famous individuals) may not recover damages in a libel action against the press or other offending party for false and defamatory statements unless the persons who published the statements knew them to be false or made them in reckless disregard of their possible falsity.[8] Holding the speaker liable for making statements believed to be true could inhibit "wide open and robust debate" about issues of public interest and importance, a hallmark value of the First Amendment.

A fourth important principle is that the "freedom of speech" protects not only the right to speak but also the right not to speak. In other words, it forbids government actions that "coerce" speech as well as those that restrict it. The centrality of this principle is illustrated nicely by the Supreme Court's rightly famous decision in *West Virginia State Board of Education v Barnette* (1943), holding that school officials cannot compel students to salute and pledge allegiance to the flag.[9] As Justice Jackson said, "[i]f there is any fixed star in our constitutional constellation, it is that no official, high or petty, can prescribe what shall be orthodox in politics, nationalism, religion, or other matters of opinion or force fellow citizens to confess by word or act their faith therein." More recently, the Court applied the same principle in *Wooley v. Maynard* (1977), striking down a New Hampshire law requiring most automobiles to bear license plates carrying the state motto, "Live Free or Die."[10]

Finally, a fifth key principle is that government has considerably more leeway in restricting speech when it is regulating the "time, place or manner" of speech than when it is regulating its "content." In most cases, a restriction of speech based on its content is subject to the strictest scrutiny, especially when it involves political or religious speech. However, regulations of the "time, place or manner" of speech (e.g., no speech with a loudspeaker at 2:00 AM in a residential neighborhood) are permissible as long as they are content-neutral, narrowly tailored to an important nonspeech purpose, and leave open alternative channels of communication.

To test your understanding of these principles, consider some interventions that might be undertaken to prevent and reduce injuries. Local public health officials may be concerned about interrupting the emergence of "suicide clusters" in the wake of an adolescent suicide. Would it be permissible for the health commissioner to direct local news media not to publicize a suicide, essentially on the ground that doing so is necessary to prevent transmission of an "infectious idea" to a vulnerable population? Is this a regulation of the time, place, and manner of speech? Or does it regulate speech based on its content? What difference should it make that the government is trying to suppress or censor the speech in advance of the feared harm (a "prior restraint") rather than waiting to punish the dangerous speech after it has occurred? Consider also analogous problems that can arise in the context of explicit depictions of violent crimes by the entertainment media (as opposed to the news media) if courts were to hold broadcasters liable for victims of "copycat" crimes by psychologically vulnerable adolescents or young adults. This sort of liability opens up a broader question about violence prevention that is much debated in legislative hearings as well as in the scientific literature—what is the effect of exposing children to violence in the entertainment media, including video games? Are explicit depictions of violence protected by the First Amendment at all? Even if protected, is the level of protection less when targeted toward adolescents? Is it possible to design a regulatory scheme that would protect children without restricting access by adults to these forms of expression?

Commercial Advertising

The most contested domain of speech in the context of contemporary public health policy is "commercial speech" by companies that market products thought to be harmful to the public health. Until 1976, "commercial speech" was understood to be an "unprotected" category of speech due to a long tradition of regulating and even prohibiting advertising of various products or disapproved activities. However, in *Virginia State Board of Pharmacy v. Virginia Citizens Consumer Council* (1976), the Court struck down a ban on prescription drug price advertising by pharmacists based on societal value of the free flow of commercial information, both to facilitate informed consumer choice as well as to support an efficient market.[11] Although the Court made it clear that the First Amendment protects commercial speech, the opinion did not indicate what level of protection applies to such speech. If the protection accorded commercial speech were to be governed by the same rules that protect political speech, even false and misleading ads might be regarded as tolerable in order to allow "breathing room" for truthful advertising, ultimately depending on market forces rather than regulators to curtail false and misleading claims. If the rule against advance censorship were applied, any sort of pre-marketing approval of the content of advertising (as under traditional FDA regulation) would be foreclosed. Moreover, if the same rules applied to political and commercial speech, government would have to be neutral about content of commercial messages, even if the behavior being promoted were thought to be inimical to public welfare, such as tobacco use.

In *Central Hudson Gas and Electric Corp. v. Public Service Commission of New York* (1980), the Court adopted a form of so-called "intermediate scrutiny" for commercial speech rather than the stricter rules that apply to political or artistic speech.[12] Specifically, the Court said, commercial speech is protected by the First Amendment only if it concerns lawful activity and is not false or misleading (i.e., no "breathing space" for protected speech is required). However, assuming that the speech is truthful and concerns a lawful activity, it may be restricted only if the regulation "directly advances a substantial governmental interest" (i.e., it does not have to be necessary to serve a compelling interest) and if the restriction is no more extensive than necessary to serve that interest (i.e, it should be "narrowly tailored" so as to achieve a "reasonable fit" between the objective being sought and the means chosen, but it need not be the least restrictive means available).

Most of the cases decided over the past 35 years have applied the *Central Hudson* test to marketing products affecting the public health. However, it is not clear whether the *Central Hudson* test also applies to some of the other types of regulation that are regularly used in public health regulation, especially mandated disclosures of information about a particular product.

Mandated Factual Disclosures

Are mandated factual disclosures about advertised products subject to heightened scrutiny under *Central Hudson*? Should they be analogized to "coerced" speech under the First Amendment? Although the Supreme Court has not yet addressed the question, most courts have taken the view that heightened scrutiny does not apply to mandated disclosures in commercial contexts and that these regulations are constitutional if the disclosures are accurate and the challenged regulation is rationally related to a legitimate public goal. One recent example is *NYSRA v. NY City Bd of Health* (2009), in which the U.S. Court of Appeals for the First Circuit upheld New York City's ordinance requiring covered restaurants to post calorie content on menus and menu boards.[13] The Court ruled that because the provision requires disclosure of "purely factual" information, it is subject to a deferential standard of scrutiny ("reasonable relation between end and means") rather than heightened scrutiny required by *Central Hudson*.

Government Speech

As noted earlier, governments spend billions of dollars informing the people about the health consequences of their behavior and about the actions they can take to protect themselves. Even a cursory look at *Healthy People 2020* reveals the stunning scope and intensity of the national government's efforts to prod state and local governments and private organizations to inform, persuade, and cajole individuals, groups, and organizations to promote healthy and safe behaviors and discourage unhealthy and unsafe ones.[14] That media campaigns are a common feature of all these efforts can easily be seen by looking at agency websites and public service advertising on buses, billboards, newspapers, magazines, television, movies, and video games. There is no doubt that governments at all levels have the authority to spend public funds to promote the public health. It is also clear that government's expenditures on media campaigns to disseminate its message do not restrict anyone else's speech or compel anyone to do anything. A media campaign does not "abridge" anyone's "freedom of speech." To the extent that some citizens disagree with the government's message (encouraging use of condoms, declaring zero tolerance for marijuana use, criticizing the deception by the tobacco companies, or ridiculing parents who feed their children "junk food"), they may well feel aggrieved, but the remedy, according to traditional constitutional understanding, is for those who disagree with the government's message to contest that message in the marketplace of ideas and to organize voters to turn the offending government out office. Whether government speech should be curtailed is ordinarily to be decided in the political process, not in the courts. This is settled law.

AGGRESSIVE TOBACCO CONTROL: NEW FRONTIERS OF THE FIRST AMENDMENT

Public health officials and advocates have become increasingly focused on the difficulty of encouraging healthy behavior in the face of massive industry promotion of unhealthy behavior. The challenges have been emphasized in a series of reports from the Institute of Medicine (IOM) on tobacco control as early as 1994,[15] as well as on food marketing, especially to children, and alcohol marketing to youth and young adults and to minority populations with high rates of alcohol abuse. This chapter uses tobacco as a case study because it provides a unique historical context for exploring the use of aggressive measures for restricting and counteracting industry marketing practices.

For most of the 20th century (characterized by Alan Brandt as the "cigarette century" in his book with that title[16]), the tobacco industry's promotional activities were virtually unregulated. The first significant step was the mandated package warning required by Congress in 1965 in the wake of the pivotal report of the Surgeon General in 1964.[17] Congress slightly strengthened these warnings in 1969, required them in print advertising, and also banned tobacco advertising on radio and television. However, in retrospect, the tobacco industry is seen to have achieved two major victories in the 1969 legislation. First, Congress preempted any regulation of advertising "based on smoking and health" by state and local governments. Second, by ending broadcast advertising, Congress also ended the highly effective antismoking ads that broadcasters had been required to air by the Federal Communications Commission under its "fairness doctrine." Although the legally required warnings were strengthened again in 1984, industry-sponsored promotional expenditures rose exponentially over the rest of the century, reaching $15 billion in 2005.

In the 1990s, the tobacco industry came under heavy fire for advertising and other promotional activities targeting youth. These activities were reviewed and criticized by the Surgeon General and the IOM in major reports in 1994 and they, in turn, undergirded an important regulatory effort by the FDA to assert jurisdiction over tobacco products, restrict sales to persons under 18, and to restrict promotional activities targeting youth. Although the FDA's 1996 Tobacco Rule was eventually invalidated by the Supreme Court in 2000,[18] the industy agreed to substantial restrictions on youth-oriented promotions in the Master Settlement Agreement (MSA) in 1998. These included bans on use of cartoon characters and billboard advertising and restrictions on industry sponsorship of various concerts and other public events. Proceeds from the MSA were also used to support a major public education effort, including an antismoking media campaign.

The Institute of Medicine's landmark report, *Ending the Tobacco Problem: Blueprint for the Nation* (2007) identified components of an aggressive strategy for reducing tobacco use from its current adult prevalence of about 20% to a level at which it "no longer constitutes a public health problem."[19] The IOM committee endorsed unprecedented restrictions on the tobacco industry's promotional activities (**Table 9.1**).

In addition to these restrictions on the marketing and promotion of tobacco products, the IOM also recommended government support of large and sustained antismoking media campaigns to discouraging initiation and promote cessation. All these aggressive measures were justified, according to the IOM committee, by the dangerous characteristics of tobacco products, and a unique history of cynicism and deception by the tobacco industry. The IOM committee noted that the tobacco industry initially denied and hid information about tobacco's addictiveness and adverse health consequences, as it shaped a public rhetoric focused on consumer choice and anti-paternalism. Ethical justifications for government action became stronger and the public's perception of the issues shifted, however, as scientific evidence about tobacco's harms and the industry's deception emerged in court rulings and legal proceedings. Questions to have in mind when studying the following materials are

TABLE 9.1 IOM Tobacco-related Recommendations (Selected)

Tobacco advertising by manufacturers and retailers be restricted to a black-and-white text-only format;
Manufacturers and retailers be required to accompany all product marketing with "corrective advertising";
Use of "light," "low-tar," and other misleading terms be banned in tobacco advertising and on packaging;
Manufacturers be forbidden to target youth in any channel of communication;
Manufacturers increase the visibility and force of package warnings, including use of graphic images.

Data from: IOM (Institute of Medicine). 2007. Ending the tobacco problem: A blue-print for the nation. Washington, DC: The National Academies Press.

whether these measures are justified in the context of tobacco control and, if they are, whether they are permissible in other commercial contexts, including efforts to address obesity.

Restrictions on Tobacco Advertising

In a 5-4 decision in *Lorillard v. Reilly* (2001), The Supreme Court struck down a Massachusetts statute banning all outdoor tobacco advertising on billboards and at point of sale within 1000 feet of schools.[20] Applying the *Central Hudson* test that governs regulation of commercial speech, the majority opinion assumed that the state's declared interest in preventing tobacco use by minors was important and that the ban would "substantially advance" that interest; but a majority of the Justices held that the ban was not adequately tailored to serve the state's interest in preventing use by minors and that it unduly burdened the interests of adult smokers in receiving information from tobacco manufacturers and retailers.

In *Lorillard v. Reilly* and other recent commercial speech cases, several Justices have suggested that truthful, non-misleading commercial speech should have stronger constitutional protection (more demanding scrutiny) than *Central Hudson* requires. For this reason, most tobacco control advocates assume that any significant restriction of tobacco advertising (unrelated to truthfulness of a claim) that reaches the Supreme Court will be struck down. However, other observers believe that some of the Justices who want to apply stricter scrutiny are mainly concerned about bans on advertising of *information.* Persons holding this view concede that the First Amendment protects the right to receive information about commercial products and services ("this drug can be purchased for this price") and the rights of businesses to convey that information to consumers. However, they argue that the First Amendment should not be read to provide heightened protection for the purely *promotional* features of advertising (i.e., advertising not intended to provide information but that is rather intended to encourage use of the product). These features of advertising should be subject only to a weaker version of *Central Hudson* test so as leave the government adequate flexibility to regulate commercial messages that promote behavior inimical to the public health.

In the context of tobacco advertising, this is a very important distinction because very little tobacco advertising conveys information; instead, most of the billions of dollars spent by the tobacco companies aims to create a positive affective connection with the product and the brand. The test case for this basic approach is the FDA's newly re-issued regulation limiting tobacco advertising to a text-only, black-and-white format. The agency's 1996 Tobacco Rule, which banned magazine advertising with greater than 15% youth exposure, was revived by the 2009 federal tobacco bill. Under this rule, manufacturers and retailers are permitted to state the price, brand, and product information, but would no longer be able to use images of cowboys or slim women to create positive associations with the product and with smoking, or to thereby "suggest" that tobacco use is beneficial without saying so. In its 2007 Report,[19] the IOM recommended this approach for *all* tobacco advertising, including advertising directed at adults. In the IOM's view, government also has a powerful interest in encouraging cessation, and most tobacco company expenditures on promotion are by their nature designed to detract from the government's efforts to help addicted tobacco users quit. However, the FDA rule is grounded only in the state's interest in preventing initiation of smoking by minors. The IOM Report also emphasized that *images of the product* itself should be permitted in the companies' ads because these depictions are designed to inform consumers about product characteristics relating to potential health risks; failure to include this exception in the FDA rule may be a fatal flaw.

Proponents of the text-only approach argue that it accords full protection to informational advertising and provides a "reasonable fit" between means and the objective of suppressing tobacco use. They have emphasized that the government has the constitutional power to prohibit sale of tobacco altogether (which no one contests), and that the "greater power" (to prohibit) should include the "lesser power" (to allow the product to be sold, while banning advertising). From this viewpoint, disabling government from suppressing promotional marketing creates a constitutional contradiction because it forces the government to choose between prohibiting the product altogether or allowing it to be aggressively promoted, with no regulatory space in between. Critics of the black-and-white text-only advertising rule, who favor greater constitutional protection of commercial advertising for any lawful activity, respond that the language of the First Amendment refers to the "freedom of speech," not simply to dissemination of "information." If the government's power to restrict advertising of lawful products is more constrained than its power to regulate the product, that "contradiction" is created by the First Amendment itself. Moreover, critics of the rule also argue that the regulatory distinction between words and pictures is not workable, even in conveying information. After all, an effectively crafted picture may be "worth" (convey information equivalent to) one thousand words.

The tobacco advertising restriction has not fared well in the courts. A federal district court in Kentucky invalidated it, as being unconstitutionally overbroad, "[b]ecause Congress could have exempted large categories of innocuous images and colors—e.g., images that teach adult consumers how to use novel tobacco products, images that merely identify products and producers, and colors that communicate information about the nature of a product, at least where such colors and images have no special appeal to youth."[21] The federal Court of Appeals for the Sixth Circuit unanimously affirmed the district court's judgment in *Discount Tobacco City and Lottery, Inc. v. FDA* (2012)[22]; the arguments presented to the Court, summarized in its judgment, were as follows:

> The government maintains that the tobacco industry's history of targeting juveniles through colorful and graphic advertising justifies the breadth of the restriction. ... The government asserts that "[t]he industry's campaign to attract minors is not waged with tools of rational persuasion that invoke the 'merits' of taking up tobacco use. Instead, the industry relies on peripheral cues and irrational associations to distract would-be users from the fact that tobacco products are lethal and addictive." The evocation of "irrational associations," reinforced through color and image, the government argues, is more effective with juveniles than with adult consumers. The government further argues that this provision of the Act is properly tailored, as it "does not apply to advertising that appears in an adult publication. ... [and i]t does not affect the packaging of tobacco products." Furthermore, "[t]he restriction does not constrain a manufacturer's ability to communicate product information through text."
>
> Addressing the argument that the Act could impose less restrictive prohibitions on advertising, the government argues that any further exceptions to the ban on color and graphics would create loopholes that "would easily be exploited by the tobacco industry." The government asserts that, "Congress was not required to replicate a scheme that is demonstrably subject to evasion. Ample evidence supports Congress's determination that a 'less restrictive and comprehensive approaches have [sic] not and will not be effective' in reducing underage tobacco use."
>
> [The tobacco companies] counter that the ban effectively prevents the tobacco industry from communicating with adult consumers; attracting attention and differentiating their products in the retail environment; communicating useful commercial information about their products to consumers, including how to use novel products; and "depicting in advertising their products' packaging or their packaging's distinctive logos and colors." [They] further respond that the provision is not properly tailored, because the ban on imagery extends to direct mail to adults, certain magazines that are "primarily directed to persons 21 years of age and older," most tobacco retailers, and taverns that allow juveniles "to enter for meals with their parents or during restricted times." Lastly, [they] argue that the provision is overly burdensome to the industry because it requires [them] to verify the youth readership of a magazine in order to meet the criteria of the "adult publication" exception. ...
>
> [T]he government contends that the tobacco industry's graphic color advertisements are deceptive because "[t]obacco imagery ... seeks to distract potential users from the fact that tobacco products are lethal and addictive." See 2007 IOM Report:[19 (p. 322)] "The images used in tobacco marketing associate smoking with lifestyles and experiences that appeal to young people, and these positive associations tend to displace or override risk information in adolescent decision making." Consequently, the government's claim is not that tobacco advertisements make deceptive or misleading claims, but that they create positive associations in the minds of consumers, such as linking the use of tobacco products to "part of a desirable lifestyle that includes activities such as mountain biking, tug-of-war, and sex," along with concepts such as "fun" and "relaxation."
>
> [The companies] respond that, "if the Government were correct, it could similarly ban attractive advertisements for *all* age-restricted products, including beer, R-rated movies, lottery tickets, and fast cars, simply because those advertisements are appealing, not just to the adults at whom they are aimed, but to youth who happen to see them." These advertisements, too, undoubtedly attempt to entice consumers by creating desirable lifestyle associations, not by dryly conveying informational content.

> [The companies] fail to appreciate that there are ways for a person to drink beer, watch R-rated movies, buy lottery tickets, and drive fast cars, that do not necessarily cause harm to that person. In contrast, there is no method by which a person can smoke a cigarette or use smokeless tobacco in a manner that is health-neutral. ... [Nonetheless] product advertisement always seeks to create positive associations between the product and certain lifestyles or symbols. Perfume and cologne do not make people more beautiful, chewing gum does not make them more athletic, coffee does not make them more intelligent or urbane. By the same token, though the government would have us believe otherwise, using tobacco does not necessarily preclude a person from mountain biking, playing games, or engaging in romantic relationships. ...
>
> All use of color and imagery in tobacco advertising, of course, is not deceptive or manipulative. [S]ome advertising ... is largely informational. Other tobacco advertising is used to reinforce consumer preference "by simply showing the package" of the customer's preferred brand. Finally, some uses of color imagery are simply attention grabbing in a crowded marketplace, letting consumers know that their preferred brand or product is available at a particular retailer. Furthermore, there are surely certain color graphic tobacco ads that have nominal to zero appeal to the youth market. Each of these forms of advertising has great expressive value for the tobacco industry, and its suppression would be an undue burden on [their] free speech. ...
>
> Instead of instituting a blanket restriction on color and graphics in tobacco advertising, the government may instead restrict only the speech necessary to effect its purposes. "To the extent that studies have identified particular advertising and promotion practices that appeal to youth, tailoring would involve targeting those practices while permitting others. As the district court correctly stated, instead of instituting such a sweeping and complete ban, "Congress could have exempted large categories of innocuous images and colors—e.g., images that teach adult consumers how to use novel tobacco products, images that merely identify products and producers, and colors that communicate information about the nature of a product, at least where such colors and images have no special appeal to youth."
>
> There is no doubt that identifying and targeting certain advertising practices will be more arduous than banning all color and graphics in tobacco advertising. ... But this is the exact work required by the First Amendment. And, "so long as the sale and use of tobacco is lawful for adults, the tobacco industry has a protected interest in communicating information about its products and adult customers have an interest in receiving that information."[20]
>
> ---
>
> 674 F.3d 509 (2012) United States Court of Appeals, Sixth Circuit.

The Supreme Court will eventually have to confront these unsettled issues about the status of tobacco advertising (and commercial speech in general) under the First Amendment. How it does so is likely to have implications for other health-based restrictions on promotional advertising, including regulations aiming explicitly to suppress consumption of certain foods or alcohol (by youth only or by adults as well). Depending on what the Court says, it may have implications even for more narrowly drafted regulations that focus exclusively on preventing child exposure to messages that are inherently manipulative and deceptive (as with food advertising).

Aggressive Package Regulation

As noted earlier, mandatory disclosures and warnings are commonplace in health and safety regulation. These warnings typically are required to appear in advertising and on packaging. A particularly aggressive form of package regulation is a key element of the IOM's blueprint for "ending the tobacco problem" and of the FDA's regulatory initiatives under the 2009 Tobacco Control Act[23]—a requirement that packages contain large, colorful, graphic images depicting the harmful effects of tobacco use. (See examples from http://www.fda.gov/TobaccoProducts/Labeling/ucm259214.htm.) This regulation raises fundamental questions of public health ethics and constitutional law: Can the government require the manufacturer to devote the entire space on the package to the government's warnings? Can the government require the package to carry colorful and biologically explicit graphic warnings to make them more salient? Does government's authority to regulate advertising and labeling of a lawful product go beyond requiring the manufacturer to include accurate information? Is discouraging consumption of the product a permissible basis for regulating the package or for directing the manufacturer to convey the government's message?

What about requiring so-called "plain" packaging—only black-and-white text conveying the brand name and the required warnings? Plain packaging is a logical extension of the FDA's effort to take the color out of advertising: anything that is attractive about the tobacco package sends a misleading message about the virtues of the product; conversely, the message being conveyed by the plain, generic package is that "this is a product with no benefit." What are the outer limits of government's authority to "commandeer" the package for its own messages?

Graphic warnings are required in at least 30 countries and plain packaging has been proposed by the government in Australia. The justifications for these initiatives were reviewed by the IOM in *Ending the Tobacco Problem*:[19]

> The tobacco industry has long used cigarette packaging to identify and market its products, and governments have long used cigarette packaging to convey messages about tobacco risk and exposure. As legal restrictions have increasingly reduced or eliminated media advertising, the importance of the package as a vehicle for promotion has increased. The packages carried by smokers serve as mobile advertisements for particular products. Promotional displays of packages in retail outlets are also key marketing tools. In response to the increasing importance of the package in [tobacco use] promotion, governments have begun to exert more control over packaging characteristics for the dual purposes of reducing this form of marketing [by the companies] and communicating directly with consumers.
>
> Among the reasons for regulatory interest in tobacco packaging are:
>
> - communicating product information to consumers and potential consumers,
> - warning consumers about hazards and thereby discouraging consumption,
> - communicating other health information (e.g., cessation hotline numbers),
> - preventing smuggling (by requiring documentation of excise tax payment),
> - preventing misleading messages by tobacco companies and providing corrective information to counteract previous deceptions,
> - preventing promotional messages by tobacco companies as other avenues of advertising are curtailed, and
> - "denormalizing" tobacco products
>
> The use of packages to convey tobacco-related health risks has a number of potential advantages over other forms of communication. The frequency of exposure is high. The messages are delivered at the moment a smoker desires another cigarette. The messages on packages also communicate information to the public at large, and not merely the consumer.
>
> [Although] Congress first required health warnings on cigarette packages in 1966 ... U.S. package warnings are still not prominent and are located on the side of the package in small print. In 1994, a previous IOM committee made the following observation about this country's tobacco health warnings:
>
> > The adequacy of the current cigarette warnings has been repeatedly questioned by public health specialists. Moreover, in the committee's view federal cigarette labeling legislation has reflected an unsatisfactory compromise between the public's health and the tobacco industry's desire to avoid concurrent state regulation and to reduce its exposure to tort liability. Negotiations in the legislative process have tended to favor the industry. ... The inadequacy of current labeling policy is clearly revealed in the declaration of congressional purpose in the Comprehensive Smoking Education Act of 1984: *It is the purpose of this Act to provide a new strategy of making Americans more aware of any adverse health effects of smoking, to assure the timely and widespread dissemination of research findings, and to enable individuals to make informed decisions about smoking.* It is time to state unequivocally that the primary objective of tobacco regulation is not only to promote informed choice but rather to discourage consumption of tobacco products, especially by children and youths, as a means of reducing tobacco-related death

> and disease. Even though tobacco products are legally available to adults, the paramount public health aim is to reduce the number of people who use and become addicted to these products, through a focus on children and youths. The warnings must be designed to promote this objective. In the committee's view, the current warnings are inadequate even when measured against an informed choice standard, but they are woefully deficient when evaluated in terms of proper public health criteria."[15 (pp. 236–237)]

> ... Although federal law has remained unchanged for more than 20 years, evidence regarding the ineffectiveness of the prescribed warnings has continued to accumulate. [T]he U.S. package warnings have served the tobacco industry well by reducing their liability exposure while communicating ineffectively with smokers and potential smokers. The basic problems with the U.S. warnings are that they are unnoticed and stale, and they fail to convey relevant information in an effective way. ... They therefore have little effect on decision making or behavior.

As recommended by the IOM, the 2009 Tobacco Control Act strengthens package warnings and empowers FDA to strengthen them further by increasing size and visibility and by using graphics (Section 202[d]):

> The Secretary may ... adjust the format, type size, color graphics, and text of any of the label requirements, or establish the format, type size, and text of any other disclosures required under the Federal Food, Drug, and Cosmetic Act, if the Secretary finds that such a change would promote greater public understanding of the risks associated with the use of tobacco products.

The FDA promulgated regulations exercising this authority in 2011,[24] including nine images (one for each warning statement). Not surprisingly, Section 202(d) and the FDA regulations have been challenged on First Amendment grounds. How would you frame the constitutional issue? Should the graphic images be characterized as similar to mandated factual disclosures? Or are they analogous to being "coerced" to salute the flag? However they are characterized, should they be upheld?

Let's try out the argument both ways. On the one hand, assume that the justifying purpose of the graphic images is to increase the salience of the warnings, compared to the existing textual warnings, in order to enhance the prospective consumer's awareness of the dangers of smoking and to offset the accumulated effects of decades of industry deception. So understood, the new warning requirements might sensibly be characterized, in constitutional terms, as a corrective "mandated disclosure" (using pictures as well as words) necessitated by the tobacco industry's history of deceiving consumers and the failure of the previously required package warnings to communicate the health effects of tobacco use effectively. If this is the justifying interest, the regulation might be subject to the more deferential standard of judicial scrutiny applied to factual disclosures—like the calorie counts on fast food menus upheld in *NYSRA v. NY City Bd of Health* (2009).[13] If viewed in this way, should the pictorial warnings be upheld? Are they "reasonably related" to the government's interest in effectively conveying the negative health consequences of smoking to consumers? A divided panel of the U.S. Court of Appeals for the Sixth Circuit upheld Section 202(d) under this standard because pictorial images could be designed to convey information effectively and should be subject to the same level of deferential scrutiny as textual disclosures or warnings. (This decision did not address the FDA rule itself or the actual images required by the FDA in the rule.)[22]

On the other hand, assume that the regulation is characterized as an effort to dissuade people from starting to smoke and to persuade current smokers to quit, as the IOM insisted. The tobacco industry argues that if the pictorial warning requirements are seen this way, the aim is not really to convey information but rather to force the companies to subsidize the government's persuasive message by posting it on the company's channel of communication with consumers (i.e., the package). When seen in this way, it is analogous to requiring a person to affix a license plate to a motor vehicle saying "Live Free or Die" and should be subject to strict judicial scrutiny and invalidated, as was the New Hampshire license requirement in *Wooley v. Maynard* (1977).[10]

A panel of judges on the Court of Appeals for the District of Columbia Circuit—reviewing the images actually required in the FDA rule—embraced the second approach:

> The Companies contend that, to the extent the graphic warnings go beyond the textual warnings to shame and repulse smokers and denigrate smoking as an antisocial act, the message is ideological and not informational. "[B]y effectively shouting well-understood information to

> consumers," they explain, "FDA is communicating an ideological message, a point of view on how people should live their lives: that the risks from smoking outweigh the pleasure that smokers derive from it, and that smokers make bad personal decisions, and should stop smoking." In effect, the graphic images are not warnings, but admonitions: "[D]on't buy or use this product." No one doubts the government can promote smoking cessation programs; can use shock, shame, and moral opprobrium to discourage people from becoming smokers; and can use its taxing and regulatory authority to make smoking economically prohibitive and socially onerous. And the government can certainly require that consumers be fully informed about the dangers of hazardous products. But this case raises novel questions about the scope of the government's authority to force the manufacturer of a product to go beyond making purely factual and accurate commercial disclosures and undermine its own economic interest—in this case, by making "every single pack of cigarettes in the country [a] mini billboard" for the government's anti-smoking message.
>
> Even assuming the Companies' marketing efforts (packaging, branding, and other advertisements) can be properly classified as commercial speech, and thus subject to less robust First Amendment protections ... how much leeway should this Court grant the government when it seeks to compel a product's manufacturer to convey the state's subjective—and perhaps even ideological—view that consumers should reject this otherwise legal, but disfavored, product?[25]
>
> *R.J. Reynolds Tobacco Co. v. Food & Drug Administration*, 696 F.3d 1205 (D.C. Cir. 2012).

Compelling a person to endorse or utter a statement with which he does not agree and to become a mere instrument of the government's message seems deeply antithetical to the very essence of individual liberty. Thus, when viewed in this way, the graphic warnings are likely to be struck down—and, not surprisingly, the U.S. Court of Appeals, District of Columbia Circuit did strike them down in a 2-1 judgment in *R.J. Reynolds v. FDA* (2012).[25]

You should ask, though, whether the analogy between tobacco companies' interest in controlling their packages is really equivalent to freedom of political expression at issue in *Wooley*. Some might find somewhat peculiar the implicit comparison between an individual claim of conscience and the interest of a global corporation in encouraging people to use a dangerous product that is inimical to the public health (one that the government could and would prohibit if it were feasible to do so). Of course, the government may not suppress the company's billboard claim "the Government should leave smokers and their cigarettes alone!" or even that "the Government is exaggerating the dangers of cigarettes!" These statements lie at the core of political expression protected by the First Amendment. But do the companies have the right to use a cigarette package for political statements? The package is a vehicle for conveying a highly regulated, dangerous product to a consumer. Does the company have a constitutional right to use the package to encourage smoking? Does this channel of commercial communication (i.e., the package) "belong" to the company?

Perhaps neither of these two characterizations (mandated factual disclosure or "coerced speech") is apt. A third approach is possible: the graphic warnings could be characterized as persuasive speech (not as a mandated factual disclosure) by the government aiming to counteract highly persuasive commercial speech by the tobacco companies, using a well-established form of commercial product regulation (packaging and labeling) as a channel of communicating with consumers. Under this analysis, the graphic warnings would be subject to the intermediate scrutiny identified with the *Central Hudson* test. The question then would be whether the required warnings "substantially advance" an important governmental interest. The heart of the policy issue is then clearly exposed: Is the government's interest in reducing tobacco use important? Does the evidence show that these warnings are likely to reduce tobacco use and, as a result, reduce tobacco-related disease and death? So understood, the philosophy of John Stuart Mill and freedom of conscience recede to the background, and the interests of the actual stakeholders in this controversy come to the foreground. What are those interests? Whose interests are being served by the regulation? What interests are being protected by the First Amendment?

One final puzzle should be noted. How deferential should a court be to FDA's judgment about the available evidence? Graphic warnings are a regulatory innovation. Little evidence has yet accumulated regarding their effects on initiation and cessation. How should policymakers and courts proceed in the face of a plausible, but unproven, assumption about the effects of this rule? Does the government have to conduct studies regarding the effects of these images on smoker behavior before it can adopt the regulation?

How would it do that? Or may it require the package warnings based on consumer reactions to them in laboratory studies?

Government-Supported Media Campaigns

In 1988, the voters of California approved Proposition 99,[26] a statewide ballot initiative also known as the "Tobacco Tax and Health Protection Act of 1988."[27, 28] The Act imposes a 25-cents-per-pack surtax on all wholesale cigarette sales in California and directs that the revenue be used for specific purposes, including health education programs, tobacco-related disease research, and medical care for uninsured patients. In 1999, the California Assembly directed the Department of Health Services to establish a health education program, including a media campaign to raise public awareness of the deleterious effects of smoking, to effect a reduction in tobacco use. California's anti-tobacco media campaign consisted of radio, television, billboard, and print advertising, which portrayed smoking as dangerous and undesirable, and presented the tobacco industry and its executives as deceptive. In several of the television ads, actors playing tobacco executives were shown discussing how to lure more people into smoking or were portrayed as being elusive about smoking's health effects. One round of television commercials featured an actor playing a public relations executive for the fictional cigarette brand "Hampton," detailing for viewers his unseemly methods for getting people to start smoking. The ads end with the tagline, "Do You Smell Smoke?" implicitly referencing both cigarette smoke and a smoke-and-mirrors marketing strategy. Another ad portrayed tobacco executives discussing how to replace a customer base that is dying at the rate of 1,100 users a day. Some of the ads end with images of mock warning labels such as: "WARNING: The tobacco industry is not your friend." or "WARNING: Some people will say anything to sell cigarettes." Several spots suggested that tobacco companies aggressively market to children. In one particularly striking television ad entitled "Rain," children in a schoolyard are shown looking up while cigarettes rain down on them from the sky. A voice-over states "We have to sell cigarettes to your kids. We need half a million new smokers a year just to stay in business. So we advertise near schools, at candy counters. We lower our prices. We have to. It's nothing personal. You understand." At the conclusion, the narrator says, "The tobacco industry: how low will they go to make a profit?"

Several tobacco companies sued California's Department of Health Services to curtail the ads. The companies claimed that the media campaign amounted to "compelling" them to speak, in violation of their rights under the First Amendment, because the campaign was funded by a tax on wholesale cigarette sales—and thus was extracting money from them to fund a campaign to "vilify" the companies and discourage use of the industry's products.[a]

United State District Court Judge Karlton rejected this argument in *R.J. Reynolds v. Bonta* (2003)[29] on the ground that using funds derived from an otherwise properly imposed tax to fund an otherwise permissible media campaign does not make the messages proclaimed by the campaign attributable to the industry (and therefore "compel" them to communicate a disagreeable message). Each of the challenged advertisements was identified as "Sponsored by the California Department of Health Services." Every viewer understood that the message being conveyed was the government's message, not the companies' message. This case did not really encompass a "coerced speech" claim. Instead, the real question raised by the California media campaign is whether there is any constitutional constraint on the government's power to use revenues derived from tobacco excise taxes to criticize the tobacco industry and to discourage use of tobacco. Judge Karlton ruled that the answer is no, and the Ninth Circuit Court of Appeals affirmed this judgment, succinctly explaining its ruling in *R.J. Reynolds v. Shewry* (2005),[30] as follows:

> [I]f the tobacco companies were permitted to object to government speech simply because they pay an excise tax used to fund speech contrary to their interests, the result could be not only to reduce government's ability to disseminate ideas but also an explosion of litigation that could allow private interests to control public messages. There are numerous taxpayers who contribute disproportionately through excise taxes to government speech with which they disagree. If each were to have a similar right to challenge what it may deem government "propaganda," the government's ability to perform crucial educational and public health activities in the interests of all citizens would be hampered.
>
> *R.J. Reynolds Tobacco Co. v. Shewry*, 423 F. at 911 (2005).

In the course of their respective opinions, District Judge Karlton and the Ninth Circuit panel each took the occasion to engage

[a] Although most surtax payments are made by cigarette wholesalers, not the manufacturers themselves, the manufacturers also sell or provide small quantities of cigarettes directly to smokers, and the companies claimed that they collectively contributed approximately $2,800 in 2002. Approximately $25 million annually was spent on the challenged advertisements.

in a little hand-wringing about the possible constitutional constraints on "government speech." They expressed concern that, in some contexts, the government, by virtue of its sheer size and resources, could "drown out" a dissenting viewpoint. Given the fact that the tobacco industry spends almost $15 billion a year on marketing, this hypothetical concern is clearly inapplicable in the context of tobacco advertising; the risk in this context, proven by history, is the reverse—that tobacco promotion will drown out the government's message. However, Judge Karlton properly asked whether there might be more concern about the limits of the government's power to conduct a heavy-handed campaign when those who are targeted do not have the money or the power to fight back. Consider, for example, physicians who perform abortions and women who choose to have them. What if the government were to launch a campaign to vilify the doctors and cajole the women? The Supreme Court has held clearly that the government may attempt to discourage abortions by denying funding for them and by refusing to fund family planning services that do not comply with its prescribed script. What about using its powerful voice to galvanize opposition and discourage complicity? Abortion is undoubtedly a special case, but Judge Karlton's opinion properly invites ethical discussion about the limits of government's efforts to dissuade people from engaging in unsafe or unhealthy behavior. That is the subject to which we now turn.

ETHICAL DIMENSIONS OF GOVERNMENT COMMUNICATION

To inform, educate, and empower people about health is one of the 10 essential services of public health articulated and embraced by the public health profession and by officials in practice.[31] To emphasize its central role, public health departments even measure and hold themselves accountable for these services through their accreditation process.[32] Government communication about health is animated by a number of the moral considerations at the core of public health, particularly those considerations we propose in our framework that fall under the broad norm of beneficence (producing benefits; avoiding, preventing, and removing harms; and producing the maximal balance of benefits over harms and other costs). For example, infectious diseases that constitute a public health threat, such as the flu, warrant governmental action to protect the public, given the risk of outbreaks and epidemics. Therefore, communication strategies to inform, educate, and empower the public to get immunizations that provide protection for individuals and the population are clearly supported by moral considerations related to population benefit, preventing harm, and utility.

In addition, at least two other moral norms we propose for public health are implicated in health communication and promotion strategies: disclosing information as well as speaking honestly and truthfully (often grouped under the concept of transparency), and respecting autonomous choices and actions, including liberty of action. These two moral norms provide support and guidance for the way particular health communication campaigns should be designed and used, although they could serve also as constraints for particular communication strategies. Not all potentially effective interventions—in this case, messages—that produce benefits are meritorious, and U.S. public philosophy establishes presumptions in favor of those that respect liberty, transparency, and the like. That said, however, informing, educating and empowering people through communication strategies are among the least restrictive of potential public health interventions, as compared to other tools that might be used—for example, legal penalties or school requirements to encourage immunizations.

Providing Information

What then, if any, might be constraints on government health communication strategies, and what types of communication are most compatible with the moral considerations? (Recall that our legal context provides little constitutional constraint on government speech, as described in Parts 2 and 3 of this chapter.) Let us consider, as an example, a potential public health communication campaign to promote flu vaccination, based on a case described in the literature by Faden.[33] Public health officials are uncertain about which strain of flu (A or B) will circulate in a community in the upcoming season, and therefore uncertain about the overall level of effectiveness of the vaccine they will be promoting. Since the vaccine is effective for strain A only and not strain B, public health officials have a number of options for a short communication campaign: (1) the message could emphasize that the vaccine will cut an individual's chance of getting the flu in half (since it is not clear at this point which strain, A or B, will circulate), or (2) the message could emphasize that the vaccine is 100% effective against strain A and not mention the possibility that strain B, rather than strain A, may circulate in the upcoming season. Faden points out that a consideration of the options should take into account their likely effectiveness based on relevant social science data about decision making and the biases people often have when they make decisions. For example, pseudo-certainty and certainty effects suggest that "people are more willing to take protective action to eliminate risks than reduce risks, even if the amount of reduction in risk is identical in both cases. Thus, a protective action which reduces the probability of a harm from 1% to zero should be more attractive than an action that reduces the probability of the same harm from 2% to 1%."[33] Does the message provided in options 1 and 2 respect individuals' liberty interest and enhance their ability to make a good choice? Is the information in either or both options presented truthfully?

An ethical perspective might offer the following assessment: If social science data suggest option 2 may "produce more benefit" than option 1 (with benefit defined as informing and influencing more people to get the vaccine in the upcoming season), then from the perspective of short-term population benefit, option 2 arguably may be the better choice. However, since option 2 is misleading in the way it presents information, the other public health moral norms—disclosing information honestly and truthfully, respecting autonomous choices and actions, and building and maintaining trust—are in tension with and would trump the moral norm of producing benefit as defined in this case. (See **Table 9.2** for distinctions offered by Faden.)

One important constraint on government communication, then, is that public health information must be carefully designed so as not to be deceptive or misleading through the use of exaggerated or partial information. Such "manipulation of information," according to Faden, compromises autonomy because it undermines people's understanding of the situation and of their options. The essential public health service to "inform, educate, and empower people" is not only an instrumental goal (to produce population benefit) but also can be a primary goal—to provide information in a way that enhances people's capacity to make reasoned choices. Even for communication that is informational, such as where, why, and how to gain access to immunizations or other preventive services, the health messages should be presented in ways that minimize any unintended negative consequences, such as fear or misunderstanding; are proportional, i.e., the probable benefits outweigh the potential negative impact for this particular situation; and are impartial, in that particular groups that receive targeted messages are not stigmatized or blamed.

TABLE 9.2 Persuasion versus Manipulation

Persuasion: the intentional and successful attempt to induce a person(s), through appeals to reason, to freely accept—as his or her own—the beliefs, attitudes, values, intentions, or actions advocated by the influence agent.
Manipulation of Information: a deliberate act that successfully influences a person(s) by nonpersuasively altering the person's understanding of the situation, thereby modifying perceptions of the available options. Includes manipulation by deception, such as lying, withholding of information, and misleading exaggeration where people are led to believe what is false.
Psychological Manipulation: a catch-all classification that includes any intentional act that successfully influences a person(s) to belief or behavior by causing changes in mental processes other than those involved in understanding. Includes subliminal suggestion, flattery, and other appeals to emotional weaknesses, inducing of guilt feelings.

Data from Faden R (1987). Ethical issues in government sponsored public health campaigns. Health Education Quarterly, 14(1), 27–37.

Persuading With and Without Explicit Reasons

Public health also engages in communication campaigns not only to inform but also to promote healthy behaviors and discourage unhealthy behaviors. These campaigns can manage health information by flooding the information environment to increase the sheer quantity of information available to the public on a topic and/or can use other communication techniques that "redefine or frame the issue" so that the particular health topic gets more attention or seems more important to the targeted audience.[34] Campaigns designed to influence individual behavior change carry an implicit message that one "ought" to do something or act in a certain way. Are these types of communication messages compatible with respecting autonomous choices and actions in that their goal is not to inform people about options, but rather influence them to choose a particular option? In some cases, the answer seems simple. Given the evidence that wearing seatbelts saves lives and that laws require the use of seatbelts, public health communication campaigns designed to influence individuals to wear seatbelts are clearly compatible with respecting autonomous choices. Messages to encourage or persuade people to buckle up "because it saves lives" or that picture powerful images of individuals harmed in car crashes are based on data and truthful information about consequences, and therefore the reasons for wearing seatbelts are communicated either explicitly or implicitly in the messages. (See **Exhibit 9.1** for another example of recommended themes and evidence of effectiveness for campaigns to reduce alcohol-impaired driving.)

Communication techniques, however, sometimes include the use of implicit messages, powerful images, or analogies that are not designed to convey or build on information; instead, they aim to appeal to emotion in order to create and associate positive or negative reactions with a behavior. Consider an example described by Rossi and Yudell, that aims to discourage teen pregnancy with the

EXHIBIT 9.1 Mass Media Campaigns

Mass Media Campaigns: Recommended to Reduce Alcohol-Impaired Driving

Common campaign themes: fear of arrest; fear of injury to self, others, or property; and characterizing drinking drivers as irresponsible and dangerous to others.

Evidence of effectiveness when: carefully planned and well executed; adequate audience exposure; and implemented in settings that have other ongoing alcohol-impaired driving prevention activities.

Systematic Reviews of Research:

- Total alcohol-related crashes: median decrease of 13% (interquartile interval: 6% to 14% decrease; 7 studies)
- Injury-producing alcohol-related crashes: median decrease of 10% (interquartile range: 6% to 14% decrease; 6 studies)
- Proportion of drivers who had consumed alcohol: net decreases of 30% and 158% (2 studies)

Reproduced from the Guide to Community Preventive Services. Reducing alcohol-impaired driving: mass media campaigns. www.thecommunityguide.org/mvoi/AID/massmedia.html. Last updated September 24, 2013.

statement "Before you be a mother: be a woman."[35] This message does not appear to be designed to convey information and is not therefore misleading or deceptive. However, it also does not fall clearly under definitions of persuasion either, which generally refer to inducing or influencing others, *through reasons,* to act or adopt a position voluntarily.

Ethical concerns are raised about messages with emotional content such as this that may intentionally employ techniques for psychological manipulation. An advertisement described by Tengland, for example, encourages women to explore their risk of breast cancer with their physician by picturing a woman with barely covered breasts and suggesting that men notice a woman's bosom. These types of health messages use marketing techniques to attract attention and/or exert influence, not by providing reasons, but through appeals that arouse emotion and that may be designed to even bypass reason. Assuming that such messages are effective in increasing the number of women who get breast screenings, are there any ethical constraints on their use by public health? A possible constraint offered by Rossi and Yudell involves assessing whether such an emotional appeal is so strong that it becomes a controlling influence. In other words, messages may not be ethically justifiable if the images or ideas exert such a powerful influence that peoples' ability to reason or make choices freely is not respected and instead is actually undermined.

Another ethical concern is psychological manipulation. An example might be a health campaign to discourage parent co-sleeping that pictures a baby in bed next to a big knife and compares that image to parents sleeping with their children. "Because of the protectiveness that parents feel about their children, and the sense of moral responsibility and culpability that the message is likely to create, it seems plausible to say that (regardless of intention) this kind of appeal to emotion is likely to detract from the audience's ability to reason effectively about this issue," explain Rossi and Yudell.[35]

How should we go about judging whether campaigns with strong emotional appeals, like the co-sleeping campaign, or use of so-called "scare tactics" in general, are ethically defensible? Drawing on the justificatory conditions, such an assessment would depend in part on the following: empirical data, from pretests and focus groups, of whether the message is effective in a particular situation; whether the negative impact, if any, on the target audience (e.g., parents) can be minimized; whether any harm from the messages is proportional to the magnitude and significance of the benefit it produces; whether its effect is impartial and does not stereotype particular groups; and whether it is the least restrictive in that it exerts the least controlling or manipulative influence when compared to other effective campaign strategies.

Other relevant considerations include information about the socioeconomic, cultural, and demographic features of the particular community: What public health problems, needs, or concerns are most salient in this context? For example, does co-sleeping occur because parents are unaware of the potential risk, or they lack family support needed after childbirth, or do not have resources to purchase infant beds? The appropriate goal of the communication campaign would depend on this type of information. Another relevant question: Which features of the social-cultural-historical context are relevant? If, for example, a particular community continued to have a higher than average prevalence of parent co-sleeping after a previous communication campaign provided information about free cribs and about the risks and harms of co-sleeping, then the need for an emotionally powerful communication message as described above might be justifiable in that it was necessary and the least restrictive alternative, given that other information messages had been tried unsuccessfully.

Marketing Health

The use of marketing techniques to promote socially beneficial behavior (called social marketing) has grown dramatically in public health in recent years. It involves planning and implementing a marketing campaign for a public health issue, using commercial marketing concepts, such as audience segmentation, exchange theory (that identifies the benefits or costs that are exchanged) and the marketing mix that analyzes such factors as a "product" or benefit that the target audience will value.[36] The VERB™ campaign coordinated by the CDC to encourage youth between the ages of 9 and 13 to be physically active illustrates the successful use of social marketing techniques, according to Grier and Bryant.[37] Social marketing messages were tailored for different segments of the audience based on such factors as age, ethnicity, and interest in physical activity. (See **Figure 9.2** for an example of a targeted VERB™ campaign message.) Research also is used to identify what the targeted audience finds appealing, so, for instance, the VERB™ program identified and pictured physical activity as a way "to have fun, spend time with friends, and gain recognition from peers and adults rather than to prevent obesity or chronic disease later in life."[37]

While typical health education programs aim to inform and persuade people by increasing their understanding of the benefits of adopting healthy behaviors, social marketing influences behavior by offering people alternative ways of viewing a choice. It "creates an environment more conducive for change by enhancing the attractiveness of the benefits offered and minimizing the costs," explain Grier and Bryant. Social marketing in public health is subject to a number of ethical challenges, however. Focusing on reducing obesity through individual behavior change arguably misplaces responsibility. Wymer believes, for example, that social marketing needs to shift focus from obesity as an individual disorder to the "unhealthy context" of obesity, which includes "industry marketing activities; the increased availability of junk food; increased portion sizes, food advertising, fast-food promotion, and the low cost of high fat, high calorie foods."[38]

Others raise concerns related to the behavioral change techniques used in social marketing and the potential for manipulation of individuals and of society, given the "power differentials that contribute to an unequal playing field" between marketers and the people they are attempting to influence.[37] The use of social marketing to change social norms, for example, does so without the traditional "techniques of social and political discourse, grassroots action and so forth," according to Brenker,[39] who raises concerns that the people social marketers target "are not given a voice in the sense of being accorded various participatory rights." He suggests that this "raises ethical questions about the effects of social marketing on self-determination and democracy." To address these types of concerns, some believe that consumers should be included in the entire communication process "from the beginning of the social marketing design to its implementation and evaluation."[37]

In justifying government's role in altering attitudes, choices, and social norms, Sunstein[40] also points to the need for public support for government's activities and for government transparency. He reminds us that while social norms can reduce individual freedom, they also can solve collective action problems by inducing people to do things they otherwise would not do. He states: "If government changes the social meaning of smoking, has it acted illegitimately? What if most people, or most smokers, would, on reflection, want smoking to have a different meaning.... Surely the consequences of the change matter; surely it matters if the change is supported by (most or all of those affected).... The justification for government action is firm if all or almost all people support it as a means of solving a collective action problem."[40]

Empowering Health

In contrast to top-down informational or social marketing campaigns that rely on cognitive or behavioral psychology and related analytic approaches, empowerment is a collaborative process emphasizing that individuals and communities should draw on their internal assets, resources, and capacity to catalyze social and political change, and that the client, group, or community should own and control the change processes they are involved in.

A cornerstone of ethics for the field of health promotion, which includes health communication, is the *Ottawa Charter for Health Promotion*,[41] which focuses on both individual and community empowerment. In addition, the charter,

FIGURE 9.2 Targeted Messages

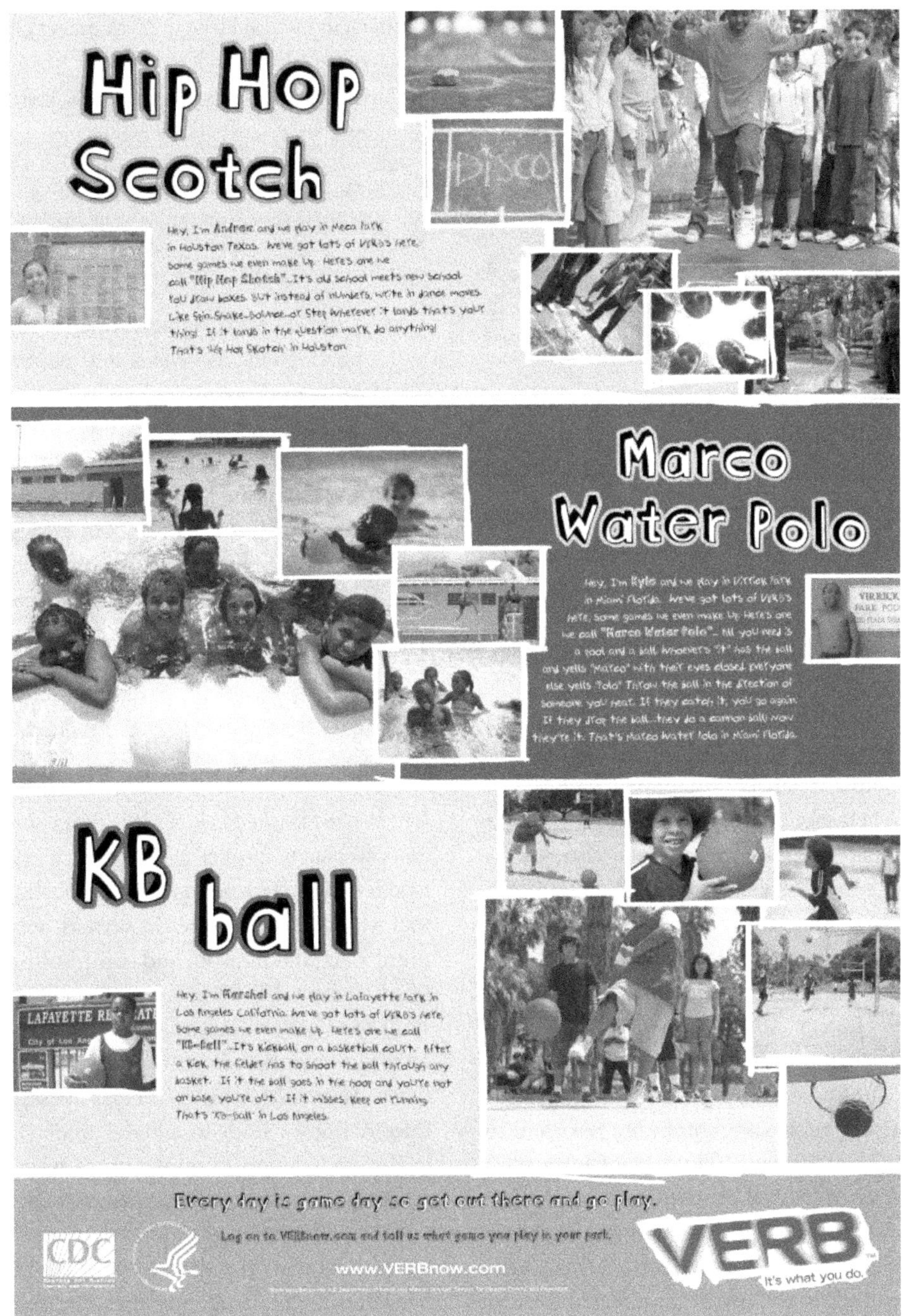

Reproduced from: CDC http://www.cdc.gov/youthcampaign/advertising/african_american/PDF/school_poster_3.pdf Accessed 4/28/13

which was developed and adopted in 1986, endorses a broad socio-ecological perspective on health. Its definition of health extends well beyond the absence of disease and instead is "a positive concept emphasizing social and personal resources, as well as physical capacities." Since then other charters and professionals in the field have expanded their activities beyond the provision of information to individuals to a focus that encompasses individual and community empowerment to achieve health equity and human rights.[3] Tengland explains that health information per se is not unimportant. But because individuals and groups vary in their capacity to understand and act on information, "even if some people will benefit from information campaigns, and the average (aggregated) health might increase in the population, there is also a risk of increasing health inequalities."[6]

Thus, in the context of health promotion, an ethic of empowerment supports strategies that encourage, persuade, inspire, and/or liberate people to make better choices themselves about health. The Ottawa Charter specifies that health promotion "supports personal and social development," in part by enhancing life skills. "By so doing, it increases the options available to people to exercise more control over their own health and over their environments, and to make choices conducive to health."[41]

What does an ethic of empowerment in health promotion require? In contrast to health campaigns of the past, which were based on a relatively simplistic understanding of a direct link between communication and behavior change, some think that "empowerment"—and also, for our purposes, the moral consideration "respecting autonomous choices and actions, including liberty of action"—can be better interpreted as health literacy. Nutbeam[42] specifies three levels of health literacy (see **Table 9.3**) in this context:

1. Functional health literacy, which "reflects the outcome of traditional health education based on the communication of factual information on health risks and on how to use the health system." This type of approach is geared to provide individual benefit; an example might be communication campaigns that provide data about health risks of smoking or the need for a flu vaccine.
2. Interactive health literacy, which is "directed towards improving personal capacity to act independently on knowledge, specifically to improving motivation and self confidence to act on advice received." This type of approach also focuses on individuals; an example might be campaigns that demonstrate skills, such as a media campaign featuring empowered, attractive teens modeling how to say no to drugs or tobacco.

TABLE 9.3 Health Literacy Levels and Foci

Functional health literacy: factual information on health risks
Interactive health literacy: development of personal skills to act independently on knowledge
Critical health literacy: cognitive and skills development to support social and political action
Data from: Nutbeam D (2000). Health literacy as a public health goal: A challenge for contemporary health education and communication strategies into the 21st century. Health Promotion International, 15(3), 259–267.

3. Critical health literacy, which is "oriented towards supporting effective social and political action, as well as individual action." Critical health literacy is linked to population benefit and might include health education or communication that aims to improve "individual and community capacity to act on social and economic determinants of health." An example might be a health campaign that points out the role of powerful corporate practices that undermine health, such as tobacco or food corporate policies, in order to mobilize regulatory change. Or one that features a social gathering, perhaps a community fair, where people modeling healthy behavior, such as nutritious eating or group physical exercise, in order to build social capital.

When framed as health literacy, Nutbeam suggests, empowerment implies a goal of achieving "higher levels of health literacy among a greater proportion of the population" that will have social benefits, such as "enabling effective community action for health and contributing to the development of social capital."[42] Thus a consideration of the ethical dimensions of a health communication campaign might include not only the potential effects on individual autonomous choices (such as whether this particular message provides truthful information or leads to a better understanding of the risks). It also includes an examination of whether the focus of the campaign is geared to the appropriate health literacy level.

Consider again the video described in the introduction to this chapter. The mother is pictured preparing to inject her child with a drug, and then the child is pictured eating "junk" food, suggesting that a mother who feeds her children junk food is comparable to one who injects her child with illegal drugs. Is the use of this level 1 strategy focusing on the mother's behavior for an issue such as childhood obesity effective in providing information—that junk food is harmful for children? Does it blame, shame, or stigmatize individuals, in this case mothers? Would a level 2 strategy

EXHIBIT 9.2 Informational Message

We Can!™ **(Ways to Enhance Children's Activity and Nutrition)** is a fast-growing national movement of families and communities coming together to promote healthy weight in children ages 8 through 13 through **improved foodchoices, increased physical activity, and reduced screen time.**

MORE INFO: wecan.nhlbi.nih.gov
866-35-WE CAN (866-359-3226)

Reproduced from: We Can! Ways to Enhance Children's Activity & Nutrition, a program of the NHLBI, accessed on 4/21/13; http://www.nhlbi.nih.gov/health/public/heart/obesity/wecan/downloads/mediatoolkit_diagram.pdf

that engages or invites participation or skill-building of the targeted audience be more ethically justifiable? Or would a level 3 strategy that builds political consensus for new zoning regulations to address "food deserts" or that features health-related social behavior be more ethically justifiable because they would focus on social or political action to address the social or environmental determinants of obesity? (See, as an example, messages of the "We Can" campaign in **Figure 9.3** and **Exhibit 9.2** that features positive images of parents and children together and practical information about ways to increase parenting skills.)

Empowerment and health literacy, as goals, suggest that communication campaigns are most effective, and ethically justifiable, when undertaken as part of a comprehensive health promotion approach that includes other complementary level 2 and level 3 interventions. Examples include the

FIGURE 9.3 Empowerment Message

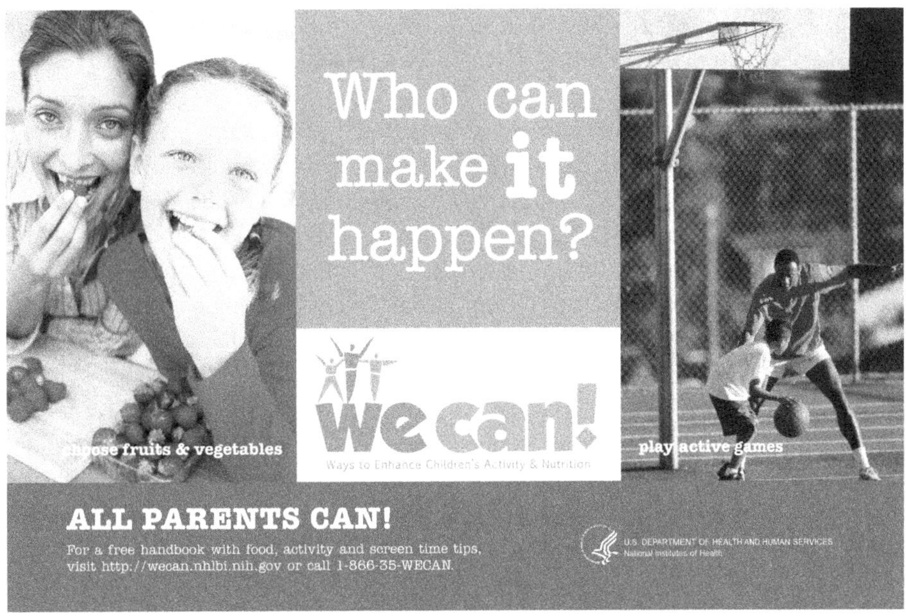

Reproduced from: We Can! Ways to Enhance Children's Activity & Nutrition, a program of the NHLBI, accessed on 4/21/13; http://www.nhlbi.nih.gov/health/public/heart/obesity/wecan_mats/ad_half_bw_en.pdf

availability of skill-building tools, like food preparation lessons, opportunities to participate in related group activities that build social capital, such as community gardens, and campaigns to support policy tools such as taxes, advertising restrictions, and other regulatory responses.

CONCLUSIONS

Public health communication that increases the availability of information, persuades the public to adopt healthy lifestyle choices, and influences community-level, ecological factors in the environment such as social norms are, in principle, compatible with moral considerations in public health in that they aim to produce benefit and enhance informed decision making. More evidence, however, is needed about the effectiveness of particular communication strategies. New evaluation methods must address value-laden questions about the appropriate goals of particular communication campaigns, what counts as evidence of effectiveness, and what measures should be used to identify unreasonable or manipulative approaches that fail to manifest proper respect for the autonomy and liberty of action of the intended audience.

Some have suggested, for example, that evaluation metrics might set a threshold for harms, so that certain negative effects on individuals or communities could never be judged "proportional" to population benefit. One commentator notes that two ethical aspects are particularly relevant in this regard—concerns about coercion and stigmatization. She suggests that even a marketing campaign can exhibit a manipulative or coercive character, insofar as it aims to change behavior and does so often with vast resources at its disposal. And others point out that even if the use of blame or stigmatization is effective in achieving a particular goal, it may be "inherently *unfair* if the targeted groups do not *deserve* to be blamed or stigmatized." Highlighting anti-obesity ads, like the one focusing on mothers providing junk food described in the introduction to this chapter, Carter et al argue that policy makers must attend to the risk of reinforcing negative stereotypes and of encouraging self-harm that already accompanies obesity in society, or, as others point out, that deflect attention from the ecological factors that shape behavior and contribute to obesity.[43]

CDC Director Dr. Thomas Friedan highlights government's important role in information management and in reducing "the likelihood that misinformation or hidden information will endanger health," using the example of anti-tobacco advertising to encourage smoking cessation. According to Friedan: "Pack warnings convey clear information about the health effects of tobacco use, creating a visual and visceral counter to the aggressive and often misleading information spread by tobacco companies, which have been convicted of deliberately deceiving the public about the health effects of tobacco." He argues that anti-tobacco advertising is necessary to counter industry "efforts to undermine science and its massive marketing expenditures."[44]

The FDA's proposed graphic package warnings provide a suitable context for summarizing several key themes developed in this chapter. The messages conveyed in the explicit images are intended both to inform and to persuade. They intentionally invite affective responses in order to increase salience and to reinforce motivation to quit. Whether they have these intended effects can be ascertained only in real time, but available evidence on the initial reactions of smokers and on the impact of other media campaigns on smoking prevalence is encouraging. However, whether the content of the images crosses an important ethical boundary between persuasion and manipulation is a question that can be fully addressed only by looking at the images themselves. The view of the authors is that they do not, especially in comparison with images that have been used in package warnings in other countries and given the strong scientific consensus that the previous textual warnings have been ineffective.

Assuming that the content of the graphic warnings is ethically acceptable, additional ethical and legal questions can be raised about the channel of communication being used by the federal government to convey these warnings. To the extent that the government buys space on billboards, social media, or other channels of mass communication, the pertinent constraints are essentially political—is the anti-smoking campaign supported by the public, and does its anticipated benefits justify its costs? However, the innovations in the FDA rule are that the federal government is using the tobacco package itself as the channel of communication, is requiring the tobacco manufacturers (and eventually tobacco consumers) to bear the cost of the communication, and is doing so for the explicit purpose of reducing use of the unhealthy product.

Whether this communication strategy is legally permissible will be determined by the courts. However, we may ask whether it is ethically appropriate. Does it restrict the autonomous choice or liberty of action of tobacco consumers? Does it represent an unduly intrusive use of government power to promote healthy behavior? Is it adequately grounded in community consent about "ends" of public health (what counts as a goal? what are the priorities?) as well as "means" (acceptable strategies to achieve better health)? Government transparency and democratic public processes about both the ends and means are necessary to provide legitimacy for government communication and to ensure that health communications undertaken by and required by the government and its private partners are morally justifiable.

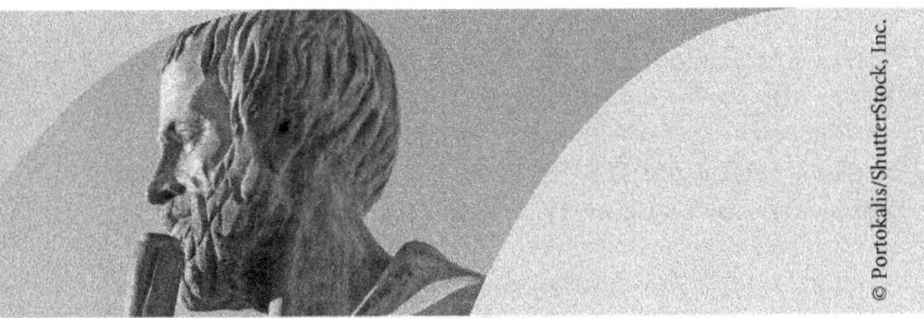
© Portokalis/ShutterStock, Inc.

Discussion Questions

1. Malcolm Gladwell's book, *The Tipping Point*, explores the significant role of innovators or trendsetters in spreading ideas that become influential throughout society. Should public health officials engage superstars in health communication campaigns? Should government public health programs provide funding to television producers to include public health messages in the scripts of their shows—for example, so that characters in programs talk about the need to eat healthy food or practice safe sex?

2. A community obesity task force, co-sponsored and partially supported by the local health department, decided the community needed to give more attention to childhood obesity, given that the community's childhood obesity prevalence is higher than the rest of the state and appears to be increasing. The task force, therefore, voted to initiate an anti-obesity communication campaign featuring images of (unidentifiable) overweight children. For example, one pictures a group of children running in a race, with an overweight child struggling behind everyone else, with a tag line that says, *Childhood obesity, it's no fun*. How should the health department assess the communication campaign? Is it informational, persuasive, or manipulative? What level of health literacy does it address? What are the ethical dimensions, if any, of the communication?

3. What arguments were useful in justifying the regulation of tobacco advertising and use of graphic antismoking ads? Given the obesity epidemic, do public health approaches used for the prevention and cessation of tobacco use serve as a good model for obesity? If you were a member of a community task force on obesity, what health communication approaches would you suggest, based on the ideas in this chapter?

REFERENCES

1. Centers for Disease Control and Prevention. *Winnable Battles.* Atlanta, GA: CDC. Available at http://www.cdc.gov/winnablebattles/tobacco/index.html (accessed April 13, 2013).

2. Department of Health and Human Services, Centers for Disease Control and Prevention. Health marketing for a healthier nation and a healthier world. Atlanta, GA: CDC, 2008. Available at http://www.cdc.gov/healthcommunication/successstories/hmmreport2008.pdf (accessed April 13, 2013).

3. World Health Organization. Milestones in health promotion. Statements from global conferences. Atlanta, GA: CDC, 2009. Available at: http://www.who.int/topics/health_promotion/en/ (accessed September 9, 2013).

4. Best Ads on TV. *Childhood Obesity: Break the Habit* [video]. Available at http://www.bestadsontv.com/ad/31653/Childhood-Obesity-Break-the-Habit) (accessed August 23, 2013).

5. Colgrove J. The power of persuasion: Diphtheria immunization, advertising, and the rise of health education. *Public Health Reports,* 2004;119(5):506–509.

6. Tengland P. Behavior change or empowerment: On the ethics of health-promotion strategies. *Public Health Ethics,* 2012;5(2):140–153.

7. *Gravel v. United States,* 408 U.S. 606 (1972). Available at http://scholar.google.com/scholar_case?case=2739100783028836019 (accessed August 23, 2013).

8. *New York Times Co. v. Sullivan,* 376 U.S. 254 (1964). Available at http://supreme.justia.com/cases/federal/us/376/254/case.html (accessed August 23, 2013).

9. *West Virginia State Board of Education v. Barnette,* 319 U.S. 624 (1943). Available at http://www.law.cornell.edu/supct/html/historics/USSC_CR_0319_0624_ZO.html (accessed August 23, 2013).

10. *Wooley v. Maynard,* 430 U.S. 705 (1977). Available at http://supreme.justia.com/cases/federal/us/430/705/case.html (accessed August 23, 2013).

11. *Virginia State Pharmacy Board v. Virginia Citizens Consumer Council,* 425 U.S. 748 (1976). Available at http://www.law.cornell.edu/supct/html/historics/USSC_CR_0425_0748_ZS.html (accessed August 23, 2013).

12. *Central Hudson Gas & Electric Corp. v. Public Service Commission of New York* 447 U.S. 557 (1980). Available at http://www.law.cornell.edu/supct/html/historics/USSC_CR_0447_0557_ZO.html (accessed August 23, 2013).

13. *New York State Restaurant Association v. New York City Board of Health,* 556 F.3d 114 (2d Cir. 2009). Available at http://caselaw.findlaw.com/us-2nd-circuit/1189180.html (accessed August 23, 2013).

14. *Healthy People 2020.* Available at http://www.healthypeople.gov/2020/default.aspx. (accessed April 22, 2013)

15. Institute of Medicine. *Growing Up Tobacco Free.* Washington, DC: The National Academies Press, 1994. Available at http://www.nap.edu/catalog.php?record_id=4757 (accessed April 29, 2013).

16. Brandt A. *The Cigarette Century: The Rise, Fall, and Deadly Persistence of the Product That Defined America.* New York: Basic Books, 2007.

17. U.S. Department of Health and Human Services. The Health Consequences of Involuntary Exposure to Tobacco Smoke: A Report of the Surgeon General. Atlanta, GA: U.S. Department of Health and Human Services, Centers for Disease Control and Prevention, Coordinating Center for Health Promotion, National Center for Chronic Disease Prevention and Health Promotion, Office on Smoking and Health, 2006. Available at http://www.surgeongeneral.gov/library/reports/secondhandsmoke/index.html (accessed August 23, 2013).

18. *FDA v. Brown & Williamson Tobacco Corp., 529 U.S. 120* (2000). Available at http://supreme.justia.com/cases/federal/us/529/120/case.html (accessed August 23, 2013).

19. Institute of Medicine. *Ending the Tobacco Problem: A Blue-Print for the Nation.* Washington, DC: The National Academies Press, 2007. Available at http://www.iom.edu/Reports/2007/Ending-the-Tobacco-Problem-A-Blueprint-for-the-Nation.aspx (accessed September 9, 2013).

20. *Lorillard v. Reilly,* 533 U.S. 525 (2001). Available at http://scholar.google.com/scholar_case?case=5243407339487774276 (accessed August 23, 2013).

21. *Discount Tobacco City & Lottery, Inc., et al. v. U.S. et al.,* 678 F.Supp.2d 512 (6th Cir. 2010). Available at http://www.ca6.uscourts.gov/opinions.pdf/12a0076p-06.pdf (accessed August 23, 2013).

22. *Discount Tobacco City & Lottery, Inc., et al. v. U.S. et al.,* 674 F.3d 509 (6th Cir. Appeals 2012). Available at http://www.leagle.com/decision/In%20FCO%2020120319119 (accessed August 23, 2013).

23. Family Smoking Prevention And Tobacco Control Act, Public Law 111–31–June 22, 2009. Available at http://www.gpo.gov/fdsys/pkg/PLAW-111publ31/pdf/PLAW-111publ31.pdf (accessed August 23, 2013).

24. U.S. Food and Drug Administration, Tobacco Products, Rules & Regulations http://www.fda.gov/TobaccoProducts/GuidanceComplianceRegulatoryInformation/ucm283974.htm (accessed April 13, 2013).

25. *R.J. Reynolds Tobacco Co. v. Food & Drug Administration,* 696 F.3d 1205 (D.C. Cir. 2012). Available at http://www.leagle.com/decision/In%20FCO%2020120824144 (accessed August 23, 2013).

26. California Department of Public Health. Legislative Mandate for Tobacco Control—Proposition 99. Available at http://www.cdph.ca.gov/programs/tobacco/Pages/CTCPLegislativeMandateforTobaccoControl-Prop99.aspx (accessed August 23, 2013).

27. Traynor MP, Glantz SA. California's tobacco tax initiative: the development and passage of proposition 99. *Journal of Health Policy & Law,* 1996;21(3):543–585.

28. Balbach ED, Traynor MP, Glantz SA. The implementation of California's tobacco tax initiative: the critical role of outsider strategies in protecting Proposition 99. *Journal of Health Policy & Law,* 2000;25:689–716.

29. 272 F. Supp. 2d 1085 (E.D. Cal. 2003), *affd sub nom. R.J. Reynolds Tobacco Co. v. Shewry,* 423 F.3d 906 (9th Cir. 2005). Subsequent to the tobacco companies' appeal to the Ninth Circuit, Ms. Bonta left the Department of Health Services. On appeal, the case was renamed *R.J. Reynolds Tobacco Co. v. Shewry* to account for the newly named Director of the Department of Health Services, Ms. Shewry.

30. *R.J. Reynolds Tobacco Co. v. Shewry* 423 F.3d at 911 (2005).

31. Centers for Disease Control and Prevention. The Public Health System and the 10 Essential Public Health Services. Available at http://www.cdc.gov/nphpsp/essentialservices.html (accessed August 23, 2013).

32. Public Health Accreditation Board. Standards and Measures. Available at http://www.phaboard.org/wp-content/uploads/PHAB-Standards-and-Measures-Version-1.0.pdf (accessed August 23, 2013).

33. Faden R. Ethical issues in government sponsored public health campaigns. *Health Education Quarterly,* 1987;14(1):27–37.

34. Randolph W, Viswanath K. Lessons learned from public health mass media campaigns: Marketing health in a crowded media world. *Annual Review of Public Health,* 2004;25:419–437.

35. Rossi J, Yudell M. The use of persuasion in public health communication: An ethical critique. *Public Health Ethics,* 2012;5(2):192–205.

36. U.S. Department of Health and Human Services. Health Communication & Social Marketing. Available at http://www.thecommunityguide.org/healthcommunication/index.html (accessed April 13, 2013).

37. Grier S, Bryant C. Social marketing in public health. *Annual Review of Public Health,* 2005;26:319–339.

38. Wymer W. Rethinking the boundaries of social marketing: Activism or advertising. *Journal of Business Research*, 2010;63:99–103.

39. Brenkert G. Ethical challenges of social marketing. *Journal of Public Policy & Marketing*, 2002;21(1):14–25.

40. Sunstein CR. Social norms and social roles. *Columbia Law Review*, 1996;96:903–968.

41. Ottawa Charter for Health Promotion (1986). Available at http://www.phac-aspc.gc.ca/ph-sp/docs/charter-chartre/pdf/charter.pdf (accessed April 13, 2013).

42. Nutbeam D. Health literacy as a public health goal: A challenge for contemporary health education and communication strategies into the 21st century. *Health Promotion International*, 2000;15(3):259–267.

43. Carter SM, Rychetnik L, Lloyd B, Kerridge IH, Baur L, Bauman A, Hooker C, Zask A. Evidence, ethics, and values: A framework for health promotion. *American Journal of Public Health*, 2011;101(3):465–472.

44. Frieden TR. Government's role in protecting health and safety. *The New England Journal of Medicine*, 2013;368:1857–1859.

© Portokalis/ShutterStock, Inc.

CHAPTER 10

Public Health and the Environment

by Alan L. Melnick

Learning Objectives

By the end of this chapter, the reader will be able to:

- understand ways that public health ethics can inform the use and/or regulation of materials in the environment
- develop ethical justifications for public health environmental interventions aimed at improving community health and addressing health risks and harms
- provide information about the complex and significant roles that numerous community stakeholders, including individuals and organizations, play in environmental health regulation
- assess the ethical dimensions of harms and risks related to environmentally influenced health disparities

INTRODUCTION

"It is critical to incorporate human health concerns into environmental policy-making."[1]

"Healthy environments promote individual and community health; unhealthy environments can create substantial morbidity, mortality, and disability, in addition to sapping the economic welfare of societies."[2]

The relationship between the environment and public health is complex, interdependent, and often politically charged. Consider the national political debate about the potential health and environmental effects of hydraulic fracturing or "fracking," a drilling method using water, chemicals, and sand that creates fractures in underground shale formations to extract natural gas. While a few states have allowed the practice and are reaping economic benefits that flow from developing new sources of energy, other states such as New York are embroiled in a raging public controversy.

New York has struggled for years with a decision about whether to allow fracking, and if so, how to regulate it. Since 2008, the state has had a moratorium on the practice; in 2013, it again postponed a decision about whether to allow fracking, unleashing public outcry on both sides of the issue.[3] One news report suggested that Governor Andrew M. Cuomo was "becoming Hamlet on the Shale,"[4] as environmental activists, public health advocates, landowners, industry, and others staked out strong conflicting positions on such issues as harms to population health,[5] environmental stewardship, benefits of economic development, and property rights. New Yorkers Against Fracking founder Sandra Steingraber, for example, reportedly stated: "We expect that Governor Cuomo will listen to scientists and medical experts and let evidence dictate whether or not to lift our state's moratorium, and we further expect that he will wait for national studies and a real New York-specific study."[3] Meanwhile, conservative business mogul Donald Trump reportedly posted on Twitter: "NY should frack now. What's the hold up? Is Albany opposed to creating jobs and making gas cheaper for middle class?"[4] Others echoed the belief that the economic benefits for some regions far outweighed any potential health concerns and suggested that politics, not science, was the barrier to sound policy.[3]

The state's health commissioner, Dr. Nirav R. Shah, recommended in 2013 that the decision be postponed until his agency completed an assessment of the potential health effects of drilling and whether the state's Department of Environmental Conservation's plan on fracking adequately protected health.[6] A *National Geographic* news article on the debate summed up New York's public health dilemma thus:

> Shah's decision isn't likely to settle the contentious debate, but the state's inclusion of health

effects in its decision-making process adds relatively new complexity to an already thorny issue.

While several studies have examined the environmental impact of fracking—from its ability to cause earthquakes to the potential contamination of drinking water by methane gas or industry fluids—the direct impact on health has received only limited scientific attention so far. The chief concerns: how drinking water, air quality, and ambient noise levels might be affected by the processes and chemicals used in fracking, and in turn how they might affect human health, said Robert Jackson, a professor of environmental sciences at Duke University. Some health experts say there simply isn't enough evidence yet to judge whether the drilling process could harm those who live or work near natural gas wells. The studies on health outcomes that have been done are small and not very rigorous, said Madelon Finkel, professor of clinical public health at Weill Cornell Medical College in New York City. "People are coming in and saying, 'I have this, this and this, and I didn't have that condition before fracking, so it must be from that,'" she said. "Without properly done epidemiological studies, it becomes a he-said, she-said [situation]. We really do need well-designed studies to focus on a multitude of factors." Finkel and her colleagues are trying to obtain funding for a study of health outcomes in southwestern Pennsylvania.

A lack of money has been one of the obstacles to studying the health effects of fracking, said Jackson, who co-authored 2011 research and policy recommendations for fracking. Another stumbling block has been determining what exactly to study. An uptick in asthma symptoms, for example, would be apparent very soon after changes in air quality. But other conditions, such as cancer, would take years after exposure to develop, were they to occur, Jackson said. And some conditions are so rare that it would require very large studies to detect any increase.[6a]

[a] Reproduced from: Hobson K. New York State's review of high-volume hydraulic fracturing has taken more than four years—and it's not over yet. National Geographic (2013, April 1). Retrieved from http://news.nationalgeographic.com/news/energy/2013/04/130401-new-york-fracking-health-questions/. Courtesy of NG Creative.

Effective environmental policies and interventions, grounded in utilitarian justifications, require that public health officials protect and promote the common good of health in ways that cannot be achieved, or that would be unduly burdensome to achieve, by individuals acting alone. The fracking controversy illustrates some common dimensions of the public health–environmental tensions that make utilitarian analysis complex, such as scientific uncertainty about both the short-term and long-term health impact of the environmental activities in question; the economic interests and property rights of industries and other stakeholders who have an interest in the issue; the challenges of undertaking research on community environmental activities[7]; and the number and political visibility of government and community stakeholders with different moral claims engaged in decision making. Ethical tensions also often involve questions about the decision-making process, such as the level of scientific evidence needed about benefits and harms and which stakeholder group or government agency bears the burden of proof on any one issue. For example, should industry be allowed to practice fracking until adverse health effects are proven, or should those who favor fracking bear the burden of proving the practice is safe before it is allowed (as might be suggested by those invoking the precautionary principle)? And who should participate in and make the decisions about whether and how to permit and regulate an environmental activity such as fracking? Other ethical tensions involve equity, in that exposures to environmental hazards often disproportionately affect particular populations or geographical regions that are already disadvantaged or that have existing higher health risks.

In addition, public health efforts that involve environmental issues can entail ethical questions about respect for the environment as well as whether and/or how ethical norms apply to our relationships with and responsibilities for natural creatures and objects such as animals, plants, air, water, soil, land formations, and ecosystems. For decades, environmental ethicists have debated among themselves the respective norms, values, and ethical considerations related to the natural world.

In this chapter, we do not address or advance features of these debates regarding intrinsic environmental value or the consequences of anthropocentric approaches to environmental ethics. Rather, we focus on the importance of attending to ethical considerations that arise from environmental sources that affect ***human*** health, and in particular the process through which the multiplicity of stakeholders with different moral claims are engaged in the decision-making processes regarding public health policy. In Part 2 of the chapter, we explore the way public health officials address ethical tensions that arise in day-to-day practice.

Public health environmental efforts seek not only to ameliorate harms caused by substances in the environment but also, at times, to promote public health through introducing and regulating substances beneficial to the health of the public. Whether introducing or extracting materials from the environment, both actions will have particular unavoidable and sometimes unanticipated environmental and health impacts, however slight, and will often require public deliberation and justification that takes into account ethical considerations and competing moral claims of stakeholders.

PART 1: ETHICAL PERSPECTIVES ON ENVIRONMENTAL POLICIES: WATER FLUORIDATION AND LEAD

Environmental public health issues often are related to human use of naturally occurring resources—renewable and nonrenewable—as well as to the public health impact of a wide range of society's patterns of activities—e.g., energy production and delivery, food production and consumption, corporate and residential construction, and public drinking water treatment and waste-water management.

Water Fluoridation: Too Much or Too Little?

Fluoridation has been among the most highly touted public health interventions. The Centers for Disease Control and Prevention (CDC) heralds it as one of the 10 great public health achievements of the 20th century, alongside other feats such as vaccination and the recognition of tobacco as a health hazard.[8] Fluoride is a mineral that occurs naturally in soil and water, and fluoridation is the natural or artificial introduction of fluoride to a community water supply (CWS). This process aims to set the fluoride concentration at optimal levels for public health, balancing the potential benefits and burdens in a cost-effective manner for the common good.

Precisely because of the enormous health successes and benefits, and not only because of alleged health risks from too much fluoridation, community fluoridation interventions pose ethical challenges and require careful attention to the criteria of ethical justification, particularly necessity and least infringement. In part, fluoridation is appealing to communities because it is easy to implement, wide-reaching, reasonably equitable, and cost-effective. It is thought to be especially beneficial for communities that are economically disadvantaged, which tend to have a disproportionate prevalence of dental caries and less access to dental care. Thus, fluoridation is held up as "a classic example of clinical observation leading to epidemiologic investigation and community-based public health intervention."[9] Critics of fluoridation, however, cite potentially damaging public health effects, and, importantly, a lack of public health necessity. As one commentator put it, "Fluoridating public water in an attempt to target children whose permanent teeth are still developing is like using a shotgun to shoot an apple off someone's head; sure, you hit the apple, but the side effects are undesirable."[10] Ethical perspectives about fluoridation policies in other developed nations also question whether fluoridation of public drinking water satisfies such ethical criteria as necessity and least infringement.[11] For example, an ethical analysis of Australian policies by Awofeso challenged the effectiveness and cost-effectiveness data that are used to support fluoridation policies and argued that fluoridation was unjustified for a number of reasons, including necessity. The author states, "Given the increasing awareness of the various sources of fluoride in the community, it would appear that artificial water fluoridation is not a necessary tool for assuring optimal fluoride levels among community members. Indeed, the consistent caries decline in both communities where water is fluoridated and those with no water fluoridation indicate that multiple sources provide adequate water fluoridation, thus making it unnecessary to artificially fluoridate water."[11 (p. 167)] Awofeso also argues that community fluoridation is not the least restrictive alternative and additionally fails the precautionary principle test: "The easy and widespread availability of other fluoride delivery channels that infringe less on individual autonomy bodily integrity and community health—perceived or real—impairs the ethical justification of water fluoridation."[11 (p. 168)] Thus, the evolving story of water fluoridation demonstrates the ongoing need for surveillance, research, and public justification of public health policies.

Fluoridation History and Trends

In 1901, Dr. Frederick McKay of Colorado Springs observed an unusual prevalence of brown stains on his patients' teeth, known at the time as "mottling" and now called "fluorosis." McKay discovered that patients with mottled teeth were less susceptible to cavities, or dental caries. After dentist F. L. Robertson of Bauxite, Arkansas made similar clinical observations, newly developed mass-spectrometer technology determined that the cause of the staining and reduction of dental caries was an unusually high concentration of fluoride occurring naturally in the local water supplies. A series of studies beginning in the 1930s confirmed the association of increased fluoride with decreased tooth decay and increased discoloration, or fluorosis. Subsequently, researchers determined that most public drinking water supplies contained insufficient concentrations of fluoride to inhibit dental caries, and that Colorado Springs and Bauxite were unusual environments in which fluoride concentrations in excess of 10 ppm both inhibited caries and led to fluorosis. A mean concentration of 1 ppm, it was discovered, promised to reduce significantly the occurrences of caries without increased incidence of fluorosis.

In 1945, a first experimental trial introduced artificial fluoridation processes to the CWS in Grand Rapids, Michigan. This community-based public health intervention reduced the rate of caries among children by 60%. The results were quickly publicized and embraced as such a success that the population in the experiment's control city, Muskegon, insisted upon introducing fluoride to its own community water system. In 1962, the U.S. Public Health Service produced a recommendation that all communities seek to regulate fluoride to achieve levels between 0.7 ppm and 1.2 ppm (well above the naturally occurring levels in most communities, but far less than in others). In 1974, the U.S. Congress passed the Safe Drinking Water Act (SDWA)—an enforceable regulation that set a maximum contaminant level goal (MCLG) for fluoride at 4.0 ppm and a nonenforced regulation that set a secondary maximum contaminant level (SMCL) at 2.0 ppm. The SDWA did not mandate that communities fluoridate their drinking water apart from the requirement that the level of fluoride remain below the MCLG. Decisions about whether to enforce the SMCL continue to be taken up at state and local levels under SDWA, often resulting in public disputes about the merits and potential dangers of fluoridation. These debates, though often contentious, manifest the sort of ongoing, deliberative public rationalization and justification that are properly central to public health policy and ethics.

Ever since the original Grand Rapids experimental trial, the U.S. has seen a growth in the number of communities adding fluoride to their drinking water in efforts to decrease dental caries in a cost-effective manner. In 1951, 5 million people (3.3% of the U.S. population) were receiving fluoridated water. By 2008, that number had increased to 196 million (64%), including 100% of the Washington D.C. population and about 95% of persons in Maryland, Kentucky, Minnesota, North Dakota, Georgia, and Illinois. These state and local fluoridation practices are in sharp contrast to others, however, as less than 9% of those who are on public water systems in Hawaii and less than 25% in New Jersey receive fluoridated water.[12]

Two federal agencies, the Department of Health and Human Services (HHS) and the Environmental Protection Agency (EPA), provide recommendations on fluoride that also continue to evolve, based on scientific data. In January 2011, HHS lowered the recommended level of fluoride in drinking water from the range set in 1962 to a single target rate of 0.7 ppm. (The EPA uses the scientific assessments to set the maximum amount of fluoride allowed in drinking water to prevent adverse health effects.) Reasons cited for the change included updated data about child water consumption and the prevalence of other fluoride sources in various consumer products, such as toothpaste and mouthwash.[13] This change demonstrates that regulations about levels of various environmental substances, like all public health policies, warrant continual monitoring through surveillance and regular review of health and ethical concerns. While federal recommendations provide guidelines, however, water fluoridation decisions are generally local and state public health responsibilities, carried out in the exercise of their police power.

Courts have upheld the authority of governments to fluoridate water systems when challenged by community members who oppose fluoridation. For example, in a 1954 case in the state of Washington, *Kaul v. Chehalis*, the court upheld a locality's fluoridation policy and ruled that even though dental caries are neither infectious nor contagious, "this does not detract from the fact that it is a common disease of mankind" and thus within the state's authority to prevent and exterminate. The court ruled that the public health decision on fluoride was beyond judicial control, unless the decision violated some constitutional right, which it did not: "We fail to see, however, where any right of the appellant (who challenged fluoridation), guaranteed by the constitution, has been invaded. The instant situation is vastly different from one where appellant is required to take affirmative action

TABLE 10.1 Water Fluoridation: Ethical Considerations

Principles in favor of water fluoridation
Reduction of risks of ill health
Special care for the health of children
Reducing health inequalities
Principles against water fluoridation
Not intervening without consent of those affected
Minimize interventions that affect important areas of personal life
Not coercing ordinary adults to lead healthy lives

Data from: Public health:ethical issues, Nuffield Council on Bioethics, 2007, http://www.nuffieldbioethics.org/public-health, accessed 3/12/13.

and is subject to punishment for failure to act. The ordinance under consideration does not compel him to do anything; it subjects him to no penalty. Liberty implies absence of arbitrary restraint. It does not necessarily imply immunity from reasonable regulations imposed in the interest of the community."[14] Decisions about water fluoridation, then, often occur in the political realm amidst debates about the scientific data on the benefits, harms, and costs, as well about ethical claims of bodily integrity, autonomy, and equity.

Benefits of Fluoridation

In the early 20th century, tooth decay was not only a major public health problem, but—as a reason for disqualifying American men from military service in both World Wars—it presented a potential national security interest. Within a generation, fluoridation of drinking water greatly decreased the severity of both of these concerns, changing the context of fluoridation dramatically. For some observers at the time, the significant benefits accrued by communities with water fluoridation introduced the potential for a socially recognized "right" to fluoridated drinking water, along the lines of Muskegon's response to the Grand Rapid's results.

Dental caries remains the most common chronic, preventable condition affecting children aged 6–11 and adolescents aged 12–19. Consequences of early childhood caries include early tooth loss with concomitant failure to thrive, difficulty eating, impaired speech development, increased school absence, distraction and poor concentration at school, poor school performance, and decreased self-esteem. Not surprisingly, poor oral health is associated with poor school performance, impaired social relationships, and a reduced likelihood of success.[15, 16]

Importantly, there is a significantly greater prevalence of caries among children of vulnerable, lower socioeconomic populations. Those most susceptible to dental caries are those least empowered to protect their health interests in the public arena by voicing these concerns for themselves. Of course, it is this reality of the unique needs and vulnerability of children, particularly those from less affluent families, that advocates cite in justifying fluoridation and in celebrating its successes. To a significant degree, the public health benefit of community water fluoridation has been distributed in such a way that the most vulnerable are included in this public good. As Neidell observes, fluoridation "appears to have led to a lasting improvement in racial and economic disparities in oral health."[15]

This is not to say that children and the poor are the only beneficiaries of fluoridation. Studies indicate that adult tooth loss also decreases as a result of water fluoridation from a young age. Other studies have found the financial cost of fluoridation favorable in comparison to the medical costs of treating the averted dental decay.[16] As this total financial burden is lessened, it is shared across the tax base rather than borne by the most vulnerable populations, a reality of no small consequence to policy debates.

Opposition to Fluoridation

Fluoridation measures undertaken to promote public dental health have not gone unchallenged. A powerful anti-fluoridation subculture has developed that has argued with significant success against this public health intervention, citing economic, medical, environmental, and ethical reasons.[17] Fluoridation has been attacked variously as "illegal, a communist plot, immoral, and unconstitutional. It has been blamed for cancer, birth defects, osteoarthritis, kidney disease, premature aging, allergies, Alzheimer's disease and AIDS."[18] There is no shortage of allegations; the negative consequences alleged are quite severe, and some of the critics serve in prominent public roles.

Some critics even compare fluoridation of drinking water to the worst historical violations of informed consent by invoking images of Nazi coercion.[19] Others point out that because dental caries are a minor and easily treatable health risk, and because decay affects primarily children under the age of 9 years, at any point in time the population targeted by this intervention is a minority subset of the entire population accessing drinking water, which nonetheless is exposed to the fluoride and receives no obvious benefit.[10]

While anti-fluoridation groups claim purported associations of fluoridation with negative health outcomes such as malignant skeletal side effects, bone cancer, increased hip fractures, and autoimmune diseases,[20, 21] none of these associations has been verified in the peer-reviewed literature. In fact, government health agencies have undertaken studies and disclaim such evidence.[22] However, given the seriousness of the negative health consequences that critics attribute to fluoridation, compared to the public's perception of the importance of the health impact of childhood caries and the disparate impact on stigmatized populations, a portion of the public is cautious about accepting the public health assessment of the risk-benefit trade-off and reticent to embrace this public health intervention.

Concerns about the environmental impacts of community water fluoridation have also given rise to numerous studies of the effects of CWS fluoridation upon soil, streams, plants, and animals. These studies have found minimal environmental impact.[23] The changes to naturally occurring fluoride levels in the environment as a result of fluoride regulation in a CWS is often below the amount detectable through current technologies.[24] Nevertheless, the delicacy of diverse ecosystems warrants continued diligence in surveillance of environmental impacts toward assessing whether fluoridation continues to meet the least-infringement criteria, not only in terms of its respect for the public, but also the environment.

Perhaps the most compelling ethical arguments against the justification of fluoridation come from detractors who argue fluoride treatments and toothpaste are sufficient and preferable as a lesser infringement than fluoridation. Brushing and treatments are primarily topical, directly fighting tooth decay, whereas fluoridated drinking water is ingested, leading to increased fluoride exposure to the entire body. The viability of these sorts of lesser infringements is evident in European countries that do not modify the fluoride content in CWS. To follow such an approach in the U.S., where fluoride treatments are not currently available universally to children and patients through the healthcare system, however, would not provide the protective public health benefits that fluoridated CWS provides to many of our communities.

Vulnerable populations who benefit most from fluoridation would be those most affected, and there currently may not be sufficient public will or financial resources to ensure that alternative programs would provide the health benefits that community fluoridation currently achieves. It is worth noting the difference between active and passive measures from a population perspective. Fluoridation of CWS as a collective action activity essentially allows for an opt-out, with the costs borne by those who choose to purchase nonfluoridated water for consumption. Alternately, when CWS are not fluoridated, the costs are born by those *seeking* fluoridation. From a societal perspective, this raises additional justice questions. Studies examining which communities fluoridate and how fluoridation decisions are made have shown correlations based less on ethical criteria or need than on social structures and power dynamics within those communities.[24, 25] These trends warrant consideration and continued investigation in assessing fluoridation's implications for communities served by well water or those that do not fluoridate their CWS. From a procedural and distributive justice perspective, there are important ethical questions about ensuring appropriate representation in public forums and political processes to ensure that all perspectives are represented in assessing the benefits and burdens of fluoridation and how they are distributed among subpopulations and geographical regions.

Continuing Deliberation

Evaluating the ethics of environmental regulations such as fluoridation entails more than the necessary utilitarian assessment of the financial and public health benefits and burdens. Overriding the general moral considerations of respect for persons—fluoridating CWS against the wishes of an anti-fluoridation contingency, however small—requires ongoing efforts by public health officials to demonstrate that fluoridation is likely to improve the public's health, remains necessary and a least infringement, is proportional and impartial, and is the result of ongoing public deliberation. Public education, as we have stated before, will constitute an important component of ethical public health interventions. Education respects persons by providing accurate, unbiased, up-to-date information on the impacts of fluoridation upon public health. The financial and health benefits and burdens of fluoridation may change with time and will certainly require attention to the particular demographics and facts in each community. If there are more cost-effective and/or less intrusive means for achieving the same goal—treating those populations most vulnerable to dental caries—in a manner that does not expose the larger public to even minor risks, then alternative practices may come to appear increasingly attractive, as some advocacy groups are currently suggesting.

Regardless of the scientific evidence of the effectiveness and safety of fluoridation, continuing resistance to fluoridation illustrates the potential for public backlash when constituencies impacted by public health measures are subjected to what they consider paternalistic interventions—that is, policies justified by appeals to beneficence and enacted against their wishes. Community water fluoridation provides an important case study for public health ethics, not only because of the need to balance risks and benefits to public health itself, but also because it illustrates the need for continuing public engagement and procedural justice that includes deliberation about benefits, burdens, and fairness of collective action interventions. Public health ethics can provide an invaluable resource by providing the language, tools, and justifications for helping policy makers think through *whether* and *how* such policies are enacted in the most ethical manner possible.

Lead: Too Much for Some

Like fluoride, the amount of lead in the environment has increased as a result of intentional human activities, and like fluoride, the justification for its use initially was grounded in utility. The harms of exposure to lead, however, were documented as early as the mid-1920s; despite efforts since then by consumer activists, environmental protection agencies, and public health advocates, lead poisoning remains a major public health problem, particularly for children.[26] Primary mechanisms historically responsible for dangerous environmental lead exposure have been leaded gasoline and lead-based paint. Lead in gasoline was reduced beginning in the 1970s and banned altogether in 1995. Lead-based paint remained legal in the United States until 1978, and it continues to constitute a primary source of acute lead poisoning in children—particularly among low-income communities and in poorly maintained urban environments with older homes that still contain the lead-based paint. A known neurotoxin, lead is particularly harmful to young children while their nervous systems are still developing, and they suffer a higher risk of ingestion due to their normal "hand-to-mouth" behavior.

Lead poisoning illustrates the challenges of addressing environmentally caused public health problems, in part because of the complicated relationship of science and politics. In her seminal 1997 article, "Preventing Lead Poisoning in Children," Ellen Silbergeld describes how prevention efforts were stymied for decades because of the "actions and expressed opinions of some biomedical researchers considered experts in their day" who were "retained by the lead industry in its organized campaign to control the discourse on lead poisoning."[26]

> The history of lead must induce careful reflection: The natural and laudable bias of scientists toward vigorous skepticism can be exploited to support inaction on the basis of uncertainty. In public health, giving the "benefit of the doubt" to a potentially toxic substance like lead runs the risk of denying a margin of protection to its victims. In the case of lead, the expressed uncertainties about low-level lead exposures (a relative term that changed over the course of this history, as described below) provided not only repeated excuses for inaction but, more dangerously, justifications for new and expanded uses of this toxic metal. By the time these uncertainties were reduced to a level to support a new consensus on lead's hazards in the early 1980s, thousands of tons of lead had been dispersed into the environment. The responsibility for this catastrophic mistake (to use the terms of Carl Shy) must be shared among industry, government, and academic researchers.[26]

As attention to social justice and awareness of the plight of urban populations rose in the 1960s, surveillance data showed additional strong correlations of lead poisoning with poverty, poor nutrition, and dilapidated housing that still contained lead paint. Many now emphasize the need for primary prevention that focuses not only on screening children who live in high risk geographical areas, but also on screening and treating high-risk older housing units.[27]

Once a high-risk property is identified, however, significant ethical issues center on how to clean up older housing units, given that limited government funds are available and the front-end financial investments for clean-up efforts are substantial. Corporate urban landlords and private rental property owners have a short-term disincentive to ameliorate lead levels when the costs are greater than the current property values. Who should be responsible? Landlords? Taxpayers?—and if so, local, state, or federal taxpayers? Paint manufacturers? Paint consumers? Perhaps even a multiparty superfund? These policy questions demonstrate the need for multitiered strategies that include government funding and regulations, as well as the engagement of many stakeholders.

A basic moral problem, however, is what to do when environmental screening reveals that the baseline housing conditions are unjust, and there is no funding capacity or commitment in the short term to provide complete abatement. From one perspective, the moral baseline is that every child has a right to safe housing. Under this view, any policy that aims for less than total lead abatement in every home is problematic because it allows the perpetuation of injustice and relieves political pressure. But, on the other hand, if there is little prospect that total abatement can be achieved in the short run, is allowing landlords to provide varying levels of partial abatement a morally justifiable option? Would it be ethical to provide less costly alternatives if there was evidence that showed these alternatives provided some health benefits?

A 2001 case in the Maryland Court of Appeals, *Grimes v. Kennedy Krieger Institute*,[28] highlighted the challenges of undertaking community research to gather data about policy options to address environmental conditions, such as low-income housing that contained health risks, particularly when children or other vulnerable participants are involved. The case involved a lead repair and abatement study by the Kennedy Krieger Institute of Johns Hopkins University to evaluate the effectiveness of different low-cost lead abatement measures in homes in which children resided. The court opinion provided the following description of the study:

> The research study included five test groups, each consisting of twenty-five houses. The first three groups consisted of houses with a considerable amount of lead dust present therein and each group received assigned amounts of

maintenance and repair. The fourth group consisted of houses, which at one time had lead present in the form of lead based paint but had since received a supposedly complete abatement of lead dust. The fifth group consisted of modern houses, which had never had a presence of lead dust. The aim of the research study was to analyze the effectiveness of different degrees of partial lead paint abatement in reducing levels of lead dust present in these houses. The ultimate aim of the research was to find a less than complete level of abatement that would be relatively safe, but economical, so that Baltimore landlords with lower socio-economical rental units would not abandon the units. The research study was specifically designed, in part, to do less than comprehensive lead paint abatement in order to study the potential effectiveness, if any, over a period of time, of lesser levels of repair and maintenance on the presence of lead dust by measuring the presence of lead in the blood of theretofore (as far as the record of the cases reveals) healthy children. In essence, the study at its inception was designed not only to test current levels of lead in the blood of the children, but the increase or decrease in future lead levels in the blood that would be affected by the various abatement programs. It appears that this study was also partially motivated, as we have indicated, by the reaction of property owners in Baltimore City to the cost of lead dust abatement. The cost of full abatement of such housing at times far exceeded the monetary worth of the property—in other words, the cost of full abatement was simply too high for certain landlords to be able to afford to pay or be willing to pay. As a result, some lower level rental properties containing lead based paint in Baltimore had been simply abandoned and left vacant. The study was attempting to determine whether a less expensive means of rehabilitation could be available to the owners of such properties.[28]

Ericka Grimes v. Kennedy Krieger Institute, Inc. Myron Higgins, a minor, etc., et al. v. Kennedy Krieger Institute, Inc. Court of Appeals of Maryland, 3666Md. 29, 782 A.2d 807 (2001).

The research study led to a lawsuit initiated by mothers of children who were enrolled in the study. The mothers claimed that the Kennedy Krieger researchers were negligent in the way they conducted the study, contending that the researchers did not adequately inform the mothers of the risks associated with the study and that the study design placed the children in the study at an unacceptable level of risk. While the case was eventually settled out of court after preliminary court rulings, it sparked renewed interest in ethical topics relevant to both public health research and practice, such as the adequacy of informed consent and the role of community involvement and varying perceptions of risk in community interventions. The legal and ethical issues in the case were complicated (and beyond the scope of this chapter), however, a subsequent analysis of the ethical issues raised in Grimes by an Institute of Medicine (IOM) expert committee emphasized the need to involve the community and engage all stakeholders, given the particular ethical issues that may arise in community research (**Table 10.2**).[29]

TABLE 10.2 Particular Ethical Issues that May Arise in Housing Health Hazards Research

Research conducted in homes intrudes on the privacy of all residents and reveals many things about the residents that would not otherwise be apparent or shared.
The research is almost always based in the community and frequently involves community concerns about the safety and quality of local housing.
Because some hazards occur disproportionately among children in low-income families who live in poor-quality housing, they are more likely to be candidates for housing health hazards research, and disproportionate enrollment of children in low-income families may raise questions about targeting or inequitable selection of subjects.
The residents of poor-quality housing in low-income communities often face a range of housing health hazards and may be concerned about hazards other than the one being studied or may mistakenly believe that research designed to test an intervention may actually eliminate the hazard.
Parents of potential subjects and community residents may be concerned about the housing risks that persist after the research interventions and the study are completed.
Economic and educational disadvantage and limited literacy among low-income parents may place them at a disadvantage in the informed consent process.
Financial or other material incentives may present undue influences for parents in the decision to allow their children to participate in a research project.

Data from material from IOM report, see reference 29 (p. 3).

Dr. Bernard Lo, the committee chair, described two major themes in the IOM report:

> "... First, when researchers discuss a planned study with community representatives, understand their concerns and needs, and respond to them, protocols can be strengthened both scientifically and ethically. Community representatives and parents can identify problems with a project and risks to participants that researchers do not fully appreciate. Moreover, community representatives can suggest better ways to collect data, to explain the project to participants, and to recruit and retain them. Although there are problems with identifying appropriate community representatives, reasonable efforts to elicit the range of views of the community are preferable to making no attempt to engage the community. Furthermore, working with the community can help the community understand the role and value of research.
>
> Second, the informed consent process needs to be strengthened when research involves children who are vulnerable in many ways. Parents may not understand that the research is not designed to eliminate the hazards being studied and that children will still be at risk for health hazards. In particular, researchers need to take steps to ensure that parents actually understand the essential features of the research study. This requires researchers and institutional review boards to go far beyond their usual focus on describing the risks of research interventions and on refining the consent form."[29 (p. xviii)b]

The IOM report also offers an enriched understanding of the principle of justice in the context of community research. It suggests that for communities that lack economic, social, and political power, the general understanding of distributive justice may be challenged because community residents, who may be distrustful of researchers from past experiences of discrimination and abuses, "may have a different view than researchers regarding what constitutes a risk and whether a particular research project is worthwhile."[29 (p. 77)] The report describes another approach, a relationship paradigm for ethical decision making,

> that acknowledges the notion that an individual is situated in his or her social context, environment, or community. ... This paradigm acknowledges that researchers and participants may differ in their assessment of research risks and benefits and values each perspective. Researchers are encouraged to engage participants and community residents—and community residents are encouraged to proactively engage researchers—as partners in designing research that meets the needs and addresses the values of all stakeholders. In this paradigm, justice evolves into a principle that goes beyond the issues of participant selection to a principle that is related to past, present, and future distributions of power. This shift reflects the view that research is part of a broader societal context and that the conduct of research often mirrors a system in which power is unequally and perhaps unfairly distributed. Through discussion with potential and actual research participants, the respective views of researchers and community residents can be examined and a research plan can be constructed that accommodates the views and values of prospective participants, their families, and their communities.[29 (p. 77)b]

Addressing lead poisoning illustrates the challenges embedded in many environmental issues that disproportionately affect vulnerable populations and that raise unique and complex policy and research ethics issues. Questions about community involvement, justice, and conflicting assessments of risks and benefits similarly arise in day-to-day public health practice and will be explored in Part 2.

PART 2: ENVIRONMENTAL PUBLIC HEALTH PRACTICE

Introduction

Governmental health officials in practice must address similar ethical tensions to those described earlier in the background on fluoride and lead. When invoking state police powers, health officials have many interventions they can consider, with each intervention requiring them to balance individual rights and community benefits. As with communicable disease control, environmental health interventions range from providing health education to constraining individual liberties. Compared to communicable disease

[b] Reprinted with permission from the National Academies Press, Lo B, O'Connell M (Eds). (2005). Ethical Considerations for Research on Housing-Related Health Hazards Involving Children (pp. 1–216). Washington, D.C., The National Academies Press. Retrieved from http://www.nap.edu/catalog/11450.html

interventions, which sometimes constrain individual movement, environmental health measures frequently constrain individual property rights. Again, public health law, which varies from state to state, often provides little guidance for specific situations. In many contexts, legal authority related to environmental health decisions may be ambiguous, leaving public health officials without clear direction regarding actions they should take and requiring them to offer ethical justifications and reasons for their actions.

When taking measures to prevent environmental hazard exposures, public health officials must consider three factors when balancing individual rights and community benefits:

- Whether the measure used to prevent or mitigate exposure is the least restrictive of individual rights, including property rights
- Whether public health officials have attempted to reduce any negative effects of these restrictions, such as providing an alternative
- Whether the burdens involved do not disproportionately affect a minority or otherwise vulnerable population

Environmental health decisions based solely on science or on legal authority might not always have the best outcomes, and in addition there may be uncertainty about the effectiveness or even of unforeseen harms of specific interventions, either in the short-term or long-term. Public health officials should always question whether a given action is necessary, whether there are less restrictive alternatives, and whether they can justify their actions to their community constituents. In this section, we will use two cases illustrating the use of ethical analysis in helping public health officials make better decisions regarding protecting their constituents from environmental hazards.

Case Study: Lead Poisoning at a Private Indoor Shooting Range

Background

Although lead occurs naturally in the environment, most lead is present because of human activity. Over the past three centuries, human activities have increased the amount of lead in the environment more than 1000 times.[30] Lead has several qualities that make it useful as a commercial additive. Because of its resistance to corrosion, humans have added lead to dyes, ceramic glazes, caulk, and paint. Two lead compounds, tetraethyl lead and tetramethyl lead, when added to gasoline, boost its octane rating. The greatest increase in environmental lead was a consequence of its global use as a gasoline additive in the second half of the 20th century. Because lead is soft, easily malleable, and easy to combine with other metals to create alloys, industry has used lead for producing pipes, analytic weights, ammunition, and fishing weights. Current uses for lead include lead batteries (its major use), ammunition, and fishing weights. Lead is particularly attractive as ammunition for indoor shooting ranges, since soft lead shot will not penetrate unhardened walls and because it has favorable ballistic characteristics.

Lead exposure can occur through inhalation, ingestion, and skin contact. Before regulations banned the use of leaded gasoline, inhalation was the major source of exposure. Currently, the greatest risk of exposure, particularly for very young children, is ingestion of dust and chips resulting from the deterioration of leaded paint in older houses. Following ingestion, the amount of lead entering the bloodstream depends on age and stomach contents. In general, children absorb a larger amount of lead compared to adults. For adults who had recently eaten, only about 6% of ingested lead reaches the bloodstream, whereas 60%–80% does so in adults who had not eaten for a day. Children absorb about 50% of ingested lead.[31] Although inhalation is no longer a common source of exposure, it is much more efficient than ingestion, with nearly all inhaled lead absorbed into the bloodstream.[31]

Because of the diminished use of lead in gasoline and paint and other regulations targeting lead exposure, human blood lead levels (BLLs) have decreased dramatically in the United States across all age, racial, and ethnic groups. For children 1–5 years of age, the average BLL decreased from 15.0 μg/dL in 1976–1980 to 1.9 μg/dL in 2002.[32] For adults, aged 18–74, the average BLL decreased from14.2 μg/dL from 1976–80 to 3.0 μg/dL in 1988–1991 (**Figure 10.1**).[33]

Because lead serves no useful physiologic purpose, it is not a nutrient, even in small quantities. For over a century, clinicians and researchers have been aware that lead exposure damaged the brain, and for the past three decades, many studies have shown an inverse relationship between blood levels and children's intelligence quotients.[34] Continuing research has revealed that the inverse relationship between BLL and intelligence quotient persists at progressively lower lead levels. Consequently, over the past 50 years, the CDC has lowered the BLL it considered elevated, the blood level of concern, from 60 μg/dL in the 1950s to 10 μg/dL in the early 1990s (See **Figure 10.2**).

Recently, the CDC's Advisory Committee for Childhood Lead Poisoning Prevention (ACCLPP) recommended that the CDC eliminate the term "blood level of concern" based on three conclusions. First, the ACCLPP found "compelling evidence that even low BLLs were associated with IQ deficits, attention-related behaviors, and poor academic achievement." Second, it found that there was no identified BLL threshold below which these outcomes did not occur. Third, it found that the effects of lead on the brain were irreversible.

FIGURE 10.1 Timeline of Lead Poisoning Prevention Policies and Blood Lead Levels in Children Aged 1–5 Years, by Year

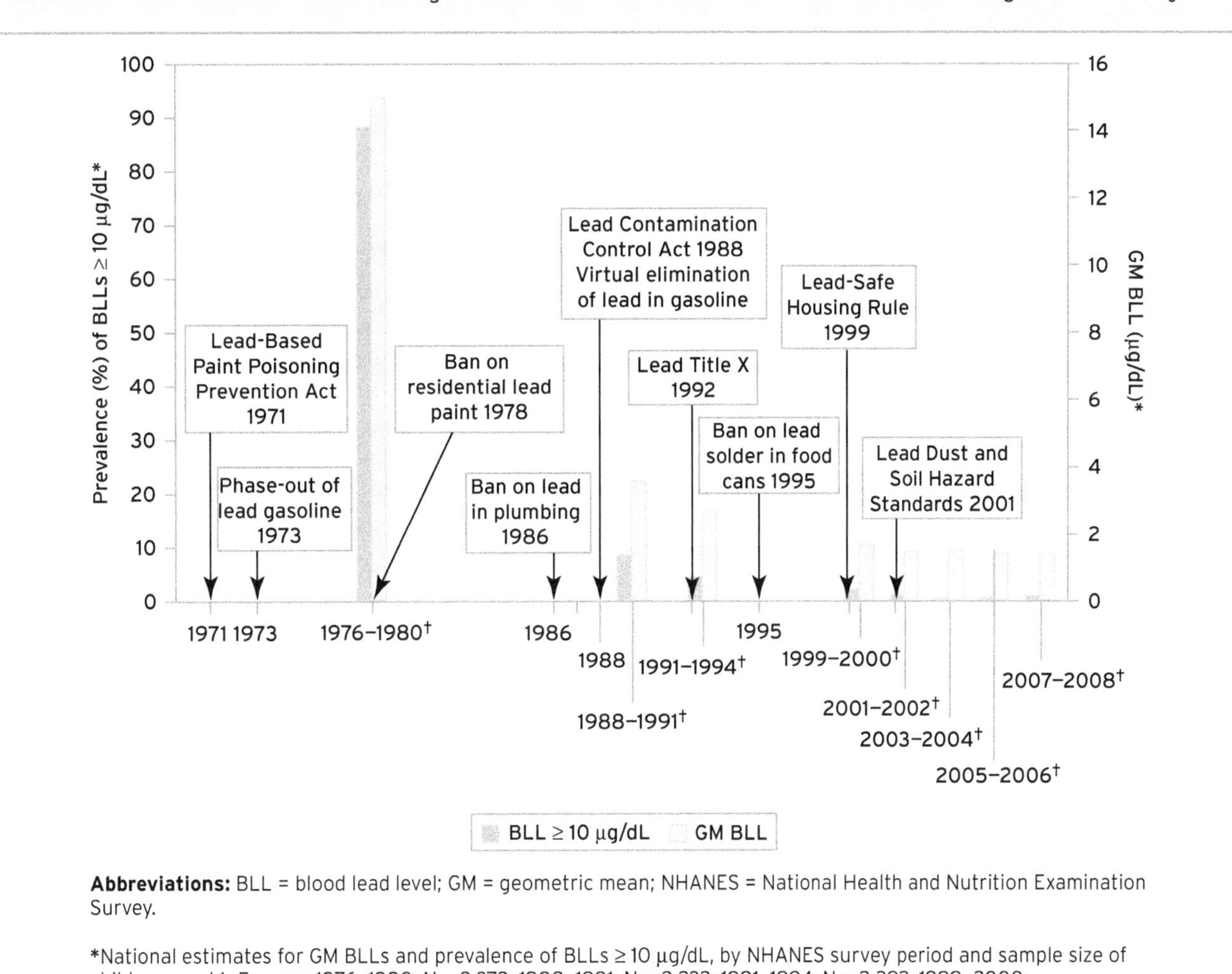

Abbreviations: BLL = blood lead level; GM = geometric mean; NHANES = National Health and Nutrition Examination Survey.

*National estimates for GM BLLs and prevalence of BLLs ≥ 10 µg/dL, by NHANES survey period and sample size of children aged 1–5 years: 1976–1980: N = 2,372; 1988–1991: N = 2,232; 1991–1994: N = 2,392; 1999–2000: N = 723; 2001–2002: N = 898; 2003–2004: N = 911; 2005–2006: N = 968; 2007–2008: N = 817.

†NHANES survey period.

Modified from: National Health and Nutrition Examination Survey, United States, 1971–2008. MMWR, Lead in Drinking Water and Human Blood Lead Levels in the United States, Supplements, August 10, 2012 / 61(04);1–9 http://www.cdc.gov/mmwr/preview/mmwrhtml/su6104a1.htm. Accessed June 6, 2013.

The ACCLPP concluded that the CDC, public health practitioners, and their clinical partners should emphasize a primary preventive strategy to prevent exposure instead of responding after the exposure had already occurred. In addition, the ACCLPP recommended using a reference value based on the 97.5th percentile of the BLL distribution among children 1–5 years old in the United States, currently 5 µg/dL. The CDC concurred with these recommendations and agreed to use the 5 µg/dL reference value for clinical follow-up recommendations for children with elevated BLLs and for identifying high-risk populations and geographic areas needing primary prevention.[35] In addition, the CDC agreed to update the reference value every four years based on the most recent population surveys for children.

Besides the neurologic effects of low BLLs on IQ, attention-related behaviors, and academic performance in children, higher levels of exposure can cause many other adverse health outcomes in children and adults ranging from mood changes to seizures, coma, and death, as well as kidney damage, hypertension, anemia, severe abdominal pain, and poor pregnancy outcomes.[30, 31]

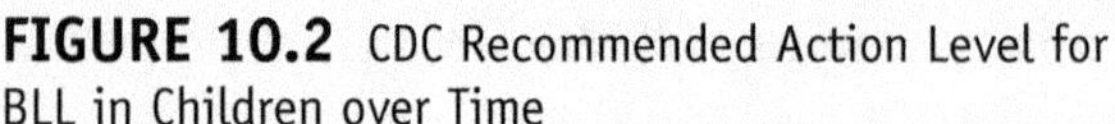

FIGURE 10.2 CDC Recommended Action Level for BLL in Children over Time

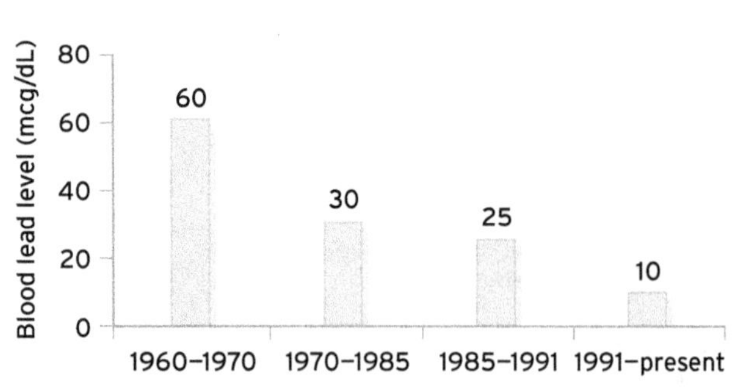

Reproduced from: Agency for Toxic Substances and Disease Registry. Case studies in environmental medicine (CSEM). Retrieved from http://www.atsdr.cdc.gov/csem/lead/docs/lead_patient-education.pdf

The Case

One local jurisdiction, characterized by having few neighborhoods with older housing, seldom received reports of elevated lead levels through the state childhood lead-screening program. In February 2010, a laboratory reported high blood lead levels, ranging between 10 μg/dL and 20 μg/dL, in three teenage males. Preliminary investigation revealed that all three children participated in target-shooting sports using lead ammunition at a local, private indoor shooting range. The three teenagers were siblings. Although the mother did not participate in shooting activities, she had visited the range several times and had noticed that dust from shooting activities was present throughout the facility. After reading about potential hazards associated with lead ammunition, she arranged to have her teenage sons' healthcare provider test them for lead. Subsequent testing revealed the high levels that the provider and lab reported to the local health department.

A private rifle and pistol club, present in the community for over 50 years, owns and operated the indoor shooting range. Only members and their invited guests could use the range. To become a member, one had to be a U.S. citizen or legal resident, able to own a firearm legally, and belong to the National Rifle Association (NRA). Membership applied to the entire household, so that immediate family members and "life partners" living under the same roof were included. Members used access cards to get into the range, which was available from 8 AM to 10 PM daily, including weekends. To promote safety, specifically to prevent hardened ammunition from passing through the unhardened walls of the range, the club only allowed lead, copper-plated, nylon-coated, or copper wash ammunition. The club would expel members found using fully or semi jacket ammunition. Besides members, the club allowed selected organizations to use the range, including (but not limited to), the Boy Scouts, Junior ROTC, and 4-H clubs. Because the private club had no employees, the State Division of Occupational Safety and Health had no jurisdiction related to club operations and safety.

During their investigation of the three reported elevated BLLs, local health officials determined that the indoor shooting range was the likely source of lead exposure and subsequent elevated BLLs in the teenagers. They approached the leadership of the private club and were able to obtain permission to inspect the range. To accommodate the club, health officials performed the inspection outside of normal business hours so that members could continue to use the facility. In addition, health officials asked the club leadership for access to contact information for members with other potentially exposed children under 18 so they could contact them and arrange for testing. At first, the club leadership had concerns about releasing names and contact information for members and asked for documentation that health officials had legal rights to ask for this information. After meeting with parents, however, the club obtained their consent to share their information with health officials, who also offered to meet with parents and answer any of their questions. To demonstrate mutual concern and collaboration, the club and the health department cosponsored a blood lead-testing clinic on site at the facility classroom and kitchen, which used a different ventilation system than the shooting range. Some of the parents chose to have their children tested at their healthcare providers' offices instead. The club asked these parents to share their children's healthcare provider information with health officials so that they could obtain the results for their investigation.

Club leadership expressed concerns about whether other governmental agencies would have access to inspection and testing reports. Health officials informed the club that they would keep confidential any information they obtained and that they would not use the club's name in any generated reports. The only agencies with information on the club were those agencies already involved in the investigation, including the local health department, the state health department, and the State Division of Occupational Safety and Health.

Subsequently, the health department obtained blood lead levels on 48 club members who participated in shooting activities. Of these, 32 were children and 16 were adults. The youngest child tested was 7 years old. Blood lead levels

TABLE 10.3 Distribution of Blood Lead Levels of Children (<18) and Adults who Participated in Shooting Activities at the Private Indoor Shooting Range

Age Group	Range	Mean	Median
Children N = 32	0.6–20 μg/dL	8 μg/dL	6.3 μg/dL
Adults N = 10	2.4–29.1 μg/dL	13.3 μg/dL	13.1 μg/dL

ranged from 0.3 μg/dL to 29.3 μg/dL, and 62.5% of children had blood lead levels of 5 μg/dL or greater (**Tables 10.3** and **10.4**) After controlling for other potential lead exposures, there was a significant ($P < 0.05$, $R^2 = 0.51$) positive linear association between amount of time spent shooting at the club and blood lead level among those surveyed.

The facility inspection included measuring airborne lead levels, sampling surfaces for settled lead, and assessing the ventilation system. The results revealed high levels of lead dust throughout the building and inadequate ventilation at the shooting range. Lead contamination was present on surfaces throughout the facility, including the classroom and kitchen. There was no measurable air movement at the firing line or at points downrange towards the exhaust system above the target area. At the firing line, lead contaminated air tended to flow backward towards the shooters. The firing range was under high pressure relative to the rest of the facility, causing lead-contaminated air to flow out of the range doors and into the classroom, kitchen, restroom, and outdoors. Additionally, the shooting range had a water-filled trough below the targets designed to trap lead-contaminated shot. Instead of taking the contaminated material to a hazardous waste facility, the club was discharging the contaminated water into the outside yard. Soil testing revealed high lead levels, which fortunately were confined to a small area near the discharge point on the facility lot. Given these findings, health officials considered several options, ranging from strongly recommending that all children under 18 and pregnant women refrain from practicing shooting at the club to ordering the facility closed pending repair of the ventilation system and elimination of environmental contamination within and without the facility. Health officials gave parents specific recommendations based on their children's blood levels (**Table 10.5**). Recommendations for blood lead levels under 20 μg/dL involved reducing lead exposure and arranging for follow-up blood testing with healthcare providers. For children with blood levels 20 μg/dL or higher, considered a moderate to severe elevation, health officials assigned a nurse case manager to ensure appropriate follow-up and care. Only one child, tested by a private healthcare provider, had a level in this range. After health officials assigned the case manager to work with the child's family, the parents notified the health department that they believed the problem was improper hygienic practices, that they had instructed their child to wash his hands after handling ammunition, and they believed the club would make improvements to the facility. Therefore, they believed their child was not at risk. In addition, they informed health department staff that the healthcare provider who performed the test told them that a level of 20 μg/dL was not a level for concern. Consequently, they told health officials they intended to have their child continue shooting at the facility, and they refused to share the name of the child's healthcare provider with the nurse case manager. Health officials were able to obtain the contact information for the child's healthcare provider through the state immunization registry. The child's healthcare provider confirmed that the child was a patient but was unaware of the blood lead tests. Health officials then discovered that the parents had taken the child to an urgent clinic for testing. Staff at the urgent care center denied telling the parents that a level of 20 μg/dL was not concerning. The lab results they shared with the parents stated, "Children with this lead level should receive environmental evaluation and remediation and medical evaluation."

TABLE 10.4 Distribution of Blood Lead Levels of Children (<18) and Adults who Participated in Shooting Activities at the Private Indoor Shooting Range

Age Group	< 5 μg/dL	5–9.9 μg/dL	10–19.9 μg/dL	≥ 20 μg/dL
Children N = 32	12 (37.5%)	8 (25%)	11 (34.4%)	1 (3.1%)
Adults N = 10	1 (10%)	3 (30%)	4 (40%)	2 (20%)

Once the child's healthcare provider was aware of the blood lead results, she contacted the parents to arrange for follow-up testing. The parents refused further testing and filed a complaint with the State Board of Health, complaining that local health officials had violated their privacy rights by sharing the test results with their child's healthcare provider. Based on concerns about the parent's expressed intention to continue allowing their child risk additional lead exposure and their refusal for follow-up evaluation, health officials contemplated whether they should report the family to Child Protective Services (CPS).

TABLE 10.5 Recommendations Health Officials Gave to Parents Based on their Children's Blood Lead Levels

Blood Lead Level (μg/dL)	What you should do for your child:
5–9	• This is a mild elevation. • You should consider removing your child from activities that could cause exposure to lead, such as indoor shooting activities that involve lead shot or lead pellets. • Whether or not you remove your child from these activities, your child's healthcare provider should repeat the blood lead level test within 3 months to ensure the level is dropping. If the level remains above 5 μg/dL, you should remove your child from these activities. In that case, your child's healthcare provider will need to repeat the blood lead level test within an additional 3 months to ensure the level is dropping.
10–19	• This is a mild to moderate elevation. • You should remove your child from activities that could cause exposure to lead, such as indoor shooting activities that involve lead shot or pellets or any other activities that involve lead exposure as identified on the form you filled out when your child was tested. • Your child should see his/her healthcare provider for counseling and follow-up. • Your child's healthcare provider will need to repeat the blood lead level test within 3 months to ensure the level is dropping.
20–44	• This is a moderate to severe elevation. • You should remove your child from any activities that could cause exposure to lead, such as indoor shooting activities that involve lead shot or pellets or any other activities that involve lead exposure as identified on the form you filled out when your child was tested. • Your child should see a healthcare provider immediately for a medical evaluation, counseling, and follow-up. • We will assign a nurse case manager to work with you and your child's healthcare provider to ensure appropriate follow-up care and additional environmental assessments as necessary, especially if there are other sources of exposure. • Depending on the level, your healthcare provider will need to repeat the blood lead level test within 1 week to 1 month, and your child will need follow-up testing every 1–2 months to ensure the level is dropping.

Based on CDC recommendations.

At this point in their investigation, health officials had three concerns. First, what actions should they take regarding the shooting range, given that interventions could range from providing guidelines and recommending remediation to ordering closure of the facility pending improvements? Second, should they report the outdoor soil contamination to the responsible state environmental agency? Third, what actions should they take regarding the parents' refusal to cooperate with follow-up for their child?

Ethical Framework

Step 1: Analysis of the Ethical Issues

The analysis includes the following considerations:

- What are the public health goals?
- What are the public health risks and harms of concern?
- What are the ethical conflicts and competing moral claims of stakeholders in the situation?
- Is the source or scope of authority in question? Are laws and regulations relevant?
- Are precedent cases or the historical context relevant?
- Do professional codes of ethics provide guidance?

As in our other examples, this case illustrates that local health officials should first carefully identify their public health goals, some of which might or might not be compatible, and clarify any potential risks or harms for any decision. In this example, is the primary public health goal to protect the environment, to prevent lead exposure or to prevent complications from lead exposure such as developmental delay? As in our other cases, health officials must address these questions to provide justification for their interventions.

Requiring the club to close until environmental conditions are improved creates potential risks and harms for club members, because it forces them to seek alternative venues for shooting that may be less safe. For example, some of the members could choose to practice shooting in their garages, where ventilation might be inadequate, where injury might be more likely, and where it might be more difficult to identify children at risk for exposure. In addition, by moving their shooting activities to other sites, including their homes, club members could spread lead contamination elsewhere in the community. Given that lead remains stable in the environment, widespread contamination could pose a risk to future community residents. On the other hand, allowing the club to remain open without any mitigation certainly puts members, particularly children and pregnant women, at risk for complications from lead exposure. In addition, allowing the club to remain open conveys a message that lead exposure does not pose a serious health concern.

In this case, stakeholders include club members, parents and children, club leadership, including board members, organizations that support and sanction the club, including the National Rifle Association and the public who expects the health department to promote health and protect the community, including the most vulnerable members of the community, from illness. Regarding moral claims, the club leadership has expectations that they have the freedom to operate their private shooting range without governmental interference and that it is their responsibility to ensure that the shooting range provides a clean and safe environment for their members. Adult club members have expectations related to access to the range based on their membership agreements and their own conclusions about the safety of the shooting range environment. Members who are parents have expectations regarding respect for parental rights, including their freedom to weigh the health benefits and risks while deciding whether to allow their children to participate in shooting activities in the range or elsewhere, respect for privacy, and respect for their decisions regarding what sort of medical care their children require.

Sponsoring organizations, such as the National Rifle Association, have expectations that the public has access to gun ownership and safe environments in which to practice shooting. However, as in other cases, these claims are not absolute, and competing moral claims can supersede them. Children have moral claims that could compete with their parents' claims, specifically their expectations that their parents will protect them from harm. Club members have expectations that environmental conditions within the shooting range protect them and their children from harm. Sponsoring organizations, such as the National Rifle Association, have expectations that their affiliate organizations understand that their members are to be protected, that "proper housekeeping is not only good for business, it is required by law," and that "there is much less likelihood of overexposure and cross contamination on a range that is properly maintained."[36] The public has a moral claim based on two expectations: first, that the health department will protect them from environmental contamination, and second, that club members will protect their neighbors by ensuring that they minimize release of lead contamination into the environment around the shooting range as well as around their homes.

Like other cases, health officials must consider any interventions within a particular community that has a unique history and culture. Frequently, the health officer's scope of authority is not completely clear. According to state statute, the health officer has statutory power to:

- Take such action as is necessary to maintain health and sanitation supervision over the territory within his or her jurisdiction;
- Control and prevent the spread of any dangerous, contagious, or infectious diseases that may occur within his or her jurisdiction;
- Prevent, control, or abate nuisances detrimental to the public health;
- Take such measures as he or she deems necessary in order to promote the public health.

Although the health officer might have the statutory authority to close the shooting range, it is not clear whether doing so would achieve the goals stated earlier, nor is it completely clear that the health officer could order this private club closed. Given that the environmental contamination has been present for some time, closing the club might cause the club to delay environmental cleanup or even vacate a contaminated building. In addition, because the contamination is contained within the building and within a small area outside, it is not clear the range poses any dangerous condition or nuisance for anyone other than the members and their families.

Regarding reporting the outdoor soil lead samples to the state environmental agency, health officials had informed the club that they would keep inspection and testing reports confidential and not report the results to other state agencies. However, health officials made this claim before they had become aware that the facility was discharging lead contaminated water into the ground surrounding the facility. In this case, state administrative code states "any owner or operator who has information that a hazardous substance has been released to the environment at the owner or operator's facility and may be a threat to human health or the environment shall report such information to the department within ninety days of discovery." The code further states that "persons should use best professional judgment in deciding whether a release of a hazardous substance may be a threat or potential threat to human health or the environment." The code contains a list of examples of situations requiring reporting, including "any contaminated soil or unpermitted disposal of waste materials that would be classified as a hazardous waste under federal or state law" (WAC 173-340-300).

Regarding the decision to report the family refusing to cooperate with follow-up for their child to CPS, state statutes related to child abuse and neglect and state statutes requiring reporting abuse and neglect might apply. State statute defines child abuse and neglect as:

> the injury, sexual abuse, or sexual exploitation of a child by any person under circumstances which indicate that the child's health, welfare, or safety is harmed, or the negligent treatment or maltreatment of a child by a person responsible for or providing care to the child. An abused child is a child who has been subjected to child abuse or neglect as defined in this section.

Paragraph 5 of the statute defines neglect as:

> (5) Negligent treatment or maltreatment means an act or a failure to act, or the cumulative effects of a pattern of conduct, behavior, or inaction, on the part of a child's parent, legal custodian, guardian, or caregiver that shows a serious disregard of the consequences to the child of such magnitude that it creates a clear and present danger to the child's health, welfare, or safety. A child does not have to suffer actual damage or physical or emotional harm to be in circumstances which create a clear and present danger to the child's health, welfare, or safety. Negligent treatment or maltreatment includes, but is not limited, to:
>
> (a) Failure to provide adequate food, shelter, clothing, supervision, or health care necessary for a child's health, welfare, or safety. Poverty and/or homelessness do not constitute negligent treatment or maltreatment in and of themselves;
>
> (b) Actions, failures to act, or omissions that result in injury to or which create a substantial risk of injury to the physical, emotional, and/or cognitive development of a child; or
>
> (c) The cumulative effects of a pattern of conduct, behavior or inaction by a parent or guardian in providing for the physical, emotional, and developmental needs of a child's, or the effects of chronic failure on the part of a parent or guardian to perform basic parental functions, obligations, and duties, when the result is to cause injury or create a substantial risk of injury to the physical, emotional, and/or cognitive development of a child.

State statute defines reporting requirements as follows:

> (1)(a) When any practitioner, county coroner or medical examiner, law enforcement officer, professional school personnel, registered or licensed nurse, social service counselor, psychologist, pharmacist, employee of the department of early learning, licensed or certified child care providers or their employees, employee of the department, juvenile probation officer, placement and liaison specialist, responsible living skills program staff, HOPE center staff, or state family and children's ombudsman or any volunteer in the ombudsman's office has reasonable cause to believe that a child has suffered abuse or neglect, he or she shall report such incident, or cause a report to be made, to the proper law enforcement agency or to the department.
>
> (3) Any other person who has reasonable cause to believe that a child has suffered abuse or neglect may report such incident to the proper law enforcement agency or to the department of social and health services as provided in RCW 26.44.040.

On the other hand, it is not clear whether this particular situation presents a clear and present danger to the health, welfare, and safety of the child. At a BLL of 20 μg/dL, the child has no symptoms. Although lead is a neurotoxin at any age, most of the studies showing an inverse association between BLLS and IQ studied children under 10 years of age. All studies related to childhood lead exposure have been observational, allowing confounding between age and magnitude of exposure. In addition, animal models have revealed different effects depending on timing of exposure. Consequently, research has not identified a discrete age during which brain development is particularly vulnerable to lead exposure.[37] At this level of lead poisoning, there is no recommended treatment other than removal from the source of the exposure. The decision to report the case to

CPS would be more straightforward if the parents were withholding a specific medication or treatment from the child. The father told health officials that he was continuing to have his child shoot at the range before the club began cleanup; however, health officials did not have any proof this was occurring.

The American Medical Association (AMA) Code of Ethics provides some direction for what the health officer, as a physician, should do regarding reporting the family to CPS[38]:

> Medical decision making for pediatric patients should be based on the child's best interest, which is determined by weighing many factors, including effectiveness of appropriate medical therapies, the patient's psychological and emotional welfare, and the family situation. When there is legitimate inability to reach consensus about what is in the best interest of the child, the wishes of the parents should generally receive preference. ... Parents and physicians may disagree about the course of action that best serves the pediatric patient's interests, including how much to tell the child about his or her health status, when and how to do so, and who should lead the discussion. When disagreements occur, institutional policies for timely conflict resolution should be followed, including consultation with an ethics committee, pastoral service, or other counseling resource. If a health care facility does not have policies for resolving conflicts in a timely manner, physicians should encourage their development. Physicians should treat reversible life-threatening conditions regardless of any persistent disagreement.[38]

However, the health officer is not the patient's physician and the disagreement with the family is not over treatment but instead over potential future exposures and medical follow-up. Regardless of how state statutes and administrative codes give direction regarding what the health officer could do, the Public Health Code of Ethics again provides some guidance for deliberation about what the health officer should do. Most of the 12 principles in the Code (**Table 10.6**) are relevant to interventions addressing the shooting range operations and decisions related to reporting the parents to CPS. In addition, consideration of these principles is relevant for Steps 2 and 3 of the framework.

TABLE 10.6 Principles of the Ethical Practice of Public Health (Public Health Leadership Society)

1	Public health should address principally the fundamental causes of disease and requirements for health, aiming to prevent adverse health outcomes.
2	Public health should achieve community health in a way that respects the rights of individuals in the community.
3	Public health policies, programs, and priorities should be developed/evaluated with community members' input.
4	Public health should advocate and work for the empowerment of disenfranchised community members, aiming to ensure that the basic resources and conditions necessary for health are accessible to all.
5	Public health should seek the information needed to implement effective policies and programs that protect and promote health.
6	Public health institutions should provide communities with the information they have that is needed for decisions on policies or programs and should obtain the community's consent for their implementation.
7	Public health institutions should act in a timely manner on the information they have within the resources and the mandate given to them by the public.
8	Public health programs and policies should incorporate a variety of approaches that anticipate and respect diverse values, beliefs, and cultures in the community.
9	Public health programs and policies should be implemented in manner that most enhances the physical and social environment.
10	Public health institutions should protect the confidentiality of information that can bring harm to an individual or community if made public. Exceptions must be justified based on the high likelihood of significant harm to the individual or others.
11	Public health institutions should ensure their employees' professional competence
12	Public health institutions and their employees should engage in collaborations and affiliations in ways that build the public's trust and the institution's effectiveness.

Reproduced from: Public Health Leadership Society (2002). Principles of the ethical practice of public health version 2.2. New Orleans, LA. PHLS.

TABLE 10.7 Principles of the Ethical Practice of Public Health (Public Health Leadership Society)

Moral Considerations in Public Health	Code of Ethics Principles Relevant for Lead Poisoning at the Shooting Range Case
• Producing benefits • Avoiding, preventing, and removing harms • Producing the maximal balance of benefits over harms and other costs (often called utility)	1, 2, 4, 5, 6, 7, 8, 9, 10, 11
• Distributing benefits and burdens fairly (distributive justice) and ensuring public participation, including the participation of affected parties (procedural justice)	2, 3, 4, 6, 7, 8, 9, 12
• Respecting autonomous choices and actions, including liberty of action	2, 3, 4, 6, 7, 8, 9, 10, 12
• Protecting privacy and confidentiality • Keeping promises and commitments • Disclosing information as well as speaking honestly and truthfully (often grouped under transparency) • Building and maintaining trust	2, 3, 6, 8, 10, 12

Reproduced from: Public Health Leadership Society (2002). Principles of the ethical practice of public health version 2.2. New Orleans, LA. PHLS.

Step 2: Evaluate the Ethical Dimensions of the Public Health Options

The case evaluation, directed at determining whether one or more public health decisions/actions are more justifiable ethically than other decisions, includes the following moral considerations with the corresponding principle(s) from the Code of Ethics.

Although state statutes and rules might permit the health officer to order the private club closed, it is not clear that this would be the best action to take. Many of the club members and their leadership believe that closing the club would be a violation of their legal rights, autonomy, and privacy. While closing the club would remove the immediate source of exposure, parents could set up shooting ranges elsewhere, including their homes, thereby increasing the risk of exposure, increasing the risk of injury, and increasing the spread of lead contamination elsewhere. Likewise, although state administrative code appears to require the club to report the outdoor soil contamination to the state environmental agency, and might allow the health officer to do the same, it is not clear that this is the best action to take, at least in the short term. At this point, only the area close to the building contains any lead contamination and neighboring yards are not at risk. Given the context, closing the club and/or reporting the contamination might reduce trust between the private club and the public health officials, making the ultimate clean-up less likely.

The decision to report the family refusing to cooperate with follow-up for their lead-poisoned child presents a different challenge. Given the risk to the child from further exposure to lead, and given the parents' earlier refusal to seek follow-up for their child, is there any justification for *not* reporting the case to Children's Protective Services? On the other hand, the family's perspective is that requiring them to comply with public health recommendations is a violation of their parental rights, autonomy, and privacy. The family has no record of child abuse or neglect. Given the parents state strongly that they love their child, have only his best interests in mind, and that their main concern is privacy, is there any justification for *not* trusting the parents and allowing them to arrange for medical follow-up on their own?

When deciding whether to close the club, whether to report the soil contamination to the state environmental agency and whether to report the family to CPS, health officials might focus their deliberations on the following questions the framework raises:

1. Do these actions produce a balance of benefits over harms?
2. Are the benefits and burdens distributed fairly?[39]

The answers to these questions again depend on the values and relationships in each particular context, including the degree of trust and cooperation between health officials and each of the stakeholders in this situation, including the gun club leadership, the gun club members, the parents of the children with a high BLL, and the public.

When considering restrictive actions such as closing the club, health officials could mitigate potential harm and promote justice in several ways. First, health officials could meet with club leadership, and if helpful, club members, and listen to their concerns. Health officials could respond by considering less restrictive options, such as allowing the club to remain open but posting signs restricting the use to nonpregnant adult members pending mitigation of the contamination and repair of the ventilation system. In addition, the signage and other club publications could recommend that all adult members consider reducing or eliminating the amount of time they spend shooting at the range until environmental controls are completed. In addition, health officials could offer an industrial hygiene consultation that could identify problems with the ventilation system and make recommendations for improvement. Health officials could also consider postponing reporting outdoor environmental conditions to the state environmental agency if the club stops releasing contaminated water into the yard and hires a reputable contractor to remove the contamination based on a mutually agreed upon time schedule.

To address concerns about justice and fairness, health officials should use a consistent approach for parents with affected children. In this case, health officials might consider specific recommendations and requirements for follow-up evaluation based on the literature and specific lead levels found by testing. For example, health officials could require case management only for children with BLLs above a specific result, and they should ensure that the case manager they assign to work with the family is competent and professional.

Given the priority or presumption of liberty over coercion in public health measures in the United States,[39] health officials will have the burden of showing that the public health value of utility in this case (concerns about the risk to children) overrides the liberty interest of the club members and the burdens any restrictions might impose on them. This case is particularly salient because it involves a private club in which many members and leadership are concerned that government is attempting to eliminate their right to own firearms.

In addition, it is unclear whether older children are as vulnerable to the adverse developmental effects of lead compared to younger children. It might be possible to demonstrate that making closing the club or imposing less restrictive measures requiring enhanced signage warning against participation by younger children and pregnant women are both ethically defensible options. Likewise, it might be possible to demonstrate that reporting the parents to Children's Protective Services or continuing to work with them through case management are both ethically defensible. The question then becomes, "How does one choose and justify one option over another?" Step 3 of the framework poses questions to help public health decision makers justify a particular option.

Step 3: Provide Justification for One Particular Public Health Action

Justifying the final decision when several options are available includes the following questions, with the corresponding principles from the Code of Ethics (**Table 10.8**).

TABLE 10.8 Principles of the Ethical Practice of Public Health (Public Health Leadership Society)

Questions	Principle(s) Relevant for Lead Poisoning at the Shooting Range Case
Effectiveness: Is the action likely to accomplish the public health goal?	1, 5, 7, 8, 9, 10, 11, 12
Proportionality: Will the probable benefits of the action outweigh the infringed moral considerations?	1, 2, 7, 8, 9, 10
Necessity: Is it necessary to override the conflicting ethical claims to achieve the public health goal?	1, 2, 7, 8, 9, 10, 12
Impartiality: Are the burdens and benefits of the action distributed fairly?	1, 2, 7, 8, 9, 10
Least infringement: Is the action the least restrictive and least intrusive?	1, 2, 6, 7, 8, 9, 10, 11, 12
Public justification: Can public health officials offer public justification that citizens, and in particular those most affected, could find acceptable in principle?	1, 2, 3, 6, 7, 8, 9, 12

Reproduced from: Public Health Leadership Society (2002). Principles of the ethical practice of public health version 2.2. New Orleans, LA. PHLS.

Choosing one option generally means that one value, such as a public health benefit, overrides another value, such as liberty. In this case, the public health benefit involves eliminating childhood lead exposure and its complications. Liberty here includes the freedom to operate a private shooting club, the freedom for club members to participate in shooting activities, the freedom for club parents to allow their children to participate in shooting activities and the freedom to pursue (or not pursue) medical care for children without interference from authorities.

When deciding whether to impose restrictive measures, such as closing the shooting range, reporting the soil contamination to the state environmental agency, or reporting a family to Children's Protective Services, health officials should consider all possible factors that influence their effectiveness, and they should use the fewest and least restrictive measures necessary. The effectiveness of closing the shooting range, the most restrictive measure health officials could direct at the club, is uncertain. Clearly, the environmental conditions within the club pose a significant exposure risk through inhalation and ingestion of lead dust. However, because the club is private, and members can enter with a swipe card, enforcing closure might be difficult and expensive. Club members could choose to set up shooting ranges in alternative locations, such as private garages, many lacking any environmental controls, thereby increasing the risk of exposure elsewhere in the community, making it even more difficult for health officials to identify and protect children at risk of exposure, and increasing the likelihood of other health problems, including injuries.

Likewise, the effectiveness of reporting the soil contamination depends on the primary goal. If the primary goal is to protect the environment, immediately reporting the contamination to the state environmental health agency might make sense. On the other hand, if the primary goal is to prevent human lead exposure, it might be better to defer reporting and work with the club leadership to develop an indoor and outdoor mitigation plan. Likewise, when considering whether to report the family to Children's Protective Services, reporting might make sense if the primary goal is to protect children from all lead exposure. On the other hand, working more closely with the child's family and his healthcare provider might be a better option in the end if the goal is to prevent developmental delay. However, the effectiveness of this option depends on the family's willingness to follow up with the child's healthcare provider.

Comparing the three most restrictive options—closing the shooting range, reporting the environmental contamination, and reporting the family to CPS—with the three least restrictive options—requiring enhanced signage and educational materials, deferring reporting pending an environmental mitigation plan, and deferring CPS reporting—provides insight into questions about proportionality, necessity, and least infringement. Closing the range would restrict the freedom for adult members to participate and perhaps stigmatize the club in the community. In addition, members might choose alternative shooting venues in more risky locations. On the other hand, closing the facility would prevent further exposure to children at that particular site, and most parents would probably not choose to set up shooting ranges at their homes or alternative sites. Certainly, a conditional restriction related to children and pregnant women tips the scales towards the moral concerns of club members related to autonomy and fairness.

Health officials therefore considered the less intrusive option—having the club communicate to members, through newsletters and posted signage, that their children and pregnant women should not use the range until the club eliminated the environmental hazards. Health officials determined that reporting the outdoor contamination to the state environmental agency would not prevent human exposure as long as they club continued to own the property, and was unnecessary if the club agreed to stop discharging the lead waste into the ground. Consequently, health officials decided it would make more sense to defer reporting while supporting the club's efforts to hire a consultant and perform the necessary clean-up. Health officials also promised the club they would work with the state agency to perform the appropriate post-mitigation site evaluation as inexpensively as possible.

Determining whether to report the family to CPS was difficult. Given that the child had a significantly elevated lead level, health officials were concerned about potential adverse effects even though the child was a teenager. Health officials had given these parents the same recommendations they had given all the other parents; they had assigned this case to a case manager because this child was the only exposed child with BLLs 20 μg/dL or higher. After discussing the case with the parents, officials determined that the parents intended to continue to allow their child to shoot at the range *before* the club eliminated the exposure hazard. In addition, after discussing the case with the parents and the child's healthcare provider, health officials determined that the parents had decided against obtaining follow-up care and evaluation for their child. After speaking with the county attorney, the health officer presented the case, without naming the family, as a "hypothetical" case with officials from Children's Protective Services. Because CPS representatives informed the health officer that state statute and administrative code required him, as a licensed physician, to report the case, he did so.

Case Study: Banning Raw Milk Sales at Local Farmers' Markets

Americans rely on dairy products as primary sources of nutrition. The 2010 Dietary Guidelines published by the U.S. Department of Agriculture and the U.S. Department of Health and Human Services recommended inclusion of dairy products.[40, 41] Nearly all milk and dairy products for sale in the United States are pasteurized. The pasteurization process heats raw milk and maintains it at temperature for a short time, long enough to kill any bacterial pathogens that might be present. Before the advent of pasteurization, raw milk consumption commonly caused outbreaks of tuberculosis, diphtheria, severe streptococcal infections, typhoid fever, and other food-borne illnesses.[42]

By the late 19th century, commercial dairies recognized the effectiveness of pasteurization in preventing illness and began adopting its use in several cities across the United States. In 1908, Chicago passed the first ordinance requiring pasteurization of milk intended for sale, unless the milk came from tuberculin-tested cows. Forty years later, in 1948, Michigan became the first state to require pasteurization of dairy products. Since then, other states have passed laws either requiring pasteurization or allowing the sale of raw dairy products only if accompanied by warning labels. In 1987, the U.S. Food and Drug Administration (FDA) prohibited commercial distribution of unpasteurized dairy products across state boundaries. However, the FDA has had no jurisdiction within each state, and depending on individual state regulations, raw dairy products might still be available for purchase.

Recently, many American consumers have adopted a "back to nature philosophy" about raw dairy products, believing that foods produced locally with less processing or no processing taste better and are more nutritious than processed foods such as pasteurized dairy products.[42] In response to consumer demand, raw milk and other dairy products made from raw milk have become increasingly available in boutique shops, farmers' markets, and retail stores. Despite the beliefs of these consumers, the CDC and the FDA have cited research showing that pasteurization does not affect the nutritional value of dairy products and that all the nutrition found in raw dairy products is available in pasteurized dairy products. In addition, both agencies have warned that consuming unpasteurized dairy products increases the risk of food-borne illness.

Not surprisingly, the increased availability of raw dairy has led to food-borne illness outbreaks related to dairy consumption, and more than half of the cases have involved children. A CDC study of dairy-associated outbreaks of food-borne illness between 1993 and 2006 revealed that unpasteurized (raw) dairy products had been responsible for far more outbreaks than pasteurized dairy products. Sixty percent of the raw dairy outbreaks involved persons less than 20 years of age. Considering that less than 1% of the volume of dairy consumed in the United States is unpasteurized, the study concluded that the incidence of outbreaks due to unpasteurized dairy was 150 times that of pasteurized dairy. In addition, because of the pathogens present in raw dairy but not in pasteurized dairy, consumption of raw dairy products caused more severe disease, with 13% of patients hospitalized in raw dairy outbreaks compared to 1% in pasteurized dairy outbreaks. For example, *Escherichia coli* O157:H7, commonly found in cattle feces and a contaminant in raw milk, can cause hemolytic uremic syndrome (HUS), especially in young children. HUS frequently leads to kidney failure, other severe complications, and death.

Besides *Escherichia coli* O157:H7, other bacteria found in raw dairy products and associated with disease include *Brucella*, *Campylobacter*, *Listeria* (a cause of meningitis and septic abortion in pregnant women), *Mycobacterium bovis* (a cause of tuberculosis), *Salmonella*, *Shigella*, and *Yersinia*. During the milking process, even the most stringent hygienic precautions cannot eliminate the risk of contamination, and consumers cannot rely on color, smell, or taste to tell whether raw milk is safe to drink. In addition, laboratory testing cannot guarantee that raw milk is uncontaminated.

In one large local jurisdiction, a county, where state regulations allow the retail sale of raw milk accompanied by warning labels, raw milk was available in a few local retail stores. Recently, an outbreak of *Escherichia coli* O157:H7 infection due to raw milk had included a case residing within the county. The case, a 2-year-old child, had consumed raw milk purchased through a cow-share agreement with a local farm in a neighboring state. Soon after, two local organic farmers asked the county health department for a permit to provide raw milk samples and sell raw milk at local farmers' markets. The county health department had promoted the development and expansion of farmers' markets in an attempt to increase the availability of healthy foods, especially for low-income populations that live in areas of the county with minimal healthy food access. The county has been in the midst of an obesity epidemic, with 25% of 10th graders and 66% of adults either overweight or obese. Recently, the health department negotiated an agreement with several of the farmers' markets through which the markets would accept the supplemental nutrition assistance program (SNAP). The agreement, which included grant funding from the health department, required the farmers' markets to be responsible for vendor compliance with the SNAP program and allowed participants to use food stamps to purchase fruits, vegetables, eggs, meats, fish, poultry, dairy products, seeds, and plants intended for growing food. The relatively small amount of funding ($1,500 for each market) also required the markets to follow federal SNAP rules, attend trainings, and participate in surveys, outreach, and evaluation. Given the somewhat onerous SNAP requirements and the small amount of funding, local public health staff spent several years building relationships with the markets and encouraging them to participate. As a result, many low-income residents in the county formerly living in "food deserts" had access to wholesome, fresh food. However, health officials were concerned that permitting the sampling and sale of raw milk at local farmers' markets, heretofore only available in a few retail outlets, would increase accessibility to an inherently dangerous product while conveying a message that raw milk is healthy and wholesome. Although local health officials could make funding contingent on banning raw milk sales, health department staff were concerned that requiring the markets to ban raw milk might scuttle the agreement, thereby reducing access to fresh foods for low-income residents.

Ethical Framework

Step 1: Analysis of the Ethical Issues

The analysis includes the following considerations:

- What are the public health goals?
- What are the public health risks and harms of concern?
- What are the ethical conflicts and competing moral claims of stakeholders in the situation?
- Is the source or scope of authority in question? Are laws and regulations relevant?
- Are precedent cases or the historical context relevant?
- Do professional codes of ethics provide guidance?

As in our other examples, local health officials facing cases like this should first carefully identify their public health goals, some of which might or might not be compatible, and clarify any potential risks or harms for any decision. In this example, is the primary public health goal to prevent food-borne illness or to ensure the healthy food is available and affordable for low-income county residents? Public health officials will need to address these questions to provide justification for any interventions they choose.

Requiring the farmers' markets to ban raw milk sales as a condition for participating in the SNAP program creates potential risks and harms for low-income residents, who until now had limited access to fresh, wholesome foods. If the farmers' markets choose not to participate in the SNAP program, low-income residents might continue to suffer from poor access to healthy foods, which in turn might put them at increased risk for obesity and its attendant chronic disease complications. This is especially true if the farmers' markets are located in low-income neighborhoods with already limited access to affordable healthy food. On the other hand, allowing the sale of raw milk at farmers' markets puts consumers at risk for the communicable diseases associated with raw milk consumption. In addition, given that many families attend farmers' markets, the easy access to raw milk through samples and sales threatens the health of children who are particularly at risk for complications from *Escherichia coli* O157:H7 and other infections associated with raw milk. Allowing raw milk sales at farmers' markets also sends a message to the public that raw milk is a healthy, wholesome food, thereby potentially increasing consumption and the risk of infection.

In this case, stakeholders include the farmers' market boards, the farmers' market vendors, including the raw milk producers, consumers, including children, and the public who expects the health department to promote health and protect the community from food-borne illness. Regarding moral claims, the farmers' market boards have expectations that they have the freedom to negotiate agreements with vendors of their choice, and that it is their responsibility to ensure that safe and wholesome products are available in their markets. Likewise, the organic farmers, who like many other raw milk proponents believe that their product is not only safe but also healthier than pasteurized milk, have expectations of freedom to promote and sell their products at farmers' markets as long as they follow strict hygienic practices and comply with existing regulations about bottling and labeling. Consumers have expectations related to food access, including the freedom to purchase whatever food products they choose based on their own conclusions about the wholesomeness and safety of the each product. Consumers who are parents also have expectations regarding respect for parental rights, which includes their freedom to weigh the health benefits and risks while deciding whether to serve raw milk to their children.

However, these claims are not absolute and competing moral claims can supersede them. Children have moral claims that could compete with their parents' claims, specifically their expectations that their parents will protect them from harm. Consumers have expectations that food products they purchase are free of contamination and thereby safe for consumption. The public has a moral claim based on two expectations: first, that the health department will protect them from communicable disease, and second, that consumers will protect others by minimizing their risks of acquiring communicable diseases that they could subsequently transmit through person-to-person contact.

Like other cases, this particular policy question is arising in a particular community with a unique history and culture. Consequently, public health officials and community stakeholders must clarify the conflicting ethical tensions within the existing political and social context. In this case, the health officer's scope of authority, in statute and administrative code, is not completely clear. On one hand, state statute states that the local health officer, acting under the direction of the local board of health, shall do the following:

- Take such action as is necessary to maintain health and sanitation supervision over the territory within his or her jurisdiction
- Control and prevent the spread of any dangerous, contagious, or infectious diseases that may occur within his or her jurisdiction
- Prevent, control, or abate nuisances detrimental to the public health
- Take such measures as he or she deems necessary in order to promote the public health

On the other hand, even though the health officer might consider raw milk to be a potentially contaminated product, state public health administrative code states that "Grade A raw milk" products meeting state department of agriculture standards defined in statute may be sold in retail stores in the original container. State statute requires the state Department of Agriculture to adopt by rule the FDA pasteurized milk ordinance and to adopt rules establishing standards for pasteurized and raw milk that are more stringent than the FDA pasteurized milk ordinance.[43]

Accordingly, raw milk vendors must obtain a milk producer license and milk processing plant license because the state Department of Agriculture administrative code requires retail raw milk bottling to occur at the site of milk production. In addition, the state code requires that raw milk operations meet animal health requirements, including requirements for microbiologic testing, as well as sanitation requirements related to facilities, milking, production, processing, and bottling.

Furthermore, raw milk products must meet labeling requirements including the following warning: "WARNING: This product has not been pasteurized and may contain harmful bacteria. Pregnant women, children, the elderly, and persons with lowered resistance to disease have the highest risk of harm from use of this product."

The state Department of Agriculture administrative code allows vendors to sell appropriately labeled raw milk products to "end retail" consumers at grocery stores, farmers' markets, on-farm stores, and through delivery. However, the code prohibits taste-testing product sampling, consumption on premises, and the sale of retail raw milk to restaurants or institutions such as schools, long-term care facilities, and hospitals. Federal law prohibits selling raw milk products across state lines.

The state public health administrative code includes additional labeling requirements, specifically, that whenever food establishments offer unpasteurized milk and foods containing unpasteurized milk for sale, the permit holder and person in charge must ensure that:

- The product is conspicuously labeled "RAW MILK" or "CONTAINS RAW MILK"; and
- A sign is posted in a conspicuous manner near the product stating: "WARNING: RAW MILK OR FOODS PREPARED FROM RAW MILK MAY BE CONTAMINATED WITH DANGEROUS BACTERIA CAPABLE OF CAUSING SEVERE ILLNESS. CONTACT YOUR LOCAL HEALTH AGENCY FOR ADVICE OR TO REPORT A SUSPECTED ILLNESS."

Although the public health code allows raw milk sale in retail stores, and although the agriculture code considers farmers' markets as retail outlets, public health code related to temporary food establishments, which includes vendors at farmers' markets, authorizes the regulatory authority, the public health department, to impose additional requirements. These requirements, intended to provide protection from "health hazards related to the operation of the establishment," include the authority to prohibit some menu items.

While the local jurisdiction's state statute and administrative code appear to allow the sale of raw milk in retail stores and perhaps farmers' markets, statute and administrative rule in the neighboring state are much more restrictive, and do not allow retail sale. Instead, consumers must purchase unpasteurized milk through cooperatives or directly on site from the producer (farmer). These producers cannot advertise the raw milk for sale, and they cannot have more than two producing dairy cows, nine producing sheep, or nine producing goats. Nevertheless, the recent case, a 2-year-old child, had consumed raw milk purchased through a cow share in the neighboring state.

Clearly, statutes, rules, and guidelines vary from state to state, and the authority to restrict raw milk sales is unclear. It is possible that the health officer could meet the public health goal of preventing food-borne illness by making the SNAP grant conditional on restricting raw milk sales.

However, some farmers' markets might choose to forgo the grant, thereby making the farmers' market products inaccessible to food stamp holders. Regardless of how state statutes, administrative rules the grant deliverables related to SNAP give direction regarding what the health officer could do, the Public Health Code of Ethics provides some guidance for deliberation about what the health officer should do. Several of the 12 principles in the Code are particularly relevant to the decision to ban raw milk sales at farmers' markets and are relevant for Step 2 and Step 3 of the framework.

Step 2: Evaluate the Ethical Dimensions of the Public Health Options

The case evaluation, directed at determining whether one or more public health decisions/actions are more justifiable ethically than other decisions, includes the following considerations with the corresponding principle(s) from the Code of Ethics (**Table 10.9**):

Although it is unclear whether state statutes and rules permit the health officer to ban raw milk sales at farmers' markets, the health officer can probably prohibit taste-testing samples. However, given the risk to children and other consumers from unpasteurized dairy products, and given that allowing the sale of raw milk at such locations might connote that raw milk is a healthy, wholesome product, is there any justification for *not* restricting raw milk sales? On the other hand, many parents, consumers, and organic farmers believe that restriction of such a legal product is a violation of their parental rights, autonomy, and privacy. In addition, if the health officer makes restriction of raw milk sales a requirement to accept food stamps, some farmers' markets might refuse to comply, thereby limiting access to healthy food for low-income consumers. Given the already poor access to healthy food in the community, and given the risk of obesity in the low-income population, is there any justification for restricting raw milk sales given that the farmers' markets might refuse to accept food stamps?

When deciding whether to make banning raw milk sales a condition for participating in the SNAP program, health officials might focus their deliberations on the following questions the framework raises:

1. Does choosing to make banning raw milk sales produce a balance of benefits over harms?
2. Are the benefits and burdens distributed fairly?[39]

The answers to these questions would depend in part on the values and relationships in the particular context, including the degree of trust and cooperation between health officials and each of the stakeholders in this situation, including the farmers' market boards, the farmers' market vendors, the raw milk producers, farmers' market consumers, and the public. In addition, depending on the location of the farmers' markets, the benefits and harms could apply to a low-income population already suffering from inadequate access to fresh, healthy foods. When considering restrictive actions, health officials could mitigate potential harm and promote justice in several ways. For example, health officials could meet with stakeholder representatives, including the farmers'

TABLE 10.9 Principles of the Ethical Practice of Public Health (Public Health Leadership Society)

Moral Considerations in Public Health	Principles Relevant for Raw Milk Case
• Producing benefits • Avoiding, preventing, and removing harms • Producing the maximal balance of benefits over harms and other costs (often called utility	1, 2, 4, 5, 6, 8, 9
• Distributing benefits and burdens fairly (distributive justice) and ensuring public participation, including the participation of affected parties (procedural justice)	1, 2, 3, 4, 8, 9
• Respecting autonomous choices and actions, including liberty of action	2, 3, 4, 8, 9
• Protecting privacy and confidentiality • Keeping promises and commitments • Disclosing information as well as speaking honestly and truthfully (often grouped under transparency) • Building and maintaining trust	2, 3, 4, 6, 8, 12

Reproduced from: Public Health Leadership Society (2002). Principles of the ethical practice of public health version 2.2. New Orleans, LA. PHLS.

market boards, the raw milk vendors, and consumer groups, including activist organizations opposed to pasteurization, and consider their concerns. Based on input from stakeholder groups, health officials could consider other less restrictive options, such as allowing raw milk sales but providing on-site enhanced signage and educational materials that describe potential hazards associated with raw milk consumption. A more restrictive option short of an outright ban would allow vendors to sell vouchers that consumers could use to purchase raw milk products directly from farmers or from retail stores that already sell raw milk products.

In meeting with stakeholders and the public, health officials should clarify that they are recommending making SNAP participation conditional on restricting raw milk sales, not to create hardship for particular individuals or populations, but to protect the health of the public. Health officials will have the burden of showing that the utility of their decision, based on the hazards associated with raw milk consumption, especially for children, overrides the liberty interest of the farmers' markets, vendors, and consumers. This case is particularly salient because it involves access to healthy food for a low-income population, and it involves a group of raw milk supporters that distrusts government regulations. It might be possible to demonstrate that making SNAP participation contingent on banning raw milk sales or a less restrictive measure requiring enhanced signage are both ethically defensible options. The question then becomes, "how does one choose and justify one option over another?" Part 3 of the framework poses questions to help public health decision makers justify a particular option.

Step 3: Provide Justification for One Particular Public Health Action

Justifying the final decision when several options are available includes the following questions, with the corresponding principles from the Code of Ethics (**Table 10.6**).

Choosing one option usually means that one value, such as a public health benefit, preventing enteric disease, overrides another value, such as individual liberty, in this case, the freedom to purchase raw milk. When deciding whether to impose restrictive measures, such as restricting raw milk sales, health officials should consider all possible factors that influence their effectiveness, and health officials should use the fewest and least restrictive measures necessary. The effectiveness of the most restrictive intervention, making participation in the SNAP program conditional on restricting raw milk sales at farmers' markets, is fraught with uncertainty. We know that raw milk consumption is associated with enteric illness, and we know that even the most stringent hygienic precautions cannot eliminate the risk of contamination. We also know that consumers cannot rely on color, smell, or taste to tell whether raw milk is safe to drink, and that laboratory testing cannot guarantee that raw milk is uncontaminated. Clearly, restricting raw milk sales should prevent enteric disease. On the other hand, because raw milk products are legally available in retail stores throughout the county, the extent of disease protection from restricting sales only at farmers' markets is not clear. In addition, although we might believe that allowing raw milk sales at farmers' markets conveys a message that raw milk products are healthy and wholesome, there is no evidence that this would increase consumption.

TABLE 10.10 Principles of the Ethical Practice of Public Health (Public Health Leadership Society)

Questions	Principle(s) Relevant for Raw Milk Case
Effectiveness: Is the action likely to accomplish the public health goal?	1, 4, 5, 8, 9, 12
Proportionality: Will the probable benefits of the action outweigh the infringed moral considerations?	1, 2, 4, 5, 8, 9
Necessity: Is it necessary to override the conflicting ethical claims to achieve the public health goal?	1, 2, 3, 4, 5, 8, 9, 12
Impartiality: Are the burdens and benefits of the action distributed fairly?	1, 2, 3, 4, 8, 9, 12
Least infringement: Is the action the least restrictive and least intrusive?	2, 3, 4, 5, 6, 8, 9, 12
Public justification: Can public health officials offer public justification that citizens, and in particular those most affected, could find acceptable in principle?	1, 2, 3, 6, 8, 9, 12

Reproduced from: Public Health Leadership Society (2002). Principles of the ethical practice of public health version 2.2. New Orleans, LA. PHLS.

The effectiveness of the intervention also depends on the primary goal. If the primary public health goal is to ensure the healthy food is available and affordable for low-income county residents, and if the intervention results in farmers' markets refusing to participate in the SNAP program, the intervention might be counterproductive. On the other hand, while healthy food access is essential for long-term health, one exposure to contaminated raw milk could have significant morbidity and mortality.

Comparing the most restrictive option, banning raw milk sales, with perhaps the least restrictive option, requiring enhanced signage and educational materials, provides insight into questions about proportionality, necessity, and least infringement. If farmers' markets agree to restrict raw milk sales as a condition of participating in the SNAP program, small farms would have fewer places to market their products and consumers would have to travel to a limited number of retail stores to purchase a legal product. On the other hand, if farmers' markets refuse, low-income residents would have less access to fresh, healthy foods. Certainly, a conditional restriction tips the scales towards the moral concerns of vendors and consumers related to autonomy and fairness. Health officials therefore considered the less intrusive option, enhanced signage and educational materials. However, because of previous experience with *Escherichia coli* O157:H7 victims who ignored the associated warnings and educational materials, the officials remained concerned that restrictions were necessary. These officials intend to propose legislation that would restrict sales of raw dairy products through any retail outlet.

Explicitly addressing these questions is essential in explaining public health decisions to affected individuals and to the public. Public health officials should justify actions and policies with rhetorical strategies that build not only community support and trust, but also build support and trust from the individuals and families directly affected. Even if health officials succeeded in restricting raw milk sales through farmers' markets, raw dairy products would still be available at retail stores, through direct purchase from farms, and through ownership of dairy cows. Although they can possibly restrict access, health officials do not have the right to force people to consume only pasteurized products. In justifying their decisions, health officials might appeal to principles, rights, and duties, and by acknowledging that while a particular action overrides important values, the action is likely to be effective and the least restrictive infringement, given the situation.[39]

Environmental health threats often pose the same type of challenges to health officials as communicable disease outbreaks. Implementing public health measures to prevent environmental exposures requires balancing individual rights, including property rights, with community benefit. Health officials considering alternative interventions, especially interventions that restrict individual rights, must clearly address questions about effectiveness, proportionality, necessity, and fairness when justifying their decisions to affected individuals and to the public.

To build community trust, health officials must build support and trust from individuals and families directly affected. Some of those directly affected might belong to vulnerable populations, such as low-income populations or minorities, or groups already mistrustful of government. In the raw milk case, even if health officials succeeded in restricting raw milk sales through farmers' markets, raw dairy products would continue to be available at retail stores and through direct purchase from farms and through ownership of dairy cows. Although they can possibly restrict access, health officials cannot force people to consume only pasteurized products. In addition, if the farmers' markets refused to comply, low-income populations might have lost access to healthy food in their communities.

In the gun club case, although health officials could have ordered the range closed, enforcement would have been difficult, and health officials cannot prevent people from engaging in legal activities such as target shooting. If health officials had ordered the club closed, club members had alternative venues, perhaps more risky, they could have used for shooting activities. By using less restrictive interventions, specifically signage at the farmers' markets and voluntary shooting range restrictions for children and pregnant women, health officials built support and trust that protected consumers, preserved healthy food access, and that led to an effective cleanup of a shooting range now safe for use by everyone. Health officials were able to justify their decisions by appealing to principles, rights, and duties, and by acknowledging that while a particular action overrode some important values, the action was likely to be effective and the least restrictive infringement, given the situation.[10] In doing so, health officials were also able to demonstrate to the community that a restrictive action, notifying CPS, was appropriate when they determined it was necessary because a child's health was at risk.

CONCLUSIONS

As with other public health issues, the public health ethics framework provides ethical considerations to guide and provoke deliberation on environmental issues to help public health officials make and justify decisions.[44,45] The case studies on environmental health in this chapter illustrate in particular the importance of community involvement, as well as of understanding the perspectives and moral claims of different stakeholders, when public health officials assess risks, benefits, and harms of any one intervention (**Table 10.11**).

The relationship with the community is key to public health effectiveness when addressing the ethical tensions that arise with environmental health issues. While one of public health's essential services is broadly stated as "mobilizing community partnerships to identify and solve health problems," an ethics framework, along with the Code of Ethics, can provide a frame of reference for public health officials when they assess what kinds of activities constitute meaningful community partnership and involvement in a particular context. As the fluoride and lead cases suggest, seeking community consent (Principle 6) for an environmental issue is complex and would involve determining what would be respectful and ethically justifiable participation and communication in a particular context and community. These determinations might focus on metrics or questions about the type of communication (e.g., whether the communication with the community should be one way or two way), intention (e.g., whether the community involvement and communication is for education, input, or consensus) and participants (all community members, community representatives, leaders, or experts).[46] Public justification, which is fundamental to public health ethics, requires appropriate stakeholder and community engagement.

TABLE 10.11 Using Ethical Principles to Highlight Metrics for Community Engagement

Ethical Principles	Metrics: Examples
Principle 3. Public health policies, programs, and priorities should be developed and evaluated through processes that ensure an opportunity for input from community members. Principle 6. Public health institutions should provide communities with the information that they have that is needed for decisions on polices or programs and should obtain the community's consent for their implementation. Principle 12. Public health institutions and their employees should engage in collaborations and affiliations in ways that build the public's trust and the institution's effectiveness.	1. How is the "community" identified and involved? 2. In what ways are the values of the community elucidated and affirmed in the definition of the health problem; generation of solutions; implementation of the solution and dissemination of the results? 3. Is the context of the local community (for example, history, availability of key stakeholders, inclusion of underrepresented groups) reflected in the type and structure of the engagement techniques? 4. What is the public's level of trust after engagement (as measured, for example, in an evaluation of the attitudes of engaged participants or by actions taken to address stakeholder concerns)?

Data from: Public Health Accreditation and Metrics for Ethics. *Journal of Public Health Management and Practice*, 2013;12(1):8.

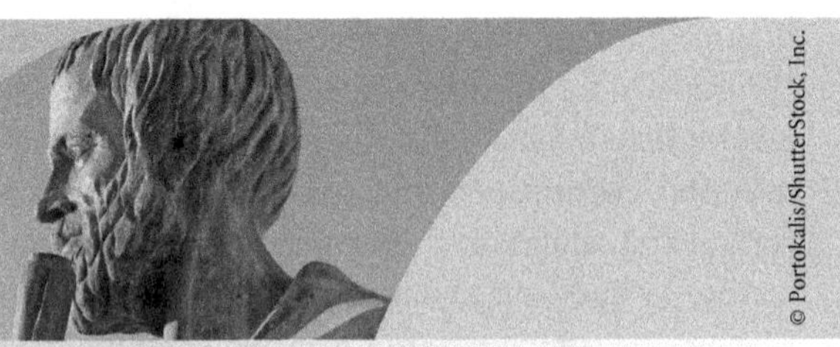
© Portokalis/ShutterStock, Inc.

Discussion Questions

1. Should water fluoridation decisions be made and funded at the local or state level of government, and why?
2. What are some examples of the challenges of developing public health policies based on science and data, and what causes the challenges?
3. How should public health officials approach issues such as fracking? How should they weigh the arguments of economically vulnerable populations who want to permit fracking in order to improve the economic opportunities in their region?
4. What are the challenges in balancing health equity with individual and property rights in daily public health practice? How can public health officials address these challenges?

REFERENCES

1. Jones R, Homa D, Meyer P, et al. Trends in blood lead levels and blood lead testing among U.S. children aged 1 to 5 years, 1998–2004. *Pediatrics*, 2009;123:e376–e385.

2. Pope A, Rall D (Eds.). Environmental medicine: Integrating a missing element into medical education. Committee on Curriculum Development in Environmental Medicine, Institute of Medicine. Washington, DC: National Academy Press, 1995.

3. Associated Press. N.Y. fracking held as Cuomo, RFK Jr. talk health. (March 2, 2013). Available at http://www.politico.com/story/2013/03/ny-fracking-held-as-cuomo-rfk-jr-talk-health-88326.html (accessed August 25, 2013).

4. Hakim D. New York governor puts off decision on drilling. *The New York Times* (February 12, 2013). Available at http://www.nytimes.com/2013/02/13/nyregion/cuomo-delays-decision-on-gas-drilling-as-health-study-continues.html?_r=0 (accessed August 25, 2013).

5. Urbina I. A tainted water well, and concern there may be more. *The New York Times* (August 3 2011). Available at http://www.nytimes.com/2011/08/04/us/04natgas.html?pagewanted=all (accessed August 25, 2013).

6. Hobson K. New York State's review of high-volume hydraulic fracturing has taken more than four years—and it's not over yet. *National Geographic* (2013, April 1). Available at http://news.nationalgeographic.com/news/energy/2013/04/130401-new-york-fracking-health-questions/ (accessed August 25, 2013).

7. Tucker C. Health concerns of 'fracking' drawing increased attention: EPA conducting studies on health effects. *The Nation's Health*, 2012;42(2):1–14. Available at http://thenationshealth.aphapublications.org/content/42/2/1.2.full (accessed August 25, 2013).

8. Centers for Disease Control and Prevention. Ten Great Public Health Achievements—United States, 1900–1999. *Morbidity and Mortality Weekly Report* 1999;48(12):241–243. Available at http://www.cdc.gov/mmwr/preview/mmwrhtml/00056796.htm (accessed August 25, 2013).

9. Centers for Disease Control and Prevention. Achievements in Public Health, 1900–1999: Fluoridation of Drinking Water to Prevent Dental Caries. *Morbidity and Mortality Weekly Report*, 1999;48(41):933–940. Available at http://www.cdc.gov/mmwr/preview/mmwrhtml/mm4841a1.htm (accessed August 25, 2013).

10. Balog D. Fluoridation of public water systems: Valid exercise of state police power or constitutional violation? *Pace Environmental Law Review*, 1997;14(2). Paper 314.

11. Awofeso N. Ethics of artificial water fluoridation in Australia. *Public Health Ethics*, 2012;5(2):161–172.

12. Centers for Disease Control and Prevention. Populations Receiving Optimally Fluoridated Public Drinking Water—United States, 1992–2006. *Morbidity and Mortality Weekly Report*, 2008;57(27):737–741. Available at http://www.cdc.gov/mmwr/preview/mmwrhtml/mm5727a1.htm (accessed August 25, 2013).

13. U.S. Department of Health and Human Services and U.S. Environmental Protection Agency. EPA and HHS announce new scientific assessments and actions on fluoride / agencies working together to maintain benefits of preventing tooth decay while preventing excessive exposure. (Release Date: 01/07/2011.) Available at http://yosemite.epa.gov/opa/admpress.nsf/3881d73f4d4aaa0b85257359003f5348/86964af577c37ab285257811005a8417!opendocument (accessed August 25, 2013).

14. *Kaul v. Chehalis*, Supreme Court of Washington, 45Wn.2d 616, 277P.2d 352 (1954).

15. Neidell M, Herzog K, Glied S. The association between community water fluoridation and adult tooth loss. *American Journal of Public Health*, 2010;100(10):1980–1985.

16. Griffin S, Jones K, Tomar S. An economic evaluation of community water fluoridation. *Journal of Public Health Dentistry*, 2001;61(2):78–86.

17. Freeze R, Lehr J. *The Fluoride Wars: How a Modest Health Measure Became America's Longest–Running Political Melodrama.* Hoboken, NJ: John Wiley & Sons, 2009.

18. Corbin S. Fluoridation then and now. *American Journal of Public Health*, 1989;79(5):561–563.

19. Cross D, Carton R. Fluoridation: A violation of medical ethics and human rights. *International Journal of Occupational and Environmental Health*, 2003;9(1):24–29.

20. Yes4CleanWater.org. Appendix D, Adverse Effect Report. Fluoridation causes and contributes to imminent and immediate harm to the public. Available at http://www.yes4cleanwater.org/Documents/Complaint%20Appendix%20D%20Harm.pdf (accessed August 25, 2013).

21. Bassin E, Wypij D, Davis R, Mittleman M. Age-specific fluoride exposure in drinking water and osteosarcoma (United States). *Cancer Causes Control*, 2006;17(4):421–428.

22. Centers for Disease Control. Community Water Fluoridation. Scientific Reviews: Assessing the Weight of the Evidence. (2010) Available at http://www.cdc.gov/fluoridation/safety/systematic.htm (accessed August 25, 2013).

23. Osterman J. Evaluating the impact of municipal water fluoridation on the aquatic environment. *American Journal of Public Health*, 1990;80(10):1230–1235.

24. Pollick H. Water fluoridation and the environment: Current perspective in the United States. *International Journal of Occupational Environmental Health*, 2004;10:343–350.

25. Smith R. Community structural characteristics and the adoption of fluoride. *Journal of Public Health*, 1981;71(1):24–30.

26. Silbergeld E. Preventing lead poisoning in children. *Annual Review of Public Health*, 1997;18:187–210.

27. Lanphear B. Childhood lead poisoning prevention. *Journal of the American Medical Association*, 2005;293:2274–2276.

28. *Ericka Grimes v. Kennedy Krieger Institute, Inc. | Myron Higgins, a minor, etc., et al. v. Kennedy Krieger Institute, Inc.* Court of Appeals of Maryland, 3666Md. 29, 782 A.2d 807 (2001).

29. Lo B, O'Connell M (Eds). *Ethical Considerations for Research on Housing-Related Health Hazards Involving Children.* Washington, D.C.: The National Academies Press, 2005:1–216.

30. Agency for Toxic Substances and Disease Registry. *Toxicological Profile for Lead.* (August 2007). Available at http://www.atsdr.cdc.gov/toxprofiles/tp.asp?id=96&tid=22 (accessed August 23, 2013).

31. Agency for Toxic Substances and Disease Registry. Case studies in environmental medicine (CSEM). Available at http://www.atsdr.cdc.gov/csem/lead/docs/lead_patient-education.pdf (accessed August 23, 2013).

32. Centers for Disease Control and Prevention. Blood lead levels—United States 1999–2002. *Morbidity and Mortality Weekly Report*, 2005;54(20):513–516. Available at http://www.cdc.gov/mmwr/preview/mmwrhtml/mm5420a5.htm (accessed August 23, 2013).

33. Centers for Disease Control and Prevention. Update: blood lead levels—United States, 1991–1994. *Morbidity and Mortality Weekly Report*, 1997;46(7):141–146. Available at http://www.cdc.gov/mmwr/preview/mmwrhtml/00048339.htm (accessed August 23, 2013).

34. Rogan W, Ware J. Exposure to lead in children—how low is low enough? *The New England Journal of Medicine*, 2003;348(16):1515–1516.

35. Centers for Disease Control and Prevention. CDC Response to Advisory Committee on Childhood Lead Poisoning Prevention. Recommendations in "Low Level Lead Exposure Harms Children: A Renewed Call of Primary Prevention" (published 2010; updated 2012). Available at http://www.cdc.gov/nceh/lead/ACCLPP/CDC_Response_Lead_Exposure_Recs.pdf (accessed August 23, 2013).

36. Giordano J. Clean as Practicable. *National Rifle Association Club Connection*, 2010;15(3):12.

37. Bellinger D. Lead. *Pediatrics*, 2004;113:1016–1022.

38. American Medical Association. Code of Ethics. Opinion 10.016. Pediatric Decision Making. Available at http://www.ama-assn.org//ama/pub/physician-resources/medical-ethics/code-medical-ethics/opinion10016.page (accessed August 25, 2013).

39. Bernheim R, Nieburg P, Bonnie R. Ethics and the practice of public health. In: Goodman RA (Ed.). *Law in Public Health Practice* (2nd edition). Oxford, U.K.: Oxford University Press, 2007.

40. U.S. Department of Agriculture/U.S. Department of Health and Human Services. *Dietary Guidelines for Americans 2010*, 7th ed. Washington: U.S. Government Printing Office; 2010. Available at http://www.health.gov/dietaryguidelines/dga2010/DietaryGuidelines2010.pdf

41. Langer AJ, Ayers T, Grass J, Lynch M, Angulo FJ, Mahon BE. Nonpasteurized dairy products, disease outbreaks, and state laws—United States, 1993–2006. *Emerging Infectious Diseases*, 2012;18(3): 385–391. Available at http://wwwnc.cdc.gov/eid/article/18/3/pdfs/11-1370.pdf (accessed August 23, 2013).

42. Centers for Disease Control and Prevention. Food Safety and Raw Milk. Available at http://www.cdc.gov/foodsafety/rawmilk/raw-milk-index.html (accessed August 23, 2013).

43. Washington State Department of Agriculture. Retail Raw Milk, A Quick Guide for Producer-Processors. Available at http://agr.wa.gov/foodanimal/dairy/docs/RetailRawMilkGuide042111.pdf (accessed August 23, 2013).

44. Bernheim R, Melnick A. Principled leadership in public health: Integrating ethics into practice and management. *Journal of Public Health Management and Practice*, 2008;14(4):358–366.

45. Kass N. An ethics framework for public health. *American Journal of Public Health*, 2001;91:1776–1782.

46. Bernheim R, Stefanak M, Brandenburg T, Pannone A, Melnick A. Public health accreditation and metrics for ethics: A case study on environmental health and community engagement. *Journal of Public Health and Management Practice*, 2013;19(1):4–8.

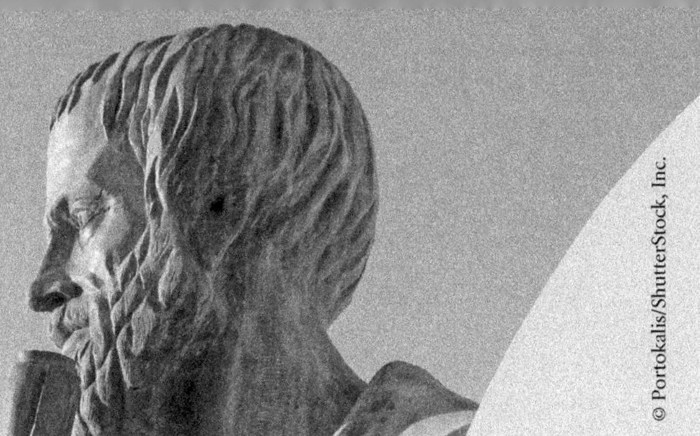

Index

Note: Page numbers followed by *f* or *t* indicate material in figures or tables, respectively.

C

D

E

F

T

CPSIA information can be obtained
at www.ICGtesting.com
Printed in the USA
JSHW012044120819
1075JS00003B/13